Neuropsychology of Learning Disabilities:
Essentials of Subtype Analysis

NEUROPSYCHOLOGY OF LEARNING DISABILITIES

Essentials of Subtype Analysis

Edited by

BYRON P. ROURKE

University of Windsor and
Windsor Western Hospital Centre

THE GUILFORD PRESS
New York   London

© 1985 The Guilford Press
A Division of Guilford Publications, Inc.

Printed in the United States of America

Last digit is print number 9 8 7

LIBRARY OF CONGRESS CATALOGING IN PUBLICATION DATA
Main entry under title:

Neuropsychology of learning disabilities.

Includes indexes.
1. Learning disabilities—Classification. 2. Learning
disabilities—Physiological aspects. 3. Learning
disabilities—Psychological aspects. I. Rourke, Byron P.
(Byron Patrick), 1939-   . [DNLM: 1. Learning Disorders
—classification. WS 15 N494]
RJ506.L4N48   1985   618.92'89   84-10860
ISBN 0-89862-644-7

Contributors

KENNETH M. ADAMS, PhD, Division of Neuropsychology, Henry Ford Hospital, Detroit, Michigan, USA

JEREL E. DEL DOTTO, PhD, Division of Neuropsychology, Henry Ford Hospital, Detroit, Michigan, USA

DONALD G. DOEHRING, PhD, School of Human Communication Disorders, McGill University, Montreal, Quebec, Canada

RHEA FINNELL, PhD, Division of Neuropsychology, North Shore University Hospital, Manhasset, New York, USA

JOHN L. FISK, PhD, Department of Neuropsychology, Windsor Western Hospital Centre, Windsor, Ontario, Canada

JACK M. FLETCHER, PhD, Developmental Neuropsychology Research Section, Texas Research Institute of Mental Sciences, Houston, Texas, USA

MICHAEL JOSCHKO, PhD, Department of Psychology, Queen Alexandra Hospital for Children, and University of Victoria, Victoria, British Columbia, Canada

G. REID LYON, PhD, Center for Language and Cerebral Function, and Departments of Neurology and Communication Science and Disorders, University of Vermont, Burlington, Vermont, USA

EDITE J. OZOLS, PhD, Department of Psychology, University of Windsor, Windsor, Ontario, Canada, and Department of Neuropsychology, St. Michael's Hospital, Toronto, Ontario, Canada

JAMES E. PORTER, PhD, Department of Psychology, University of Windsor, Windsor, Ontario, Canada

BYRON P. ROURKE, PhD, Department of Psychology, University of Windsor, and Department of Neuropsychology, Windsor Western Hospital Centre, Windsor, Ontario, Canada

PAUL SATZ, PhD, The Neuropsychiatric Institute, University of California at Los Angeles, Los Angeles, California, USA

JOHN D. STRANG, PhD, Department of Neuropsychology, Windsor Western Hospital Centre, Windsor, Ontario, Canada

JAMES E. SWEENEY, PhD, District of Parry Sound Child and Family Centre, Parry Sound, Ontario, Canada

HARRY VAN DER VLUGT, PhD, MD, Department of Developmental Psychology, University of Tilburg, Tilburg, The Netherlands

Preface

It is difficult to overestimate the crucial role that valid taxonomies play in any area of investigative endeavor where one seeks to generate models of human functioning that are meant to be heuristic for both theoretical and applied purposes. This is no less the case in the study of learning disabilities in children than it is in any other area of inquiry. Indeed, the confusion that abounds in the literature dealing with the group of clinical problems known as learning disabilities is, in many ways, a direct reflection of the failure of many scientists and practitioners in this field to acknowledge and address the heterogeneity and diversity extant among the learning-disabled population.

Claims that learning disabilities in children are caused by, result from, or are reflections of more basic attentional, mnestic, linguistic, or perceptual deficiencies abound in the literature in this area. In most cases, unfortunately, these "unitary deficit" views are defended in a manner that can best be characterized as narrow, insular, and argumentative. The self-serving, myopic rationale for such positions is also apparent among those who, with the naiveté that only studied ignorance can spawn, claim that learning disabilities in children are direct reflections of inappropriate teaching. One would be hard put to disagree with the proposition that learning-disabled children are in need of very special, sensitive, and appropriate forms of educational intervention. However, the very evident problem that remains is the determination of the precise parameters of "special," "sensitive," and "appropriate" as these apply to the educational programs designed for the individual learning-disabled child.

The authors whose work is contained in this volume are of the opinion that attempts to designate reliable and valid subtypes of learning-disabled children constitute important first steps toward the determination of the needs and propensities of such children that would serve as the basis upon which to construct appropriate methods for their habilitation or rehabilitation. But the scope of investigative efforts represented in this volume goes well beyond the immediate concerns of the academic environment to considerations of the developmental parameters of brain–behavior relationships, the action and interaction of developing human abilities, and the larger ramifications of disabled learning and its treatment in the child's attempts to adapt to his/her everyday environment.

This book has been designed to provide a coherent set of viewpoints and findings that reflect recent advances in the exploration of the parameters and implications of the subtypal analysis of children with learning disabilities. Specifically, an attempt has been made to provide perspectives on the general theory of this genre of analysis; explanations and examples of the various methodologies that have been employed in this exercise; the sorts of remedial interventions suggested by the results of several programmatic investigations; and directions for future research and applications. Although the book is not intended to serve as a manual for either methodology or intervention strategies, we have tried to provide sufficient detail in particular research and clinical domains to enable the serious student and professional to plan and pursue investigations and applications along these lines. In those instances where sufficiently detailed explanations cannot be provided within the confines of the work, references and suggestions regarding other sources are provided for consideration.

In all of this, our plan has been to provide compelling arguments that would encourage researchers and clinicians to consider carefully the specification, description, reliability, and validity of learning disability subtypes in their scientific and applied endeavors. We are particularly interested in emphasizing the role that various patterns of adaptive abilities and deficits can play in social learning, as well as in the academic areas, such as reading, spelling, and arithmetic. Another principal aim has been to point out and explain the caveats that must be borne in mind when embarking upon—and, especially, when deriving the implications of—this taxonomic enterprise.

The programs of empirical, hypothesis-testing investigations described herein have been chosen to serve as examples of the systematic scientific efforts that have been launched recently in this area. The emphasis in some of these chapters is on theory, methodology, generalization of results, and proposals for future studies. In other chapters, more emphasis is placed on the habilitational and rehabilitational implications of these and other empirical studies. Within the latter context, we have attempted to gear our explanations of both methodological and applied issues to the concerns of the practicing researcher and clinician. Thus, we expect that this work will be of interest to research-oriented as well as applied (including clinical and school) psychologists. We have also attempted to provide a framework of issues and discussions that will be germane to the concerns of pediatricians and other professionals who are actively involved in the care of learning-disabled children.

Finally, as a perusal of this volume will make abundantly clear, the specific perspectives of researcher–clinicians in child neuropsychology predominate throughout. This is to be expected, since most of the recent experimental and applied work that has emerged in this area has been carried out by individuals who are concerned with brain–behavior relationships and their developmental ramifications for the learning-disabled child. Indeed, even for those serious students of the field who do not begin with this view, it would seem that the vast majority of the researcher–clinicians in this area are of the opinion that the models and perspectives of neurobehavioral science and practice provide a multifaceted and heuristic viewpoint from which to structure the issues and data in this field. Be that as it may, it is certainly clear that the multivariate methodologies that are so crucial for investigative work in subtyping pursuits fit well with the developmental models and theories that currently hold sway in child neuropsychology.

In an edited work such as this, it is more difficult than usual to acknowledge the assistance of those persons who have been instrumental in bringing each of the contributions to fruition. As the reader will note, some of the authors have inserted their own acknowledgments in the individual chapters. What remains is for me to convey the gratitude of the authors to others who have made substantial contributions to the work as a whole. We are grateful to the editor and editorial consultants of Guilford Press for their many helpful suggestions and critiques. The work is substantially better as a result of their wise counsel. In particular, we would acknowledge the singular contribution of Dr. H. Gerry Taylor, Department of Pediatrics, School of Medicine, University of Pittsburgh, who read and commented on the entire manuscript. His perspicacity and his very helpful suggestions are very much appreciated. We are also grateful to those who, tirelessly and assiduously, pored over the preliminary and final drafts of the chapters in an effort to transform our sometimes feeble efforts at communication into readable prose. Marilyn Chedour, Eleanor Benson, and Diane Russell were particularly instrumental in this connection. Finally, as the most important "final common path" for any neurospychologist, we wish to acknowledge with deep gratitude the herculean efforts of Maria Lalli and Marilyn Frederick, who typed, retyped, and retyped our scrambled musings.

Of course, any errors or omissions that remain are the responsibility of the contributors and, ultimately, of the editor.

BYRON P. ROURKE
June 1984

Contents

xi

Neuropsychology of Learning Disabilities:
Essentials of Subtype Analysis

I

Introduction

1

Overview of
Learning Disability Subtypes

BACKGROUND FOR THE PRESENT VOLUME

There was a protracted period in the history of Western medicine when blood-letting was the preferred mode of treatment for disturbances of physiological homeostasis. This therapeutic technique gave way to other modes of intervention as it was discovered that there was more than one type of physiological disturbance and more than one etiology that could account for such disturbances. Thus, it is the case today that the overwhelming weight of opinion among medical scientists is that treatment should be differentiated insofar as necessary in view of the individual characteristics, etiology, course, and prognosis of the various subtypes of physiological disturbances.

A parallel historical process would seem to be emerging in the investigation and care of learning-disabled children. For many years, two theoretical perspectives dominated the field: those of A. A. Strauss and S. T. Orton. Each championed a univocal etiology for the disabilities in question. However, whereas Strauss and his associates proposed an equally univocal form of intervention that was thought to be consistent with their proposed etiology, Orton and his followers proposed a system of intervention that bore no resemblance whatsoever to his view of etiology (Rourke, 1981a). It remained for others (e.g., Delacato, 1963) to

Byron P. Rourke. Department of Psychology, University of Windsor, and Department of Neuropsychology, Windsor Western Hospital Centre, Windsor, Ontario, Canada.

3

propose a uniform mode of treatment that would, in their view, be consistent with Orton's etiological hypotheses.

Thus, in the late 1950s, the 1960s, and the early 1970s, "treatment" for learning-disabled children, insofar as it was seen to be "special" and etiologically based, tended to be univocal—in the sense that, once a child was identified as "learning-disabled," he/she was most often placed in a therapeutic/remedial educational program that was designed to offer all children in it the same type and sequence of habilitational experiences. The *style* of such interventions was essentially the same as that advocated by most psychoanalysts, teachers of "normal children," and behavioral therapists: namely, the programmatic administration of the proposed form of intervention in essentially the same fashion to all of those who were identified as afflicted with the disturbance.

Fortunately, there have always been those who have resisted this trend. Johnson and Myklebust (1967), for example, have maintained steadfastly for many years that there are differentiatable subtypes of learning-disabled children, whose particular patterns of abilities and deficits cry out for vastly different forms of interventional styles and strategies. Nevertheless, their admonitions went largely ignored in many circles, mostly because the bases upon which they identified their subtypes were primarily "clinical" in nature and, in consequence, difficult to understand and apply for those who were not trained extensively in these procedures. In addition, there were a great many researcher–clinicians who felt that "objective" indices of behavior must constitute the building blocks in subtypal analysis.

For these reasons, a kind of stalemate held sway during the early 1970s. On the one hand, behaviorists continued to administer behavioral therapy, dynamically oriented therapists applied their usual methods, and school-based approaches differed only along lines of offering more intensive versions of the "normal" school curriculum or univocal programs that were tied to equally univocal views of etiology. On the other hand, clinicians who had extensive familiarity—and reported successes in dealing therapeutically—with various subtypes of learning-disabled children were unable to demonstrate to the satisfaction of their hard-nosed empirically oriented colleagues either the reliability of their subtype classifications or the validity of the differential intervention strategies that they saw as flowing from the unique ability profiles of the various subtypes. Thus, to continue the metaphor, "blood-letting" remained the therapy of choice, with the added proviso that it was modified to suit the particular etiological and theoretical proclivities of the behaviorists, dynamically oriented psychotherapists, educationists, and so on. What was needed was a means of establishing a reliable taxonomy of learning disabilities that would be amenable to empirical validations and heuristic extensions. In large measure, this process began in earnest in the mid-1970s and has increased in intensity during the late 1970s and early 1980s.

This book has been designed to provide a survey of the most current investigative efforts along these lines. Specifically, it is meant to provide an up-to-date summary of the issues raised, results obtained, and modes of intervention suggested by investigations aimed at generating scientific explanations of one or more of the multifaceted aspects of this important set of problems. The reader will find that the ways in which these issues are addressed, the data studied, and the conclusions derived are quite variegated and, in some cases, are at odds with each other. This is to be expected in an enterprise that has barely begun, that has been so sorely needed, and that has been so sadly overlooked and misunderstood.

By way of preparation for this endeavor, the reader may wish to consult some of the better-known studies from the middle and late 1970s that are not examined in the depth that they deserve herein. These would include the clinical subtyping investigations of Boder (1973) and Mattis (Mattis, French, & Rapin, 1975), and the empirical, multivariate investi-gations carried out by the following investigators and their colleagues: Doehring (Doehring & Hoshko, 1977; Doehring, Hoshko, & Bryans, 1979; Doehring, Trites, Patel, & Fiedorowicz, 1981), myself (Fisk & Rourke, 1979; Petrauskas & Rourke, 1979; Rourke, 1978b, 1981b, 1983), and Satz (Morris, Blashfield, & Satz, 1981; Satz & Morris, 1981). In this connection, the reader may also wish to review some early work on the neuropsychological significance of Wechsler Intelligence Scale for Chil-dren (WISC) Verbal–Performance intelligence quotient (IQ) discrepancies among learning-disabled children (Rourke, Dietrich, & Young, 1973; Rourke & Telegdy, 1971; Rourke, Young, & Flewelling, 1971), as this work bears upon more specific examinations of learning disabilities that some view as resulting from disordered functioning of systems thought to be subserved primarily by the right cerebral hemisphere. In addition, several reviews of the subtyping research of the middle and late 1970s could be consulted with profit (Doehring *et al.*, 1981; Satz & Morris, 1981; Rourke, 1978a). Although the current volume was designed to be read and appreciated on its own, interpretation of the specific studies elaborated on, for the most part, presumes more than passing familiarity with this previous work.

OVERVIEW OF THE VOLUME

This section of the chapter contains brief summaries of the contents of the substantive chapters of this volume. It should be pointed out that the chapters have been arranged in an order that makes sense from one pedagogical viewpoint: The progression is one that extends from theory, through methodology, to descriptions of research projects on specific learning disability subtypes, and finally to considerations of validity in the widest sense. At the same time, it must be acknowledged that this sequence may not be appropriate for some. Indeed, there is good reason to maintain, for example, that the material contained and the considerations raised in Chapter 2 would make more sense for some if they were to be read at the end of the work rather than at its beginning. Be that as it may, the script as we have designed it is as follows.

In Section II, "Theory and Methodology," the aim is to explicate, within the context of models of behavior and brain–behavior relationships, issues that affect the selection of statistical and other methodological techniques and the bearing that these choices have upon the interpretation and generalizability of results in this field. In Chapter 2, the first chapter of this section, Adams raises a number of theoretical and metatheoretical issues that should be addressed in the development of any taxonomy. He relates these to the classification of children with learning disabilities, with special reference to those considerations that should be dealt with before the adoption of particular methodologies and during the interpretation of the multivariate analyses that are so frequently employed in their execution. The issues broached in this chapter are both basic and thorny. At some point, the reader would do well to consider at length these dimensions of the subtyping enterprise, because they have considerable impact upon the issues and data discussed in all of the chapters that follow.

In Chapter 3, Fletcher and Satz describe a unique approach to the search for subtypes of learning-disabled children. Their systematic program of analysis of theoretical, methodological, and content issues is described in detail. This chapter will be of particular interest to those who are considering the initiation of systematic longitudinal projects dealing with learning-disabled children. In addition, Fletcher and Satz provide a critique of their own research and that of several others in this area, with particular emphasis upon an explanation of the dimensions that must be considered critically when decisions regarding choice of methodology and dependent variables are made. Other considerations regarding populations of interest and generalizability of results are also highlighted.

In Chapter 4, Joschko and I provide an example of the application of multivariate techniques to the subtype analysis of a subgroup of learning-disabled children who exhibit a pattern of performance (the WISC Arithmetic, Coding, Information, and Digit Span—or "ACID"—pattern) that has been the subject of some empirical work and much speculation in the literature of this field (e.g., Ackerman, Dykman, & Peters, 1976). This chapter is designed to illustrate the procedures that can be followed in the analysis of this sort of problem. Those who are primarily concerned with statistical and methodological issues will find it of particular interest. In addition, the chapter includes comparisons with another group of learning-disabled children who do not exhibit the pattern in question. This type of design is a reflection of a particular approach to the analysis of subtypes among learning-disabled children that has been exploited in a number of other investigations (e.g., see Fletcher, Chapter 9, and Strang & Rourke, Chapter 8, this volume).

The comparisons of different subgroups of learning-disabled children, with consequent subtyping analysis of these subgroups, is also the focus of concern in Chapter 5. As is the case in Chapter 4, this presentation emphasizes statistical and methodological issues and procedures; in consequence, it should be of particular interest to those who wish to pursue investigations in this field and who are primarily concerned with the application of multivariate techniques for this purpose. In addition, the interpretation of the results of the investigation highlighted in this chapter should be of interest to those who are concerned with the (possibly differential) roles of hand preference and hand dominance in relation to issues of cerebral asymmetries and functional lateralization in children. It may be of interest to note that this particular approach to the analysis of learning disability subtypes has implications for theoretical issues that reach far beyond those relating to children with outstanding learning disabilities.

In Section III, "Reading, Spelling, and Arithmetic Disability Subtypes," specific examples of research programs in these three areas are presented. It may be of particular interest to note the various starting points, methodologies, and future directions proposed in these chapters.

For example, in Chapter 6, Doehring describes a program of research in the area of reading disability subtype analysis that began with rather broad-based studies of neuropsychological and reading-related characteristics of disabled readers. Its development proceeded through a consideration of subtypes based upon each of these domains separately and in conjunction with one another, to a proposal for the multi-dimensional investigation of various reading disability subtypes at what we may refer to as the "microanalysis" level. One upshot of this approach is that we can expect to find that the analysis of subtypes of reading disability in children will lead to considerable alteration in models of disabled reading, as well as in models that purport to structure the "normal" reading process. Indeed, the principal theoretical impact of advances in the taxonomy of reading disability would be expected to be the generating of models of sufficient complexity and articulation that would allow us to comprehend the manner in which word recognition and reading comprehension proceed in both normal and disordered fashions. In fact, it may very well be the case that there are different subtypes of normal readers, and that these would be better understood not only through multivariate and other forms of subtype analysis of them, but also by comparing the (possibly) different subtypes that eventuate thereby to those that have been generated in reading-disabled populations.

Sweeney and I follow a quite different approach in Chapter 7. This chapter deals with a series of studies aimed at establishing the neuro-psychological significance (i.e., the concurrent, predictive, and construct validity) of two subtypes of disabled spellers. In these studies, the subtypes were defined on the basis of the presence or absence of a pathological sign (that is, phonetically inaccurate misspelling). Specifically, one type of disabled speller (referred to as "phonetically accurate") exhibited levels of phonetic accuracy of misspelled syllables that were indistinguishable from those of normal spellers, whereas the other subtype of disabled spellers (referred to as "phonetically inaccurate") exhibited levels of phonetic accuracy of misspelled syllables that were substantially less than those of both the other subtype of disabled spellers and of normal spellers. Of note was the attempt in this series of developmental investigations to specify, with progressively greater precision, the nature and extent of the abilities and deficits of these two subtypes of disabled spellers. Thereafter, an attempt was made to suggest modes of remedial intervention that would be consistent with the differential patterns of neuropsychological abilities and deficits exhibited by these two subtypes of disabled spellers. This exercise was meant to suggest how subtype analysis may be used to generate hypotheses regarding appropriate intervention strategies.

Chapter 8, on arithmetic disability subtypes, also deals with a series of investigations of children who present with obviously impaired levels of skill in a particular academic area. In this instance, however, the feature used to differentiate the groups in question was their particular *pattern* of academic performances in reading, spelling, and arithmetic. Having differentiated the children on the basis of three distinct patterns, a series of studies was undertaken to determine the configurations of central processing abilities and deficiencies that might account for these differential patterns of academic abilities. These studies essentially constitute investigations of the validity of the particular subtypes that were identified on the basis of patterns of relative deficiency and proficiency in academic skill areas. They also illustrate how various subtypes of arithmetic disability itself can be seen to be reflections of unique configurations of central processing abilities and deficits. In addition, an attempt is made in this chapter to show how the results of various *qualitative* analyses of arithmetic calculation performance can be shown to be consistent with the hypothesized brain–behavior patterns of relationships identified in the group studies. Finally, an attempt is made to generate and explain modes and strategies of intervention that seem to flow rather directly from the findings of these subtype studies. As is the case for the remedial programs proposed in Chapter 7, it is clear that these intervention techniques must be subjected to the two types of educational validation studies that are explained in Chapter 11 by Lyon.

The next section of the work, "Validity Studies of Learning Disability Subtypes," has to do quite specifically with validation studies of learning disability subtypes. Although there is a sense in which some of the studies discussed in Chapter 6, 7, and 8 relate to validity considerations, this section, composed of Chapters 9, 10, and 11, deals in a rather more direct fashion with issues of concurrent, predictive, and construct validity.

Chapter 9, by Fletcher, outlines a number of principles and procedures that are involved in "external" validation studies, and he goes to some length to explain the rationale and importance of such studies in this area. His review of his own research and that of some others in this area is meant to provide examples of the sort of validity studies that must be carried out if advances in our understanding are to be made. It is particularly important to note that these types of studies are essentially the "acid test" of subtype analysis of learning disabilities in children. The theoretical, methodological, data-gathering, and reliability considerations that precede this particular type of investigation would be all but useless without following through with this last step. If the subtypes of learning-disabled children that are generated by the types of analyses examined in this volume do not stand up to the test of validation, there is no good reason to proceed in these fashions in pursuit of a classificatory taxonomy.

A very specific type of validity study is the focus of Chapter 10, by van der Vlugt and Satz. Specifically, these authors describe in detail a series of studies that was designed as a cross-cultural validation in The Netherlands of subtypes originally identified in the Florida Longitudinal Project. Many would expect that the differences in language, cultural patterns, and educational practices extant in these two parts of the world would have a considerable impact on the nature of the subtypes identified. However, such was not the case. In spite of the very obvious cultural differences that might be expected to eventuate in differences in the subtypes generated, a remarkable degree of similarity emerged. This certainly adds considerable weight to the contention that the patterns of central processing abilities and deficits that have been hypothesized to underlie such subtypes are, in fact, more influenced by constitutional than by cultural factors.

In Lyon's chapter on educational validation studies, a series of investigations dealing with important issues are described. This series of studies is especially instructive because it serves as an example of the manner in which such investigations evolve and how each provides impetus for the projects that follow. The problems and the vicissitudes involved in carrying out such studies are also explained. These should serve as a caveat for those who wish to embark upon such an enterprise, for it is quite clear that these issues must be dealt with and resolved, at least to some extent, before this type of investigation is mounted.

A persistent problem and pervasive concern of investigators of learning-disabled children has been and continues to be the role(s) that personality factors and socioemotional disturbances may play in such disorders. Section V, "Personality and Socioemotional Dimensions of Learning Disabilities in Children," contains chapters that address this issue. Porter and I (Chapter 12) and Ozols and I (Chapter 13) present explanations of the relevant parameters of this set of problems. In Chapter 12, one example of an approach to this issue is outlined in detail: The study described shows how the subtypal analysis of personality inventory data can be employed to address the nature and extent of personality disturbance among learning-disabled children. In Chapter 13, a quite different approach is utilized: The performances of subtypes of learning-disabled children who were identified on the basis of their differential patterns of performance on tests reflective of psycholinguistic and visual–spatial–organizational abilities are compared on a series of tasks designed to tap various dimensions of social perception and judgment. These two chapters and the final one in this section are meant to illustrate how this complex set of considerations can be approached in a systematic fashion.

The material in Chapter 14 is an extension of that dealt with in Chapter 8. Specifically, the adaptive abilities of a particular subtype of children who exhibit outstanding impairment in arithmetic calculation abilities and an associated pattern of neuropsychological abilities and deficits are examined. This in-depth analysis of the qualitative characteristics of this subtype of learning-disabled children is designed to demonstrate the potential impact of patterns of central processing abilities and deficits within the socioemotional realm, as well as the heuristic implications of such analyses. The latter considerations and the suggestions for intervention strategies and techniques explained in all three of the chapters in this section should, of course, be subjected to the sorts of empirical validation studies that are outlined by Fletcher (Chapter 9) and Lyon (Chapter 11). Indeed, the chapters in this section serve to demonstrate how one can approach problems within this field by means of a systematic program of validity studies, each of which provides suggestions for the investigations that should follow.

The concluding chapter of this volume is designed (1) to highlight some of the major findings and conclusions that emerge from the analyses contained within the preceding chapters, and (2) to suggest some avenues for future research in this field. Although attempts have been made by each of the authors of the separate chapters to integrate their own findings with those of the other contributors, this "final" statement seems necessary in order to achieve some modest degree of closure for the volume.

THE ISSUE OF INDIVIDUAL DIFFERENCES

This concludes the summary of the chapters in this volume. However, one important issue should be addressed before drawing this discussion to a close. This relates to the ideographic–nomothetic controversy that seems to be ever with us in the no-man's-land between "pure" and "applied" psychology. Within the present context, some points should be considered and clarified before the reader considers the contents of this volume. These are as follows:

The classification of children into "homogeneous" subtypes does *not* imply that the children so classified are identical. Indeed, it would appear quite likely that children classified through the use of the methods and behavioral variables employed by the authors in this work would exhibit, together with their similarities, fairly substantial individual differences. That is, although they may be quite similar to one another with respect to their pattern of adaptive abilities and deficits (and, by implication, with respect to their central processing characteristics), any number of differences in early or current environmental circumstances, reinforcement patterns, and so on would be expected to have a differential impact on the psychosocial functioning of the children. It is for this reason that predictions (prognoses) and treatments must be framed and designed as individualized amalgams reflecting common (subtypal) and unique (historical) characteristics.

In this connection, it should be borne in mind that the common (subtypal) variance is itself a reflection of a certain level of uniqueness or individuality, insofar as it differentiates each child within a particular subtype from those in the other subtypes and from those who are not classified. In addition, the ideographic formulation of the treatment plan should take into consideration the final level of individualization that is afforded by an examination and understanding of a child's unique sociohistorical milieu and characteristics. It is in this (combined) sense that we view the identification of more general clusters of learning-disabled children who share common dimensions or factors as a complementary form of individualization that (we hope) contributes to the formulation and execution of appropriate individualized educational/therapeutic plans (Fisk & Rourke, 1983; Rourke, Bakker, Fisk, & Strang, 1983).

EDITOR'S NOTE

One final editorial point: It should be borne in mind that I have assumed the primary responsibility for integrating and cross-referencing the positions, models, techniques, findings, and suggestions for remedial intervention that are manifest in this volume. Thus, any shortcomings, errors, and omissions that remain are a direct reflection of my editorial decisions. More generally, the reader, as always, must decide on the relative merits of the array of separate contributions to this volume and the implications that these have for the evaluation of previous investigative efforts and for the design of future research. A careful reading of these contributions should leave the reader in no doubt whatsoever regarding the authors' views on these matters.

To return to the metaphor outlined at the outset, it should be clear that the contributions to this volume mirror a trend in research and practice that eschews univocal answers and correctives for a set of disturbances that is multifaceted and heterogeneous. In addition, there should be no doubt whatsoever as to the tack that these authors feel should be chosen in order to extend investigative lines with respect to theory testing, model building, and interventive evaluation. The answers anticipated are deemed to result from theoretically based, empirically couched, consensually validatable investigations that are amenable to objective scrutiny and independent replication. In their view, at least, a return to blood-letting would seem to be quite out of the question!

REFERENCES

Ackerman, P. T., Dykman, R. A., & Peters, J. E. Hierarchical factor patterns on the WISC as related to areas of learning deficits. *Perceptual and Motor Skills*, 1976, *42*, 583-615.

Boder, E. Developmental dyslexia: A diagnostic approach based on three atypical reading-spelling patterns. *Developmental Medicine and Child Neurology*, 1973, *15*, 663-687.

Delacato, C. H. *Diagnosis and treatment of speech and reading problems.* Springfield, Ill.: Charles C Thomas, 1963.

Doehring, D. G., & Hoshko, I. M. Classification of reading problms by the Q-technique of factor analysis. *Cortex*, 1977, *13*, 281-294.

Doehring, D. G., Hoshko, I. M., & Bryans, B. N. Statistical classification of children with reading problems. *Journal of Clinical Neuropsychology*, 1979, *1*, 5-16.

Doehring, D. G., Trites, R. L., Patel, P. G., & Fiedorowicz, A. M. *Reading disabilities: The interaction of reading, language, and neuropsychological deficits.* New York: Academic Press, 1981.

Fisk, J. L., & Rourke, B. P. Identification of subtypes of learning-disabled children at three age levels: A neuropsychological, multivariate approach. *Journal of Clinical Neuropsychology*, 1979, *1*, 289-310.

Fisk, J. L., & Rourke, B. P. Neuropsychological subtyping of learning disabled children: History, methods, implications. *Journal of Learning Disabilities*, 1983, *16*, 529-531.

Johnson, D. J., & Myklebust, H. R. *Learning disabilities.* New York: Grune & Stratton, 1967.

Mattis, S., French, J. H., & Rapin, I. Dyslexia in children and young adults: Three independent neuropsychological syndromes. *Developmental Medicine and Child Neurology*, 1975, *17*, 150-163.

Morris, R., Blashfield, R., & Satz, P. Neuropsychology and cluster analysis: Potentials and problems. *Journal of Clinical Neuropsychology*, 1981, *3*, 79–99.

Petrauskas, R., & Rourke, B. P. Identification of subgroups of retarded readers: A neuropsychological, multivariate approach. *Journal of Clinical Neuropsychology*, 1979, *1*, 17–37.

Rourke, B. P. Neuropsychological research in reading retardation: A review. In A. L. Benton & D. Pearl (Eds.), *Dyslexia: An appraisal of current knowledge.* New York: Oxford University Press, 1978. (a)

Rourke, B. P. Reading, spelling, arithmetic disabilities: A neuropsychologic perspective. In H. R. Myklebust (Ed.), *Progress in learning disabilities* (Vol. 4). New York: Grune & Stratton, 1978. (b)

Rourke, B. P. Due modelli neuropsicologici delle incapacita' cognitive de sviluppo: Un confronto ed una valutazione. In O. Andreani (Ed.), *Aspetti biosociali dello sviluppo* (Vol. 2, *Processi cognitivi*). Milano: Franco Angeli, 1981. (a)

Rourke, B. P. Neuropsychological assessment of children with learning disabilities. In S. B. Filskov & T. J. Boll (Eds.), *Handbook of clinical neuropsychology.* New York: Wiley-Interscience, 1981. (b)

Rourke, B. P. Reading and spelling disabilities: A developmental neuropsychological perspective. In U. Kirk (Ed.), *Neuropsychology of language, reading, and spelling.* New York: Academic Press, 1983.

Rourke, B. P., Bakker, D. J., Fisk, J. L., & Strang, J. D. *Child neuropsychology: An introduction to theory, research, and clinical practice.* New York: Guilford Press, 1983.

Rourke, B. P., Dietrich, D. M., & Young, G. C. Significance of WISC Verbal–Performance discrepancies for younger children with learning disabilities. *Perceptual and Motor Skills,* 1973, *36*, 275–282.

Rourke, B. P., & Gates, R. D. Neuropsychological research and school psychology. In G. W. Hynd & J. E. Orbzut (Eds.), *Neuropsychological assessment and the school-age child: Issues and procedures.* New York: Grune & Stratton, 1981.

Rourke, B. P., & Telegdy, G. A. Lateralizing significance of WISC Verbal–Performance discrepancies for older children with learning disabilities. *Perceptual and Motor Skills,* 1971, *33*, 875–883.

Rourke, B. P., Young, G. C., & Flewelling, R. W. The relationships between WISC Verbal–Performance discrepancies and selected verbal, auditory–perceptual, visual-perceptual, and problem-solving abilities in children with learning disabilities. *Journal of Clinical Psychology,* 1971, *27*, 475–479.

Satz, P., & Morris, R. Learning disability subtypes: A review. In F. J. Pirrozolo & M. C. Wittrock (Eds.), *Neuropsychological and cognitive processes in reading.* New York: Academic Press, 1981.

II
Theory and Methodology

2

Theoretical, Methodological, and Statistical Issues

KENNETH M. ADAMS

INTRODUCTION

This chapter informs the reader of the scientific basis of the search for subtypes in learning-disabled children. Taxonomic methods have been the central *modi operandi* to date in the major research programs that have produced objective subtypes of learning-disabled children. The epistemological basis of these methods is explained, and the methodological issues necessary for a general level of understanding of taxonomic research tools are discussed. The relationship and essential complementarity of phyletic and phenetic taxonomic conceptions are also addressed. Finally, these considerations are applied to issues arising from the use of cluster-analytic/factor-analytic methodology to identify subtypes in learning-disabled children.

The plan of this chapter is to acquaint the reader with some ideas that are important in the understanding of taxonomic research as an epistemological technique in science. In doing this, I attempt to relate these general scientific problems to specific points likely to be of value in the evaluation and appreciation of classification research with learning-disabled children. The reader can then understand the various aspects of agreement and controversy arising from research programs such as those described in this volume.

Kenneth M. Adams. Division of Neuropsychology, Henry Ford Hospital, Detroit, Michigan, USA.

This approach is necessary for three reasons. First, any taxonomic approach to the classification of children's learning problems presumes a distinctive epistemological and developmental viewpoint. Second, the ways in which psychologists define and use classification diverge from the concepts and applications that natural scientists employ. Third, the ways and means by which psychologists translate the objectives of classification into studies and results have practical differences that may influence these results and their interpretation.

In pursuing the aims of this chapter, the reader will be referred to diverse concepts in research, many of which are nonpsychological in nature. This is a deliberate choice, because, while many of the problems in classification research are universal, there are many helpful perspectives and fresh insights to be gained from the particular experiences of sister sciences. I may also add here that the discussion presented in the early portion of this chapter may at first seem distant from the topic of subtypes of learning disabilities in children. However, an understanding of the foundations of the methods used in such research is of great importance if the reader wishes to gain full appreciation of the topic.

It may be useful to turn first to some basic ideas concerning epistemology, taxonomy, and the process of subtype development.

TAXONOMY AS AN EPISTEMIC TOOL

The term "epistemic" refers to the capacity to know or knowing as a type of experience. It implies a purely cognitive or intellectual value often praised as an achievement in science. "Epistemology" refers to the study of the methods and grounds of knowledge, with particular reference to its limits and validity. This is to be contrasted with gnoseology, which is concerned with the philosophy of knowledge, or ontology, which is concerned with the nature of being or existence. A rough consideration of these terms and their differences may suggest that the epistemologist may have a good deal to tell us as scholars and scientists, but this view per se does not pretend to be a full rendering of human experience.

Put more simply, it can be said that epistemology is perhaps more essential to scientific research than other philosophical areas of inquiry about knowledge and experience. The ways in which we can strive to understand nature are constrained by the degree to which we can agree to observe and express our findings. This does not mean that unique insights or private experiences are not valuable human experiences in their own aesthetic right. Rather, it means that such experiences need to be made systematic and available to others to be considered scientific.

Thus, the epistemological perspective is a crucial one. Verified knowledge of a public nature represents the common ground on which researchers meet, and the scientific method provides the protocol for this intercourse. Researchers bring much more than codified intellectual processes into play in their work, but their plans must conform to an accepted set of procedures and standards that are eminently epistemological. The expression of a theory about subtypes of learning-disabled children, petunias, zebras, or anything else must eventually leave the "hunch" stage and be left to stand on its own merit without the need for priest, guru, or expert to protect it.

Narrowing our focus, it can be seen that taxonomy is an epistemological discipline. *"Taxonomy" refers to the systematic distinguishing, ordering, and naming of types within a subject field.* In biology or zoology, these types may represent certain groupings of samples or species. Within the present context, the search for types is actually a quest for possible *subtypes* of children who have learning disabilities. Just as epistemological clarity is a central aspect of science, it is clear that taxonomy is a vital discipline within this larger search for knowledge.

Several aspects of this definition of taxonomy are important. First, there are three main tasks in taxonomy. Second, the process refers to the identification of types or subtypes, which are *groups* of subjects or observations. Third, the taxonomic search goes on within a defined "subject field." These points deserve further consideration.

1. The first point is that the taxonomic task is multifaceted. It is simply not enough to find a structure for and describe the relationships between objects or observations. Recall from the above that taxonomy consists of the description, ordering, and naming of type groups within a given field. While the tools of epistemology must be seen as broader than taxonomy alone, these three components can be seen to be parallel to the three general tasks of epistemology itself—namely, the descriptive task, the critical task, and the advisory task (Reichenbach, 1938):

Taxonomic function	*Epistemologic task*
Distinguishing	Descriptive
Ordering	Critical
Naming	Advisory

A few moments of reflection should suggest that the actual *descriptive* creation of subgroups from a sample is only the beginning of the taxonomic task. A more challenging second phase is the *critical* study of the scheme for internal consistency and external validity. Finally, the linking of a reliable and valid scheme to the corpus of knowledge requires consideration of the meaning or import of the application of the model; hence, the *advisory* nature of the task.

2. The second major point is that taxonomy is a process aimed at the identification of *groups*. This implies that the taxonomic procedures are designed to create similar *groups* of subjects or observations whose similarity may be defined on some basis. This basis may be understandable or useful in psychological terms (in the case of behavioral data), or it may not. Psychometric group data distributions include knowable test-score components of elevation, shape, and scatter, and more ephemeral ingredients of clinical comprehensibility. Even the successful production of a subgroup or subtype produces only a template or typological standard against which new *individual* observations must be compared.

A corollary of the last-mentioned point is that not all—or even a majority—of new observations need be understandable in terms of a classification scheme involving subtypes. The only requirement is that, when new observations match the subtype model, the inferred characteristics and predicted behaviors or responses must be present *on a reliable basis*. This congruence represents the successful contribution of the advisory task as described above. More concretely, this means that each object or observation thought to match a subtype can be handled or disposed of with confidence that the decision is correct.

It would also be interesting here to see the shift in definitional emphasis of these three parallel concepts described above to the case in which a typology has been established. The application and further development of the scheme would probably have the following hierarchy:

Taxonomic function	Definition	Epistemologic task
Naming	Identification of an observation as a potential fit.	Descriptive
Distinguishing	A "yes–no" decision made along objective distinctions.	Critical
Ordering	The establishment of an ordering, priority, or degree of fit with the subtypal standard of comparison.	Advisory

The rigorous use of this protocol in the individual case would—in all likelihood—reveal inadequacies and offer directions for improvements.

3. The final major point about taxonomic subtype development is that such research is conducted within a subject field. In children's learn-

ing disabilities, this has important implications for concurrent, predictive, and construct validity. If one conducts research so as to be able to find learning-disabled children from among general classroom populations, the "dysfunctional" subtypes that emerge are likely to be identified on the basis of lower aggregate levels of performance on various academic achievement or neuropsychological measures that might be used. Conversely, subtypes developed exclusively on clinic subpopulations require careful study of their prevalence in the more general classroom environment, so as to verify their distinctiveness and to determine the likelihood that children having such psychological attributes might avoid detection or perhaps even cope with the disability in some way.

Having seen how the ways in which taxonomy serves the general objectives of epistemology, we can now turn to the topic of taxonomy itself.

TAXONOMY: CLASSICAL AND NUMERICAL

The epistemological research objective and its taxonomic tool can be seen to be powerful. Accurate systems that provide discrimination, ordering, and naming of phenomena have been sought over the span of recorded history. Greek and Roman philosopher–scientists sought natural groupings of events and objects so as to bring predictability to medicine, argriculture, and astronomy.

Actual principles of taxonomy and typing reached their highest levels of development in the modern botany and zoology of the last centuries. Taxonomic principles and protocols have been the principal basis for our systems of classification of life forms. Beyond their obvious value in creating consensual systems for the identification of samples, these systems have served the heuristic purpose of stimulating research concerning the manifest and/or latent structure of these schemes.

In psychology, the use of formal taxonomic methods and strategies is relatively new; formal concepts first saw widespread use in the 1960–1970 era. The fact that psychologists are relatively recent consumers of and contributors to taxonomic theory and process is not without cause and subsequent effect. I turn next to the role of taxonomy in classification research, and the implications of psychology's embrace of numerical taxonomy.

Prior to the advent of digital computers and the use of numerical taxonomy, taxonomic research was conducted on the basis of both phyletic and phenetic agendas. That is, the two ways of understanding taxonomy were thought to be complementary and essential. The "phyletic" (or "cladistic") goal contribution is one that emphasizes the phylogenetic and developmental aspects of taxonomic classifications. Questions concerning the origin of species, appearance of adaptive forms and phases, and a number of theoretical and practical aspects of the survival and life quality of organisms are relevant in this context. The "phenetic" contribution is one of measurement, quantification, and operationalization of taxonomic classifications. In some ways this is a more identifiable or comfortable domain for psychologists, having immediate potential links to the full array of psychological techniques. For neuropsychologists, these positions can be seen as equivalent in some ways to the qualitative and quantitative perspectives on assessment so often discussed in recent forums.

The pursuit of better classification systems in natural sciences has presumed a need for both phyletic and phenetic contributions. Indeed, botanical and zoological faculties in leading universities today value expert taxonomists who are inclined toward either of these philosophical predilections.

It would be useful here to expand on the psychological importance of these terms. For example, a phyleticist would be vitally interested in the *ways* in which children attempt to read, code, and transmit information. Of even greater importance would be the relationship of these adaptive attempts to known paths or theories of development and the implications of the taxonomic system for placement of children in these frameworks. Others using this approach would seek the ways in which psychological performance could be linked conceptually to a neural substrate.

In contrast, the pheneticist would seek to objectify, quantify, and make rigorous the taxonomy, principally by the judicious use of empirical or derived mathematical models that would allow for the reliable classification of groups of children based on some framework of measurement. The most obvious framework for psychologists is that of psychological testing, although there is no particular reason why any rigorously observed behavior or set of behaviors could not be used.

Note particularly that these goals (phenetic *and* phyletic) are complementary and can be seen to relate to legitimate attempts to understand children's learning problems, from the standpoints both of models of developmental psychology and of measurement-based prediction of high reliability and validity.

Hempel (1965) defends the multifaceted view of taxonomy and the phenetic–phyletic dialectic. However, he adds another set of considerations in terms of the *kind* of types or the *objective* the types are to serve. Examples may be seen as classificatory types, extreme types, and ideal types. The reader is referred to Chapters 6 and 7 of Hempel (1965) for an excellent exposition of these types.

A good practical example offered by Hempel (1965) of the advantages of this phenetic–phyletic complementarity is that of the evolution of the periodic table of chemical elements—one of the great natural classification schemes of science, with implications for the understanding of matter that have yet to be appreciated, fully a century after its elaboration by Mendeleev. Many of the practical relationships between chemical elements (lithium, sodium, potassium, caesium, etc.) were described in objective and specific terms by scientists prior to the discovery of the table (Jevons, 1877/1958). The empirical and numerical relationships, coupled with a search for a substrate and wider context, carried knowledge forward. It may have taken scientists years to appreciate the underlying order before them, while at the same time it is unlikely that Mendeleev invented his scheme entirely from first principles.

A RECENT CHANGE

The development of sophisticated digital computers and programs to conduct advanced mathematical analysis has changed the face and thrust of taxonomy. However, the full implications of this development are not often completely understood by psychologists.

The development of numerical taxonomy is attributed to the pioneering work of Sneath and Sokal (1973). In their text and subsequent work, they fashioned a powerful case for the development of classification schemes based on the analysis of numerical data from nature. Classification rules or models could be developed from the analysis of data matrices that represented observations of events or objects.

Such systems use to maximal advantage the apparent mathematical objectivity inherent in phenetic taxonomy, and the resultant potential for the identification of natural groupings or subtypes. The creation of subtypes in numerical taxonomy is based on the employment of very sophisticated, computerized mathematical algorithms. Thus, the computer could be programmed to search for similarities, features, or recurring patterns in data that could serve as a basis for a taxonomic scheme. This is the rough sense of numerical taxonomy. The obvious value of such methodology for the issues addressed in this volume is to search psychological data for subtypes of learning-disabled children who are diagnostically different and who will respond differentially to treatment.

It seems fair to say that the availability of technology to manipulate massive amounts of data changed the ways in which many taxonomic investigations could proceed. To many, not all of the changes are advances, and many researchers of an eclectic orientation argue that numerical taxonomy minimizes a number of important phyletic aspects of taxonomy. In a thoughtful and comprehensive essay, L. A. S. Johnson (1970) has set forth in greater detail than is possible here the issues that could divide artificially the phenetic and phyletic components of taxonomy.

Can objections such as Johnson's be taken seriously? Indeed, what reply can one make to the obvious value of the impartial computer in searching for types of children that will be based on measurement, subject to verification and validation, and, *ipso facto,* objective? The answers to these questions are developed below on the basis of a simple thesis: namely, that psychology's entry into the taxonomic enterprise at the height of its new numerical elaboration has obscured our view of many of the hidden assumptions and complexities behind the application of a seemingly irresistible new technology.

SOME LIMITATIONS AND POTENTIALS FOR NUMERICAL TAXONOMY RESEARCH IN CHILDREN'S LEARNING DISABILITIES

In their classic volume, Sneath and Sokal (1973) state that the actual separation of phyletic and phenetic views of taxonomy made possible by their techniques represented an advance. For researchers seeking useful subtypes from among learning-disabled children this might be true, in that more advanced numerical taxonomy would serve to increase the quality of phenetic models. However, numerical taxonomy seeks to identify latent relationships between objects or observations taken at a particular point in time. This search for order among data is a very cross-sectional, "now" approach to what is thought to be a very complex developmental process in children. In point of fact, were one to hold a view that the problems underlying learning disabilities were developmental in nature or delayed along some continuum of healthy development or deficit, a distinctly phyletic approach would be an essential initial approach in research.

That is, prior to collecting data and subjecting them to analysis, it would be crucial to (1) develop a phyletic model of the process under study, (2) reconcile this with current theories of brain or behavioral development, and (3) select measures for the numerical taxonomy that would reflect the contribution of the first two tasks. Put another way, a phenetic classification attempt vis-à-vis learning-disabled children will be understandable and useful to the degree that its conception and growth reflect some intelligent ideas concerning the development of the brain and behavior. One corollary of this is that it is simply unlikely that an investigator will go far by selecting some amalgam of favorite or familiar measures for application to learning-disabled children without reference to a model of human development and cerebral function.

A logical rejoinder to this position might be thought to lie in the success of numerical taxonomy in and of itself. The methods of cluster analysis and allied factor-analytic equivalents are sets of algorithms that will always be solved to some "maximum" solution allowed by the data set. Few tests or standards prevent the creation of clusters or the extraction of factors; these multivariate methods are made to function in this way.

If one were to ignore the advantages of initial phyletic taxonomy development based on systematic or syndromatic knowledge of how children perform on various tasks, there would be other compelling reasons to proceed directly to numerical analysis. One such presumed reason is the objectivity with which observations are treated in numerical taxonomy. One aspect of the objectivity would be the grouping in such analysis that is based upon the use of many *equally* weighted measures reflecting different aspects of a child's psychological functioning. The equal weighting of characters or descriptors in the search for similarities in nature has its origins, in part, in the work of the 18th-century French naturalist Michel Adanson (1763). His ideas concerning empirical weighting evolved from his studies of flora in Senegal, the Azores, and Canary Islands.

In the development of learning disability subtypes, this equal weighting may actually fly in the face of theoretical or philosophical information potentially available from phyletic analysis as described above. For example, a developmental theory of neural development might state that the visual system or some other system undergoes a period of unusual development somewhere in the epoch relevant to the analysis. This would not receive weighting in a numerical analysis of a "standard" learning disability assessment unless one took pains to do so. This equal weighting of variables in classification taxonomy is a widespread practice, but, despite all of its positive origins in Adansonian philosophy, it is not an intrinsically valuable aspect of a comprehensive taxonomy.

It should be seen, too, that developmental studies offer rather obvious and substantial opportunities for the study of change scores. It is not unreasonable to consider the prospects for the creation of subtypes or a taxonomy based upon change.

A second defense of exclusively numerical methods might be seen to lie in the multivariate nature of the taxonomic classifications of children. The applicability and power of multidimensional models of behavior appear to be recognized by many leading workers in the area of children's learning disabilities. However, it is important to note that the particular selected variables that define the learning-disabled child in a particular multivariate model represent only one possible set of attributes. And, as I have suggested above, these should be derived ideally from a phyletic phase of taxonomy that has a phylogenetic or developmental emphasis.

The fact that a particular observation is defined on a multivariate basis (e.g., length, height, weight) means that objects existing in this multivariate space may be similar in terms of (these) particular attributes. Yet these points in taxonometric space may be different in a variety of other ways (e.g., color, shape, three-headedness) that not only are relevant phylogenetically in the further understanding of the problem, but may be multidimensional in and of themselves (e.g., color).

A good example of this in the field of children's learning disabilities is seen in the area of motor performance. The selection of measures for motor performance in a taxonomic scheme for the evaluation of learning problems could be guided by such considerations as (1) their consistent relationship to known effects of brain damage or injury, (2) their regular relationship to known developmental paths of motor abilities, or (3) their comprehensiveness or specific role in the capture of the wider construct of motor abilities. Note that these three concerns would be analogous to the three tasks of "internal validation" described by Skinner (1981) in his paper on classification strategies in psychiatry. Skinner views the three tasks—

namely, the evaluation of reliability, homogeneity, and coverage—as being executed once the statistical analysis is selected and the initial typology developed. I would argue strongly that Skinner's timing of such considerations is misplaced and belongs properly at the level of phyletic taxonomic development as described above, or, as Skinner terms it, at the stage of theory formulation.

To put it another way, I would relocate the tasks described by Skinner as internal validation of a multivariate taxonomic classification in their proper place at the level of theory formulation. Careful evaluation of the individual measures in terms of the qualitative and quantitative aspects of the following parameters should precede any actual analysis:

1. Relationship of the variable to known effects or syndromes of brain damage or injury.
2. Relationship of the variable to known paths of development or theoretical developmental frameworks.
3. Relationship of the variable to more general experimental psychology concepts of the construct being measured.
4. Evidence for the reliability of the variable in the widest sense.
5. Evidence for the validity of the variable in the widest sense.
6. Prospects that the variable might be adequate from the standpoint of points 1 through 5 above, but would obscure or elucidate some other relevant attribute.

The adoption of these considerations as a necessary part of taxonomic development *prior* to the consideration of any statistical analysis would do much to satisfy the broader objectives of taxonomic practice and to maximize the benefits that might accrue from numerical analysis. Another benefit would be to end the misleading distinction between internal validation and external validation (Skinner, 1981) that seems to pervade current subtype research. Strictly speaking, the concepts of reliability and validity have quite distinctive tasks that are not served by combining the respective contexts of internal consistency and conceptual justification.

The literature on the relationship of various aspects of reliability and validity makes it quite clear that demands for the satisfaction of these aspects cannot be shuttled between internal and external theaters of observation without considerable loss in the power of the concepts. For example, to speak of reliability as "internal validation" confuses the avowed purposes of reliability and validity (Kendall & Buckland, 1971):

The *reliability* of a result is conceived of as that part which is due to permanent systematic effects, and therefore persists from sample to sample. (p. 129)

Validation is . . . a procedure which provides, by reference to independent sources, evidence that an inquiry is free from bias or otherwise conforms to its declared purpose. . . . Validity is to be contrasted with consistency, which is concerned with the internal agreement of data or procedures among themselves. (p. 160, italics added)

These definitions, as well as any number of classical statistical treatments of these topics, should provide the researcher with a constant warning that internal consistency or observational constancy cannot be put forward as evidence for validity that is inherently external to the process under study or development.

This recalls an earlier point that deserves restatement. Whereas I would agree with those who view the separation of phyletic and phenetic agendas in taxonomy as an achievement, it should also be pointed out that this separation creates unrealistic pressure on those who would rely exclusively upon measurement-based (phenetic) methods to encompass phylogenetic, theoretical, and developmental concerns. The latter are the province of the thinking scientist and are not subsumed in the application of mathematical treatment.

Multivariate mathematical methods cannot serve all of the purposes of numerical taxonomy, much less the wider purpose of taxonomy of classification. Some researchers have identified the major liability of such methods as their lack of unique solutions or tests of significance. The indeterminacy of analysis is thought to be the obstacle. Even if this were not the case, "unique-solution" multivariate methods would still not suffice to deal with the wider tasks and nuances of subtype studies.

The points made above are not intended to decry the use of numerical taxonomy, but rather to place it within a fuller context of classification research and to assign it tasks that are reasonable to perform without having to confuse reliability and validity. Given too great a task, numerical taxonomy and multivariate mathematical techniques will collapse under the weight of considerations not dealt with and the need to recast external standards of evaluation (such as validity) into *ex post facto* justifications of the obtained taxonomic network.

It should be obvious that psychologists seeking to employ exclusively numerical taxonomic methods to seek subtypes of learning-disabled children (who may be at different points in the developmental elaboration of their disorders) may be using mathematical tools that are likely to obscure totally the very perspective sought. Similarly, the relationship of brain deficit to current abilities will only be made clear by careful previous attention to the biological and behavioral ontogenesis of normal and abnormal brain–behavior relationships.

APPROACHES TO THE USE OF
NUMERICAL TAXONOMY TO DEVELOP SUBTYPES

In the discussion above, an emphasis has been placed upon the use of taxonomy as a comprehensive research tool. Actual deployment of powerful methods of numerical analysis must be preceded by thoughtful development of the theoretical objective and the parametric relation of the selected variables to the wider issues of classification of children in this context.

Given that this preparation has taken place, how can one proceed to develop subtypes? There is no shortage of sophisticated mathematical tools for this task, and they are thoroughly described in some recent reviews (Blashfield & Aldenderfer, 1978; Morris, Blashfield, & Satz, 1981; Rourke & Adams, 1984). The methods usually employed for numerical taxonomic analysis require a high-speed computer of at least moderate size, the lack of which obviously hindered the widespread use of this technology before the age of computers, and the presence of which has stimulated it since to what has been described above as a potentially unhealthy degree.

Two essential tasks must be solved in any method that will identify subtypes of learning-disabled children. One task is the definition of *similarity* or *distance* in the space defined by the variable selection. That is, we must assign positions to our observations that relate to the various attributes that the variables represent.

SOME CONSIDERATIONS OF PSYCHOLOGICAL
SIMILARITY AND DISTANCE

The task of defining similarity and distance is often called "ordination" and implies the assignment of each subject on the basis of his/her test scores along many dimensions at once. This process in itself requires some implicit classification, since many behavioral attributes of children require more than one dimension, or may even be conflicting at times in their covariation (e.g., fluency vs. accuracy). The point is that the process of ordination or position selection involves implicit decisions that may obscure the phylogenetic developmental basis of behaviors or may create barriers to the understanding of how behaviors evolve.

If the clinician or researcher is alert to this possibility, variation among children classified in the same subtype because of the numerical representation of their test performances can be evaluated for its developmental significance, and the model can be adjusted accordingly. The classification of children reliably or even validly in multidimensional space does not relieve the researcher of the need to search for subtleties that may be missed because of the analytical method used.

Professionals working with these children will have their own ways and means of evaluating these subtypes. Various aspects of learning style, classroom performance, and observable socioemotional adjustment with peers will provide rich sources of observation. A study in an allied field illustrates how observation can link defined subtypes with their origin.

In a geographical study of barns in Indiana, Noble and Hosler (1977) selected variables that would identify important functional features of barns—which are the epitome of functionality in their rural settings. The sample of barns was observed and measured, and the data were cluster-analyzed to see if subtypes of barns could be developed on the basis of functional order. Not only was the analysis successful in developing stable subtypes, but the subtypes developed appeared to reflect the cultural heritage (e.g., German, Dutch, etc.) of the regions and locales in which they were placed. This exercise thus identified useful architectural subtypes based on execution of the barns, and also detected an important historical or phylogenetic aspect of the barn types and communities. It is worthwhile to note that these origins were not necessarily known to the barn owners, and the research did not identify something "obvious." This is precisely the type of discovery that can be made if the numerical analysis is preceded by phyletic development (in fact, it was not in the case of the barns) and is followed by circumspection in areas of thought other than psychometrics or mathematics.

It is also possible, then, to use numerical methods to test what *does* seem to be obvious. Certain hypothesized syndromes in learning disabilities can be investigated, and their existence can be reaffirmed or refuted.

Joschko and Rourke (see Chapter 4, this volume), for example, conducted just such an exercise in the evaluation of the Arithmetic, Coding,

Information, and Digit Span (ACID) pattern of impairment frequently observed in the Wechsler Intelligence Scale for Children (WISC) performance of learning-disabled children. Briefly, this work started with groups of learning-disabled children with and without the ACID pattern, and identified important aspects of the ways in which children could be seen to be similar in this rough psychometric sense. More important, the results of this study showed the limitations of the ACID concept and pointed to more fundamental potential classifications, based on a fuller developmental and neuropsychological analysis of performance.

Problems in defining psychological similarity or distance in mathematical terms can occur because several types of relative and absolute information are summarized in a test-score variable. Psychological test variables (or any behavioral data points) can be seen to encompass elevation, scatter, and shape. Graphically, these components can be referred to as the overall height, irregularity, and geometrical rank of a profile. As most psychologists and educators realize, these aspects of test scores have differing diagnostic and prognostic significance for the children to whom they are assigned.

It should be noted that differing methods of defining similarity or distance will accentuate various of these test-score components. For example, correlational measures of similarity will ignore absolute level-of-performance information and will amplify profile information by default. Euclidean measures will consider level-of-performance information even when it is not relevant.

For example, one key criticism in the use of correlations as ways of defining similarity is that level-of-performance differences will not enter into the mathematical classification. This liability becomes less serious if the researcher is studying learning-disabled children selected within some well-defined level-of-performance range (which may be the most careful research strategy in any case). Cattell, Coulter, and Tsujioka (1966) have examined some compromise measures encompassing similarity and distance aspects. It should be noted that their specialized metric (rp) has advantages potentially attractive to researchers seeking subtypes of learning-disabled children.

It is noted above that the employment of the process of ordination makes certain presumptions about classification research. The selection of similarity or distance measures implies no fewer implicit decisions. Metric definitions of these qualities may imply some underlying continuum of similarity, but no such continuum need be present from the psychological point of view; only discrete positions may be required. That is, the degrees of similarity defined by Euclidean distance may, correctly or incorrectly, be presumed to have psychological meaning (Johnson, 1970). It is important to know that the space we define in ordination may be different from what we understand as three-dimensional physical space in at least one of five ways:

1. It may be finite.
2. It may have more than three dimensions.
3. It may be non-Euclidean.
4. It may be nonmetric.
5. It may be discontinuous.

Consider also that, in the case of the search for subtypes of learning-disabled children, we are creating a definition of distance between test scores from children who are, by definition, exceptional. Thus, the very selection of metrics to define similarity or distance involves a wide-ranging set of assumptions that may or may not be congruent with our philosophies or objectives.

THE SECOND MAJOR TASK OF NUMERICAL TAXONOMY: CREATION OF THE SUBTYPES

Current research in subtype analysis has tended to use one of two approaches: (1) *Q*-type factor analysis or (2) cluster analysis. Each of these methods has submethods that have been described elsewhere (Morris *et al.*, 1981; Rourke & Adams, 1984).

In *Q*-type factor analysis, the emphasis is on the reduction of a correlated set of observations (between persons) to some optimal smaller set of linear composites that preserves the underlying information. That is, the process is designed to reduce the information on persons over variables. Rather than operate on a correlation matrix between tests to accomplish this dimension reduction (as in the *R*-analysis technique), the analysis loads for factors on the basis of correlations between persons over variables. The resulting factors are linear representations in spatial form, and are the basis for identifying types (Green, 1978).

In cluster analysis, the representation and analysis of data are not necessarily spatial and depend upon the evaluation of *similarity* (Gregson, 1975). The objective of this analysis is to determine an optimal solution in which clusters contain persons whose test attributes are more like one another's than they are like those of persons in other clusters.

A large body of research has developed that concerns itself with the best *ways* to combine various children's test scores, based upon the metric of similarity or distance described above. In factor analysis, there are many ways to reduce the correlation matrix, using various spatial configurations of the data through multiplanar space to provide a solution that has the greatest power to show the full underlying dimensions of the data while minimizing the number of such dimensions. In cluster analysis, many of the approaches focus upon ways to create subtypes of children whose similarity between each other will be *minimal* and whose similarity between each child in the subtypes and children in the other subtypes will be *maximal*. This is obviously a complex mathematical problem of optimalization, one that is dependent upon the variable selection and the researcher's definition of distance or similarity as described.

Despite voluminous research on various clustering metrics (e.g., Hartigan, 1975), no cogent case has been made for why psychologists should employ Q-analysis or cluster analysis. Note that by "cogent case" I mean a multilevel, sensible rationale that is psychological in focus and is not vested in the technique itself. An empirical demonstration of superiority of a method in a trial on a "known-result" task—no matter how powerful—cannot be seen as generalizable to tasks where no standard of comparison exists other than an intuitive or aesthetic one (Blashfield, 1976). A vignette of an unreflective exercise in learning disability subtype analysis will usually feature eager investigators inspecting computer-regurgitated reams of cluster solutions, attempting to find a "best" one prior to its elevation to reality, which is based on some obscure inferred relation to child development or *ex post facto* reconciliation with the reigning theory of cerebral laterality.

The applicability of Q-analysis methods in this exercise cannot be seen to be differentially better. Principal-component or principal-factor methods have been employed with psychological data, and important heuristic ideas have emerged from actual study of the components (with reference back to the original case files). Yet the employment of the Q-analysis method provides no special liability or advantage in relation to cluster analysis.

Incontrovertible proof of my points has been provided by an interesting comparative study by Del Dotto and Rourke (see Chapter 5, this volume). Using a carefully studied sample of sinistral learning-disabled children, these researchers conducted both cluster analysis and *Q*-analysis on their data, using accepted conventions and standards. The results were clear: Both methods classified children into the *same* subtypes. It is rare enough to observe complete concordance via differing methods in psychology, but, in this case, the two modes of analysis were in near-total agreement.

To many researchers of mathematical inclination, these results would be unexpected. Based upon the corpus of self-contained numerical taxonomy literature, this result should not have happened because of problems in the use of correlational similarity indices and technical problems in factor analysis (e.g., double centering). The former proved irrelevant because the children were selected for the study on the basis of the restricted range of IQ (85–115) found in the majority of learning disability studies. It is less clear why the second set of problems did not occur.

If there is any set of reasons to adopt one of these methods over another, it should be a psychological/conceptual one. Perhaps cluster analysis will develop so as to provide innovative or unique definition of similarity or distance. The particular appeal of the *Q*-analysis technique is its place in a wider factorial model for studying persons, variables, and time.

Cattell (1966) has described a multidimensional model for research that encompasses three dimensions or facets (persons, tests, and occasions). The crossing of these parameters creates a total of six possible relevant analyses. These are given letter names corresponding to the type of analysis. The best way to understand this model of research is to study its representation. Figure 2-1 shows the three facets in the form of a "data cube." The three dimensions shown provide for a total of six kinds of analysis that could be helpful in the development of subtypes of learning-disabled children.

The complementarity of these parameters is an essential feature of the system. It is apparent that the development of subtypes of learning disabilities could be facilitated by a disciplined program of exploration along these parameters.

The actual matrices that would be reduced by "factor-analytic" methods are shown in Figure 2-2. A moment's reflection will reveal the possibilities for study. In particular, changes in variables or persons over occasions can readily be investigated, providing a true longitudinal or developmental perspective that relates to the subtypes developed on the variable–person (*Q*-analysis) matrix.

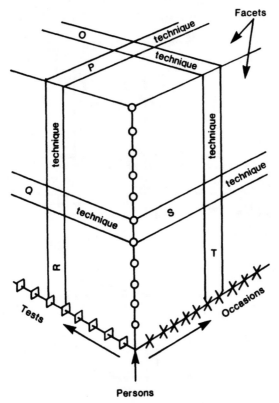

FIG. 2-1. The data cube, showing possible research strategies in subtype analysis. (From R. B. Cattell [Ed.], *Handbook of multivariate experimental psychology*. Chicago: Rand McNally, 1966. Reprinted by permission.)

These approaches could also be realized by cluster-analytic adaptations. It seems fair to say that this approach has been more completely developed at present in the context of factor-analytic methods, but there is no reason why this could not be applied to cluster-analytic methods.

The point here is that, regardless of the data-reduction method used, the primary focus should remain on the philosophy, purposes, and intent of the taxonomic research program. The vast amount of technical detail and mathematical sophistication needed for the understanding of numerical methods in taxonomy should not continue to preoccupy psychologists to the extent that their understanding of taxonomy differs in counterproductive ways from that of other sciences.

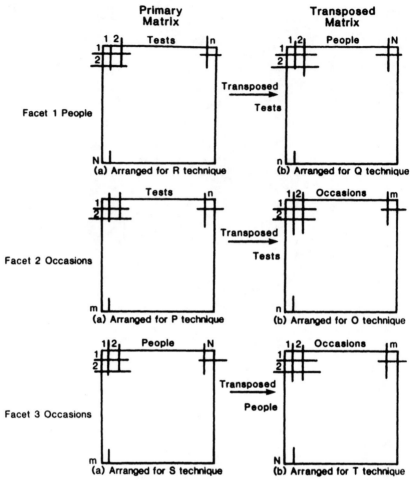

FIG. 2-2. Six major analytic matrices of potential utility in subtype research. (From R. B. Cattell [Ed.], *Handbook of multivariate experimental psychology*. Chicago: Rand McNally, 1966. Reprinted by permission.)

IN CONCLUSION

This chapter has focused on theoretical issues and important implicit assumptions in the understanding of taxonomic research. The use of taxonomic methods to identify subtypes of learning-disabled children represents an intellectual and scientific breakthrough for psychology. The uses of taxonomy to date in psychology, as described earlier in this chapter, are held to be shadows of more complete renderings done in sister sciences. To realize the benefits from other scientific attempts at classification, we must understand fully the multistage process of inter-play among theory, method, and result.

It would be worthwhile to emphasize here that this chapter is not intended to be a critical judgment of the attainments of various subtype research programs to date. This would be unwise, since taxonomic research to develop subtypes is in its infancy. To extend the metaphor, it would be fun to believe that our "learning disability subtype" baby would outgrow its primitive methodological reflexes and make rapid steps toward mature personhood. The work that follows in the ensuing chapters represents the very latest in subtype development, using powerful technology. The comparison of the admittedly ideal scientific outline offered here with the attainments described by the investigators is certain to produce ideas for research to be done or concepts that require investigation or development. This is in the very best tradition of tax-onomic research, and should not be seen as a liability.

While it has been argued here that numerical taxonomy is in-sufficient as a complete *modus operandi*, this chapter can be in no way seen as a call for a return to methods in which subtypes are developed on the basis of subjective, criterion-contaminated identification by conference-table consensus.

While clinicians have often described recurring patterns of test performance or behavior, the true brain substrates of such syndromes have rarely been explored. Rather than focusing upon the development of reliable and valid objective indicators, the development of subtypes based on the degree to which a case resembles an *ex cathedra* syndrome (e.g., Gerstmann's) is a dubious adventure of comparison against an unreliable standard. To argue that subtyping of learning-disabled children can only be done sensitively on this basis leaves us in the hands of overvalued experts whose work can never be properly emulated unless one has been in-troduced to the mysteries of this essentially private system of introspection and duly certified as a minister of its self-fulfilling prophecies. The fundamental error with this approach is that it seeks to identify dif-ferentially salient characters without the benefit of public knowledge and operational definitions. The ways in which this is inadequate have been described previously (Adams, 1980a) and apply here as well.

In closing, I can say that successful identification of subtypes requires mathematical and psychometric sophistication of the kind demonstrated in this volume. I hold here and elsewhere (Adams, 1980b) that this should not be an end in itself. The power of numerical taxonomy methods used in proper *context* is likely to produce evidence essential to the development of subtypes and to serve as a fertile source of hueristic concepts.

New work is likely to build on the kinds of subtype research seen in this volume. Inevitable questions as to the role of biological and environmental influences contributing to the subtypes, the existence of a psychological continuum linking the subtypes, and the differential responsiveness of identified subtypes to interventions in the clinic and classroom await researchers. If there is any consensus possible at this early stage of subtype research in learning disabilities, it is that we stand on the brink of a new era of scientific and clinical investigation in this vital field.

ACKNOWLEDGMENTS

This research was sponsored in part by the Fund for Henry Ford Hospital. I wish to thank Gregory G. Brown and Byron P. Rourke for their informed commentaries on draft copies of this chapter.

REFERENCES

Adams, K. M. In search of Luria's battery: A false start. *Journal of Consulting and Clinical Psychology* 1980, *48*, 511–516. (a)
Adams, K. M. The selection of appropriate multivariate analysis techniques. In S. A. Berenbaum (Chair), *Methodological and statistical issues in neuropsychological research.* Symposium presented at the meeting of the International Neuropsychological Society, San Francisco, 1980. (b)
Adanson, M. *Les familles naturelles des plantes.* Paris: Author, 1763.
Blashfield, R. K. Mixture model tests of cluster analysis: Accuracy of four agglomerative hierarchical methods. *Psychological Bulletin*, 1976, *83*, 377–388.
Blashfield, R. K., & Aldenderfer, M. S. The literature on cluster analysis. *Multivariate Behavioral Research*, 1978, *13*, 271–295.
Cattell, R. B. (Ed.). *Handbook of multivariate experimental psychology.* Chicago: Rand McNally, 1966.
Cattell, R. B., Coulter, M. A., & Tsujioka, B. The taxonomic recognition of types and functional emergents. In R. B. Cattell (Ed.), *Handbook of multivariate experimental psychology.* Chicago: Rand McNally, 1966.
Green, P. E. *Analyzing multivariate data.* Hinsdale, Ill.: Dryden Press, 1978.
Gregson, R. A. M. *The psychometrics of similarity.* New York: Academic Press, 1975.
Hartigan, J. A. *Clustering algorithms.* New York: Wiley, 1975.
Hempel, C. *Aspects of scientific explanation.* New York: Free Press, 1965.
Jevons, W. S. *The principles of science* (2nd ed.) (Ernest Nasel, Ed.). New York: Dover, 1958. (Originally published, 1877.)

Johnson, L. A. S. Rainbow's end: The quest for an optimal taxonomy. *Systematic Zoology,* 1970, *20,* 203–229.

Kendall, M. G., & Buckland, W. P. *A dictionary of statistical terms.* New York: Hafner, 1971.

Morris, R., Blashfield, R., & Satz, P. Neuropsychology and cluster analysis: Potentials and problems. *Journal of Clinical Neuropsychology,* 1981, *3,* 77–79.

Noble, A. G., & Hosler, V. A method for estimating distribution of barn styles: Indiana as a case study. *Geographic Survey,* 1977, *6,* 14–31.

Reichenbach, B. H. *Experience and prediction.* Chicago: University of Chicago Press, 1938.

Rourke, B. P., & Adams, K. M. Quantitative approaches to the neuropsychological assessment of children. In R. E. Tarter & G. Goldstein (Eds.), *Advances in clinical neuropsychology* (Vol. 2). New York: Plenum, 1984.

Skinner, H. A. Toward the integration of classification theory and methods. *Journal of Abnormal Psychology,* 1981, *90,* 68–87.

Sneath, P. H. E., & Sokal, R. R. *Numerical taxonomy.* San Francisco: W. H. Freeman, 1973.

3

Cluster Analysis and the Search for Learning Disability Subtypes

JACK M. FLETCHER

PAUL SATZ

A common paradigm for learning disabilities research is to compare groups of disabled learners and controls on a measure of some psychological construct, such as a language test. If the groups differ, then it is frequently concluded that the underlying construct (i.e., language) has some value for explaining why children have difficulty in learning. Recent reviews of research using this traditional contrasting-groups paradigm show that disabled learners differ from controls on a wide variety of neuropsychological, cognitive, and social measures (Benton, 1975; Fletcher, 1981; Rourke, 1978; Vellutino, 1978). In fact, the number of variables on which disabled learners can be differentiated is quite large, and this promotes considerable controversy concerning the underlying nature of these childhood disabilities. Controversy is an inevitable consequence of applying a research strategy based on univariate contrasting-groups methodology when the experimental group is not homogeneous and the basis for the disability is multivariate in nature. This approach, which has been termed the "single-syndrome" paradigm (Doehring, 1978), is simply not adequate for dealing with the multiple sources of variability in studies of learning disabilities (Satz & Fletcher, 1980).

The multiple sources of variability inherent in learning disability studies stem from at least two sources. The first source concerns the construct validity of the dependent variables used to investigate dif-

Jack M. Fletcher. Developmental Neuropsychology Research Section, Texas Research Institute of Mental Sciences, Houston, Texas, USA.

Paul Satz. The Neuropsychiatric Institute, University of California at Los Angeles, Los Angeles, California, USA.

ferences between disabled and nondisabled learners. These variables rarely represent pure measures of the underlying construct, so that performance is usually determined by a variety of factors embedded in the tasks (Doehring, 1978; Satz & Fletcher, 1980). The second source of variability concerns the heterogeneity of disabled learners, who can vary according to academic problems, cognitive problems, and a variety of other attributes (intelligence, socioeconomic status [SES], etc.). In an effort to deal with this intrasubject variability, several groups of researchers have attempted (e.g., Boder, 1973; Doehring & Hoshko, 1977; Fisk & Rourke, 1979; Lyon, 1982; Mattis, French, & Rapin, 1975; Petrauskas & Rourke, 1979; Satz & Morris, 1981) to develop typologies whereby disabled learners who share common attributes can be grouped together. The assumption guiding this research is that comparisons of homogeneous subgroups emerging from a typology will permit more specific delineations of the nature of childhood learning disabilities.

The purpose of this chapter is to present studies from the Florida Longitudinal Project that address the problem of classifying disabled learners (Morris, Blashfield, & Satz, 1981; Satz & Morris, 1981). The Florida Longitudinal Project was a longitudinal study of several large samples of children in Alachua County, Florida, from 1970–1978 (Fletcher, Satz, & Morris, 1984; Satz, Taylor, Friel, & Fletcher, 1978). One later objective of this project was the development of a typology of learning disabilities. In retrospect, a typology would seem to represent a starting point for this type of research. However, like most studies of learning disabilities, our research initially assumed that disabled learners were homogeneous—an assumption that later proved to be inadequate. In this chapter, we not only present the results of our classification research, but also try to illustrate why these studies were begun at a relatively late period in the Florida Longitudinal Project. Although we wrote the initial methodology for the subtyping research in 1975, the project results that led us to abandon the concept of dyslexia provide a useful introduction to our classification studies.

CONCEPT OF SPECIFIC DEVELOPMENTAL DYSLEXIA

The initial title of the grants funding the Florida Longitudinal Project concerned a clinical entity referred to as "specific developmental dyslexia." The definition of this entity was adopted from the World Federation of Neurology, as follows:

> A disorder manifested by difficulty in learning to read despite conventional instruction, adequate intelligence, and socio-cultural opportunity. It is dependent upon fundamental cognitive disabilities which are frequently of constitutional origin. (Critchley, 1970, p. 11)

What we did not recognize when we initiated the Florida Longitudinal Project was that acceptance of this definition was tantamount to adopting a theory of how learning-disabled children should be classified. When terms like "dyslexia" or "minimal brain dysfunction" (MBD) are used to identify children, the use of the criteria accompanying these labels assumes that children exist with the defining attributes. Unfortunately, a number of studies have subsequently shown that children with the defining attributes for MBD and dyslexia cannot be adequately differentiated from other disabled learners with poor intelligence, cultural deprivation, and other problems (Satz & Fletcher, 1980; Taylor & Fletcher, 1983). Concepts like MBD and dyslexia are merely hypotheses. As Rutter (1974) noted for dyslexia,

> We should not presuppose either the existence of any particular condition or the scientific value of the concept. It is not yet possible either to define dyslexia in any acceptable way or to identify cases of dyslexia. The concept of dyslexia constitutes a hypothesis. (p. 250)

We became concerned about these problems in 1974, after examining the results of our initial 3-year follow-up in 1973 (Satz, Friel, & Rudegair, 1976). In part, we were concerned because of the relatively high incidence of reading problems (12%) for an entity (i.e., dyslexia) that supposedly was fairly specific. Also, many children in the study had academic problems in areas in addition to reading (e.g., arithmetic). Consequently, a study was initiated to evaluate the concept of specific developmental dyslexia (Taylor, Satz, & Friel, 1979). For this study, the World Federation of Neurology definition of dyslexia was used to select a group of "dyslexic" disabled learners ($n = 40$) meeting the exclusionary criteria. These white male children (mean age = 8.5 years) were compared with a group of same-age "nondyslexic" disabled learners ($n = 40$) who failed to meet one or more of these criteria (e.g., low IQ, SES, etc.). Two groups of nondisabled learners ($n = 80$), similar in age to the groups of disabled learners, were also included in this study. These four groups were compared along seven dimensions on which patterns specific to the "dyslexic" group could potentially emerge: (1) neuropsychological tests; (2) other academic tests; (3) severity of reading problems; (4) reversal and letter confusions; (5)

parental reading proficiency; (6) neurological examinations; and (7) personality questionnaires. The results of this study revealed that, while both the "dyslexic" and "nondyslexic" groups differed from controls along each of these seven dimensions, there were no differences between "dyslexic" and "nondyslexic" disabled learners. Consequently, this study challenged traditional exclusionary definitions of learning disabilities, since differences between "dyslexic" and "nondyslexic" disabled learners did not emerge. Because of the null results of the Taylor *et al.* (1979) study, we initiated a program of classification research.

INITIAL CONSIDERATIONS
FOR CLASSIFICATION RESEARCH

Classification research has a long history in biology and medicine. The development of a classification system requires a number of considerations, including the nature of the population to be classified, methods by which classifications will be made, attributes to be classified, and a host of reliability and validity concerns (Cormack, 1971; Skinner, 1981). In this section, we discuss some of these issues as they pertain to our classification research.

STATISTICAL VERSUS CLINICAL APPROACHES

A major decision concerned methods for creating the classification system. Learning disability taxonomies have been developed through clinical inspection of psychometric protocols (Boder, 1973; Mattis *et al.*, 1975) and through application of such multivariate statistical methods as Q-type factor analysis and cluster analysis to psychometric protocols (Doehring & Hoshko, 1977; Fisk & Rourke, 1979; Lyon, 1982; Petrauskas & Rourke, 1979). Clinical methods were not used for our studies because of the difficulty of establishing the reliability and validity of the emergent typologies. Furthermore, visual inspection of these psychometric protocols is easily influenced by *a priori* biases and assumptions concerning learning disabilities. The presence of these assumptions runs counter to the goals of classification research, which is to discover naturally recurring subtypes (Cormack, 1971). If naturally recurring subtypes of disabled learners exist, classification studies should identify these subgroups and separate them from subgroups of children with other problems or from normal children. Hence, statistical methods were chosen so that systematic studies of the reliability and validity of the typology could be conducted. While statistical approaches carry their own set of problems and assumptions, these methods can help deal with the multiple sources of variability inherent in this type of research.

CLUSTER ANALYSIS VERSUS *Q*-ANALYSIS

When researchers choose among statistical methods, a variety of techniques are available. Two general classes of methods involve either *Q*-analysis or cluster analysis, both of which present problems. Some of these problems, which concern the reliability and validity of the measures employed, are important considerations underlying any study of disabled learners (Doehring, 1978). Other problems reflect the differences in statistical assumptions and the mathematical bases of these techniques. Some statisticians favor the dimensional representation of subjects provided by *Q*-analysis (Overall & Klett, 1972), while others prefer the flexibility provided by the multiple clustering methods (Everitt, 1980). *Q*-analysis and cluster analysis could be more or less suitable, depending on the nature of the classification problem (Fleiss & Zubin, 1969).

    Q-type factor analysis, an analogue to *R*-type factor analysis, forms correlational matrices of subjects and extracts factors that represent subtypes. While factors derived from *R*-type factor analysis represent common sources of variability across tests, the factors in *Q*-type factor analysis represent common variability shared by people. The problems with *Q*-analysis have been amply summarized (Fleiss & Zubin, 1969). Some of these problems, which involve selecting similarity coefficients and standardizing the data matrix, also apply to cluster-analytic techniques. Specific criticisms of *Q*-analysis include the need to assume that a linear model applies to a data matrix of people, which becomes a particular problem when people load on more than one factor. Another methodological problem is that the number of subtypes that can emerge will always be one less than the number of dependent variables. Consequently, if variables are carefully reduced to the least redundant set, the number of subgroups may be artificially limited. A similar problem has to do with the number of tests necessary to define a stable matrix of correlations for factor extraction. While there are no firm rules for defining a stable correlation matrix, a common guideline for *R*-type factor analysis is 100 subjects (Guertin & Bailey, 1970). One implication of this guideline is that 100 tests would be needed for *Q*-analysis. In fact, *Q*-analysis *requires* large numbers of variables. When large numbers of variables are used, interpretation of results can be more difficult. Problems with using tests that differ in reliability, particularly internal consistency, are more likely when the number of variables is increased. Finally, it is not clear that alternative *Q*-analysis methods analogous to the variety of clustering methods have been developed to permit replication across techniques, which is critical for studies of reliability (internal validity) (Everitt, 1980).

Cluster analysis represents another class of multivariate classification methods (Morris *et al.*, 1981). These methods use different algorithms and indices of similarity to accomplish a common task—forming groups of subjects that are relatively homogeneous according to a set of classification attributes. Clustering methods are complex, and many decisions must be made when these techniques are employed. There are also nuances in different software programs and some general limitations and precautions that must be applied when using cluster analysis (Blashfield, 1980; Morris *et al.*, 1981). Like all statistical techniques, cluster analysis will be effective only with reliable and valid measures. Specific criticisms include the concern that clustering methods are not built upon a clearly articulated, generally accepted statistical foundation. These techniques are best considered as heuristic. Furthermore, many cluster-analytic methods are poorly defined, and their properties have not been adequately examined. There are also many different algorithms and computer software packages, which may yield different results even when presumably similar procedures are used. Limited attempts have been made to validate cluster results; validation is especially critical because most methods will generate clusters in random data. Monte Carlo studies have raised questions about many clustering methods, as well as about *Q*-analysis (Milligan, 1981).

Attempts to compare results from *Q*-analysis and cluster analysis have met with limited success. In general, the degree to which results from these techniques replicate one another depends on the type of similarity coefficient employed and the resemblance of the clustering algorithm with factor-analytic methods. Striking replications were obtained by Del Dotto and Rourke (see Chapter 5, this volume). In this study, *Q*-analysis and two clustering methods (using correlations for similarity coefficients) perfectly replicated one another for three subtypes representing 69% of the sample. Other studies (e.g., Doehring, Hoshko, & Bryans, 1979) have experienced less success in replicating results from *Q*-analysis and cluster analysis, although the degree of replication depended on the clustering technique chosen. Since the assumptions and statistical procedures whereby subtypes are derived from *Q*-analysis and cluster analysis can be quite discrepant, divergent results would not be surprising. Monte Carlo studies comparing *Q*-analysis and cluster analysis generally fail to replicate results unless the subgroups are clearly homogeneous and are sufficiently distinct that visual inspection reveals the clusters (Morris & Blashfield, 1983). An evaluation of these different problems led us to select clustering methods for our research, largely because of (1) their flexibility, (2) the extent to which the statistical properties of some techniques had been studied, and (3) the availability of multiple methods for internal validity studies.

SIMILARITY COEFFICIENTS

A fundamental question concerns the type of similarity coefficient to be used for determining the degree of homogeneity among subtypes (i.e., the degree to which performance profiles are similar or dissimilar). Any subtype can be represented as a profile of the attributes used for classification. Profiles differ according to shape (pattern), scatter (variability), and elevation (distance). Similarity coefficients that match profiles on shape and scatter are correlation coefficients. Much of the research on learning disability subtypes employs correlations as the measure of similarity, particularly when *Q*-analysis is used. All similarity coefficients represent a tradeoff of shape and elevation information. However, correlation coefficients can present particular difficulties for this type of research. In the past, the general superiority of distance over correlation as an index of similarity has been strongly argued (Cronbach & Gleser, 1953; Fleiss & Zubin, 1969). A correlation of 0 is difficult to interpret because it cannot represent complete dissimilarity; this is represented by a correlation of -1. Similarly, it is often recognized that correlational indices can be quite similar even when profiles differ in elevation. However, it is often not recognized that high correlations do not necessarily imply similarity in the shape of the two profiles—only that the two profiles are linearly related. This latter problem presents particular difficulties for those who advocate the use of correlational indices solely on the basis of shape considerations (Rourke & Adams, 1984). Similarly, it is misleading to suggest that correlations should be used when shape is the important characteristic and distance when elevation is more important (Morris *et al.*, 1981; Rourke & Adams, 1984). Distance indices can also incorporate information about shape. However, there are situations in which distance indices can minimize shape information, usually when elevation differences are so large that they account for all the variability among profiles (Skinner, 1978).

In the future, similarity coefficients will be available that permit separation of elevation, shape, and scatter components of profiles. When these methods are available, more specific determinations of the appropriate coefficient can be made, and these will also illuminate the basis for profile differences (Skinner, 1978). For the present, the choice of coefficients depends on the classification problem.[1] To illustrate, non-disabled learners were included in the Florida studies. Since two children could have identical patterns but could differ in the severity of their problems (if any) (Fleiss & Zubin, 1969; Wiggins, 1973), distance indices, such as squared Euclidean distance, were selected as the similarity coefficients. In addition, alternative similarity coefficients were applied to the data to determine whether subtypes would change with different coefficients.

APPLYING CLUSTER ANALYSIS TO THE FLORIDA DATA

The selection of clustering techniques for the subtyping studies was based in part on our evaluation of the relative merits of *Q*-analysis versus cluster analysis. In addition, the nature of the data and our approach to classification research were more suited to cluster analysis, for a variety of reasons. First, validity studies were planned prior to the initiation of this research. There are two types of validity that a good typology should exhibit (Skinner, 1981). "Internal validity" concerns the reliability of the typology. To demonstrate that a typology is not method- or sample-dependent, results should be replicable across statistical techniques and with different samples. Additional internal validity studies should explore the adequacy of the clustering solution. The multiple methods available for cluster analysis provide an opportunity to replicate results across techniques. Similarly, split-sample and Monte Carlo studies were also conducted to address the reliability of the clustering solutions (Morris

---

1. One caveat is that, when correlational indices are employed, results should be compared with a distance index to insure that elevation information is not being overlooked.

et al., 1981). "External validity" addresses the issue of whether the subtypes are truly distinct through systematic comparisons of subgroups on variables not used to develop the typology. We had available a variety of variables that could be employed to evaluate external validity, including neurological examinations, parental reading levels, and personality questionnaires.

Second, all 236 children from the Year 6 follow-up were included (Satz *et al.*, 1978). This sample was relatively homogeneous in terms of race, sex, and SES, and had been extensively studied in previous years. The decision to include normal as well as disabled learners was critical, because it allowed us to use statistical procedures to identify the learning-disabled group. While there is nothing inherently wrong with selecting only learning-disabled children for classification studies, it seemed desirable to determine whether the clustering methods would separate disabled and nondisabled learners. This dictated the need to use similarity coefficients that incorporated elevation information.

Third, variables were carefully selected as the attributes for classification. Some studies use a large number of variables and depend upon statistical methods to deal with the dimensionality of the data (e.g., Doehring, Trites, Patel, & Fiedorowicz, 1981). Our approach was to restrict the number of variables in an effort to reduce test redundancy and increase subtype interpretability, which made use of Q-analysis less desirable. Consequently, two sets of variables were employed. The first set represented the Reading, Spelling, and Arithmetic subtests from the Wide Range Achievement Test (WRAT; Jastak, Bijou, & Jastak, 1965); these were clustered to determine whether achievement subgroups could be defined in the overall sample ($n = 236$). The second set of variables was employed with the subgroups of disabled learners that emerged from the achievement classification. According to factor-analytic studies of this sample, these variables represented measures of visual–spatial and verbal skills (Fletcher & Satz, 1980). The visual–spatial measures included the Beery Test of Visual–Motor Integration (Beery & Buktenica, 1967), a perceptual–motor copying test; and Recognition–Discrimination (Fletcher & Satz, 1984), a geometric-figure-matching task. Verbal measures included the Verbal Fluency Test (Spreen & Benton, 1969), which requires children to give words beginning with different letters of the alphabet under timed conditions, and the Wechsler Intelligence Scale for Children—Revised (WISC-R) Similarities subtest, a measure of verbal reasoning. These tests were chosen because they were the best measures of these skills in our battery and have good reliability (Fletcher & Satz, 1984).

Another important characteristic—essential for clustering methods—is that the frequency distributions of the four variables were skewed. Normally distributed variables are not consistent with the presence of subtypes in the sample (Morris *et al.*, 1981). In fact, normalization of variables through procedures such as factor scores can interfere with the derivation of subtypes, regardless of the classification method employed.

There are many other considerations that underlie the successful use of cluster analysis. These problems and the way in which they were addressed in the Florida studies were described by Morris *et al.* (1981). In the next section, a series of cluster-analytic studies based on the Florida Longitudinal Project is summarized. This research includes the initial study (Satz & Morris, 1981), along with some forthcoming cross-validation and developmental studies.

INITIAL STUDY

Subtyping research in this area, whether clinical or statistical, generally attempts to classify children according to achievement dimensions (Boder, 1973; Rourke & Finlayson, 1978; Rourke & Strang, 1978) or processing deficiencies based on a battery of cognitive–neuropsychological tests (Fisk & Rourke, 1979; Mattis *et al.*, 1975; Petrauskas & Rourke, 1979). In our initial study (Satz & Morris, 1981), we chose to attempt both types of classification by clustering first on achievement variables and then on processing-deficiency variables. All analyses were completed using CLUSTAN (Wishart, 1975), a general-purpose software package for cluster analysis.

CLASSIFICATION ON ACHIEVEMENT VARIABLES

The Reading, Spelling, and Arithmetic subtests from the WRAT (Jastak *et al.*, 1965) were subjected to a technique of average-linkage hierarchical agglomerative clustering, followed by K-means iterative partitioning in order to group individuals most similar to each other on the achievement variables. Hierarchical agglomerative techniques work by combining pairs of observations into nonoverlapping clusters on the basis of their profile similarity, beginning with a set of clusters equal to the number of subjects and recomputing successive combinations of subjects into cluster solutions. A major problem in cluster analysis is determining the optimal number of clusters. Hence, different clustering solutions were followed with an iterative partitioning method, in which subjects were reassigned to alternative clusters to determine whether the assigned subtype was the most appropriate classification for each subject. The similarity coefficient was squared Euclidean distance, which compares profiles based on shape, scatter, and elevation. From this analysis, nine clusters (subgroups) emerged, which are displayed in Figure 3-1. This figure shows the WRAT profiles for the nine subgroups, which included 230 (98%) of the 236 subjects (i.e., only six outliers).[2] The WRAT profiles are expressed in terms of z-scores based on means and standard deviations for the sample as a whole. Several patterns of reading, spelling, and arithmetic skills can be seen in Fig. 3-1. Subgroups 1 ($n = 13$) and 2 ($n = 16$) both obtained superior scores in Reading, but Subgroup 2 exhibited only average performance in Arithmetic. Subgroup 3 ($n = 25$) achieved high Reading, Spelling, and Arithmetic scores. Subgroup 4 ($n = 25$) emerged as a group with above-average Reading and Spelling scores, but average performance in Arithmetic. Subgroup 5 ($n = 12$) constituted a unique group by virtue of its average Reading, slightly-below-average Spelling, and severely depressed Arithmetic scores. Subgroup 6 ($n = 11$) showed average Reading and Spelling scores, but was superior in Arithmetic. The performance of Subgroup 7 ($n = 39$) approximated average levels in all areas. At the lower end of the achievement spectrum, Subgroups 8 ($n = 56$) and 9 ($n = 33$) each contained a large number of children severely deficient on all three WRAT subtests. Reading and Spelling scores were slightly poorer in Subgroup 9. Arithmetic scores were below average for both subgroups, but better for Subgroup 8.

The emergence of these WRAT subgroups is particularly interesting in light of research by Rourke and his associates (Rourke, 1982; Rourke & Finlayson, 1978; Rourke & Strang, 1978). In these studies, disabled learners were divided into three different groups on the basis of WRAT scores. Group 1 was uniformly deficient on all three WRAT subtests. Group 2 was poor in Reading and Spelling, but better in Arithmetic. Group 3 was composed of children who were at least average in Reading and Spelling, but poor in Arithmetic. Administration of different measures of verbal, visual–spatial, tactile, and motor skills yielded predictable

---

2. "Outliers" are subjects whose results are extremely deviant. In this instance, three children who did not belong in any real subtype were artificially placed into the sixth cluster. The children were eliminated from subsequent analysis because of the potential of outliers for distorting results.

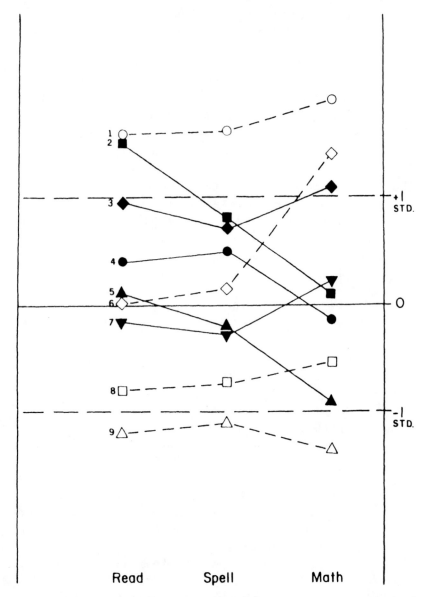

FIG. 3.1. WRAT discrepancy scores for achievement subgroups (mean based on local population). (From R. E. Tarter, *The Child at Psychiatric Risk*. New York: Oxford University Press, 1983. Reprinted by permission.)

differences among these groups. These findings are particularly interesting, since similar subgroups emerged from our cluster analyses, even though the children were not selected for learning problems. Subgroup 5 is quite similar to Rourke's Group 3. Many children in Subgroup 8 resemble either Rourke's Group 2 or Group 1, while Subgroup 9 is similar to Rourke's Group 1. The differences that Rourke and associates found in neuropsychological skills among their WRAT subtypes provides external validity for this cluster solution (see Fletcher, Chapter 9, this volume).

These cluster-analytic results have also been replicated in two independent, samples, one in The Netherlands (see van der Vlugt & Satz, Chapter 10, this volume) and one in Pittsburgh (Johnston, 1984). Both studies employed white males, but added females. In addition, a reading comprehension measure was used to improve the assessment of academic skills. Clustering procedures revealed nine subgroups in both studies. The subgroups were similar to those obtained in our study (Satz & Morris, 1981), especially for the poor achievement groups. No major changes emerged representing the additional reading measure, which is not surprising, since most standardized reading comprehension measures correlate highly with word-recognition tests (Fletcher, 1981).

CLASSIFICATION ON NEUROPSYCHOLOGICAL VARIABLES

Subgroups 8 and 9 performed approximately one standard deviation below the sample mean on the WRAT and represented most of the disabled learners ($n = 89$) in the sample. Hence, additional subtyping distinctions were explored in these subgroups. The performance of these children on the Beery Test, the Recognition–Discrimination Test, the Verbal Fluency Test, and the WISC-R Similarities subtest was subjected to cluster analysis with the same techniques used for the achievement variables. The results of this analysis are presented in Figure 3-2. Scores on the Peabody Picture Vocabulary Test (PPVT) are also presented. The PPVT was not used to classify children—only as an external variable to help illustrate subtype differences.

Figure 3-2 shows the five profiles that resulted from a six-cluster solution, consisting of five distinct subtypes representing 86 of the 89 children and 3 outliers. Using z-score units for the population ($n = 236$), Subtype 1 ($n = 27$) was found to be impaired on both of the verbal measures (Similarities and Verbal Fluency) and on PPVT IQ. In contrast,

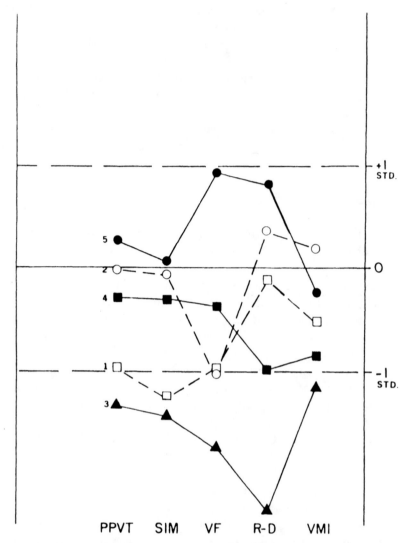

FIG. 3-2. Analysis of the performance of Subtypes 1–5 (Subgroups 8 and 9) on the Peabody Picture Vocabulary Test (PPVT), the WISC-R Similarities subtest (SIM), the Spreen-Benton Verbal Fluency Test (VF), the Recognition-Discrimination test (R-D), and the Beery Test of Visual-Motor Integration (VMI). (From R. Morris, R. Blashfield, & P. Satz, Neuropsychology and cluster analysis: Problems and pitfalls. *Journal of Clinical Neuropsychology*, 1981, *3*, 79–99. Reprinted by permission.)

performance on the visual–spatial tests was in the average range, so that this subtype represented a "general verbal" group. Subtype 2 ($n = 14$) was impaired on only the Verbal Fluency Test, and thus represented a "specific verbal" (naming) group. Subtype 3 ($n = 10$) was impaired on all of the cognitive tests (verbal and visual–spatial) and was labeled a "mixed-global" subtype. Subtype 4 ($n = 23$) was impaired primarily on the nonverbal perceptual tests, and was defined as a "visual–spatial" subtype. Subtype 5 ($n = 12$) showed no impairment on any of the neuropsychological tests, and was labeled an "unexpected" subtype.

INTERNAL VALIDITY STUDIES

In order to assess the adequacy and stability of the six-cluster solution, a variety of internal validity studies were conducted (Morris *et al.*, 1981). These studies consisted of (1) data-manipulation procedures, (2) visual graphing techniques designed to assess the generality of the six-cluster solution, and (3) Monte Carlo studies of simulated data sets. For data-manipulation studies, the data were subjected to additional clustering techniques that employed alternative similarity coefficients. Split-sample studies were also completed. Other data manipulation studies added subjects and variables to the initial solution. These studies uniformly demonstrated that the six-cluster solution was stable, despite variations in methods and samples. Graphic approaches that plotted the cluster solution in visual displays showed that there was relatively little overlap among clusters. Finally, Monte Carlo simulation studies that employed randomly generated data (i.e., containing no clusters) also demonstrated that the subtypes were probably not artifacts of the methods or sample. However, the correspondence of some simulated profiles with actual profiles raised some questions about this aspect of the study (Morris *et al.*, 1981). The van der Vlugt and Satz study (see Chapter 10, this volume) also provided partial support for the validity of the Florida subtypes in an independent cross-cultural study.

EXTERNAL VALIDITY STUDIES

Thus far, the Florida processing-deficiency subtypes have demonstrated good internal validity. In addition, results consistent with the initial

Florida study were obtained in independent samples of children. The next question concerned whether the Florida processing-deficiency subtypes could be distinguished when compared on variables not used to form the typology (i.e., external validity). A variety of criteria were available, including personality questionnaires, neurological examinations, and parental reading levels. The personality questionnaires were of interest because of the possibility that the unexpected subtype represented a group impaired in motivation or emotional adjustment. However, comparisons of the subtypes on the Children's Personality Questionnaire yielded null results. It is not likely that this subtype represents a methodological artifact (Morris *et al.*, 1981). Furthermore, Lyon (1982) obtained a similar subgroup, using more neuropsychological tasks than we used in the Florida studies. Additional external validity studies are needed to explore the basis for this subtype.

Significant differences across subtypes were found for neurological status (including birth histories) and parental reading levels. Children in the general verbal, mixed–global, and visual–spatial subtypes had a higher proportion of soft neurological signs. The specific verbal and unexpected subtypes had fewer positive soft neurological findings. In addition, the parents of the children in these latter two subtypes had higher reading scores than did the parents of children in the other three subtypes.

These external validity studies show that the specific verbal and unexpected subtypes differ from the general verbal, visual–spatial, and mixed–global subtypes. Presently, the uniqueness of all five subytpes has not been demonstrated. Such a demonstration will depend in part on the development of additional external validity studies that will identify new children into the Florida typology. We hope that comparative studies will evaluate subtype differences according to refutable *a priori* hypotheses, using variables clearly different from those employed by the initial classification research. These types of studies would constitute a rigorous approach to external validity (see Fletcher, Chapter 9, this volume).

DEVELOPMENTAL CLASSIFICATION OF DISABLED LEARNERS

The accumulation of longitudinal data on these 11-year-old Florida children made possible the investigation of ability patterns earlier in development (ages 5 and 8 years). A doctoral dissertation (Schauer, 1979) explored the earlier patterns of the Florida processing-deficiency subtypes. This study showed that ability patterns were not stable over time. In some instances, the patterns changed considerably within individual subtypes. Consequently, Morris (1982) and Morris, Blashfield, and Satz (unpublished manuscript) completed a study in which a typology was developed that classified children according to ability patterns over time.

DESIGN OF THE STUDY

The 11-year-old sample ($n = 236$) used for the initial study (Satz & Morris, 1981) was employed for this investigation. Complete testing at ages 5, 8, and 11 years was available for 222 of these children; 14 subjects were dropped because of missing data due to school absence or injury that precluded performance on part of the battery. Additional attempts to identify outliers resulted in a final sample of 200 children.[3] Eight variables available at ages 5, 8, and 11 were employed as the classification attributes, representing the four variables used in the initial cluster-analytic study and four additional measures. These attributes were grouped into measures of verbal skills (Verbal Fluency, Similarities, PPVT, and Dichotic Listening) and nonverbal skills (Beery Test, Recognition–Discrimination, Embedded Figures, and Auditory–Visual Integration), according to factor-analytic studies at each age point (Fletcher & Satz, 1980; Morris *et al.*, unpublished manuscript).

Statistical methods were derived from a successful Monte Carlo study investigating techniques for clustering longitudinal data (Carter, Morris, & Bashfield, 1983). Although several methods were used, results based on Ward's hierarchical agglomerative methods with squared Euclidean distance are reported here. Using CLUSTAN, the 24 variables (eight variables at three time probes) were clustered on the entire sample (i.e., disabled and nondisabled learners). A variety of procedures was used to determine the number of clusters. After this determination, the resulting solutions were subjected to K-means iterative partitioning methods to clarify the similarity of subgroup members.

---

3. Outliers were identified for this study by exploring univariate and multivariate data distributions, resulting in the deletion of 22 children.

RESULTS

One advantage of hierarchical clustering methods is that different levels of classification can be explored. For example, if a two-cluster solution was selected for this analysis of the longitudinal data, partitions representing subtypes of good learners and poor learners emerged. At a second level of classification, a seven-cluster solution was most appropriate, representing children in five subtypes ($n = 189$) and two small groups of outliers ($n = 11$). The five subtypes included three groups of disabled learners and two groups of good learners. Each of these subtypes showed a distinct pattern of development. Type A children ($n = 45$) were deficient in verbal and visual–spatial skills at age 5. Over time, substantial improvement in visual–spatial skills was observed; by age 11, this group resembled the general verbal subtype from the initial study (Satz & Morris, 1981). Type B ($n = 41$) was also a learning-disabled group. These children had average verbal skills and poor visual–spatial skills at age 5. By age 11, verbal skills were only slightly better than visual–spatial skills; this group thus represented a mixed subtype. The third learning-disabled group, Type C ($n = 24$), was relatively deficient on verbal and visual–spatial skills at each age. Type D ($n = 59$) represented average children with relative strengths in verbal and visual–spatial skills over time. Finally, Type E ($n = 20$) included the most proficient learners in the sample, with performance levels exceeding those of Type D.

INTERNAL VALIDITY STUDIES

Extensive studies of the reliability of the seven-cluster solution yielding the five subtypes were conducted. For example, five clustering methods were compared. A T-Rand statistic (Morey, 1981) showed that results across different methods were highly similar. Similar results were obtained by split-sample analyses. Finally, 10 Monte Carlo data sets were developed by generating random data sets with means and standard deviation vectors and a correlation matrix simulating the longitudinal clusters. These comparisons were not consistent with the hypothesis that the longitudinal clusters were artifacts of the clustering procedures (Morris, 1982; Morris *et al.*, unpublished manuscript).

EXTERNAL VALIDITY STUDIES

Several variables were available for external validity comparisons. Table 3-1 shows these variables by number, representing these domains: school achievement (1); parental achievement (2); demographic variables (3–6); teacher ratings (7–11); neurological examinations and birth history (12–13); and other neuropsychological and cognitive variables (14–18). Many differences emerged when subtypes were compared. Type A children showed poor achievement, but only their fathers had poor reading. These children had average-SES backgrounds, but teachers rated them as more active and emotionally reactive than children in the other subtypes. Type B children and their parents had poor achievement levels and came from lower-SES backgrounds. Teacher ratings were generally average for behavioral problems, but these children had a higher proportion of perinatal complications than did children in Subtypes A, D, or E. Subtype C had poor achievement, manifested more problems on teacher ratings, and had a higher incidence of neurological findings and perinatal complications than any other subtype. Consistent deficiencies on all other cognitive and neuropsychological variables were observed. Types D and E were at or above average levels on virtually all of the external variables. The difference between these latter two subtypes was one of degree: While both subtypes had similar performance levels at kindergarten, Type E developed more rapidly and had higher achievement levels than Type D by age 11.

DISCUSSION

The developmental studies suggest that results from classification studies that include children at only one age level should not be automatically extrapolated to younger or older children. Each subtype showed a different pattern of development. Types C, D, and E had relatively constant patterns of development over time, differing only in elevation. In contrast, Types A and B showed variations in ability patterns over time, with clear dissociations in the development of verbal and visual–spatial skills. At age 5, Type A had poorer verbal skills than Type B, but the two types were equally deficient on visual–spatial skills. Relative to performance patterns for the entire sample, Type A displayed more rapid development of visual–spatial skills and static development of verbal

TABLE 3-1. Performance on External Variables by Subtypes

Variables	Type A	Type B	Type C	Type D	Type E
School achievement					
1. Achievement	—	—	—	++	++
(areas)	(A on math)	(all areas)	(all areas)	(all areas)	(all areas)
Parental achievement					
2. Parental achievement					
(mother)	A	—	—	++	++
(father)	—	—	—	++	++
Demographic variables					
3. Parental education					
(mother)	A	A	—	++	A
(father)	A	A	—	++	++
4. Socioeconomic status	A	A	—	++	++
5. Income level	A	A	—	A	A
6. Number of siblings	++	A	++	A	A
Teacher ratings					
7. Activity level	++	A	++	A	A
8. Emotional reactivity	++	A	++	A	A
9. Attention span	A	A	—	++	A
10. Maturity level	A	—	—	++	++
11. Learning ability	—	—	—	++	++
Neurological examinations and birth history					
12. Neurological ratings					
(No. of problems)	A	more	more	less	less
13. Birth history					
(No. of problems)	more	more	more	less	less
Other neurological and cognitive variables					
14. Alphabet recitation	—	A	—	++	++
	(at Kg)	(all years)	(all years)	(at Kg)	(all years)
15. Right-left discrimination	A	—	—	A	++
	(all years)	(all years)	(all years)	(all years)	(all years)
16. Auditory discrimination	A	A	—	A	++
	(all years)	(all years)	(all years)	(all years)	(all years)
17. Finger tapping	A	—	—	A	++
	(all years)	(at age 8)	(all years)	(all years)	(all years)
18. Finger localization	—	—	—	++	++
	(at age 5)	(at age 5)	(all years)	(at age 5)	(all years)

Note. Symbols: A, average; —, below average; ++, above average.

skills. Type B acquired verbal and spatial skills at a slower rate than the sample as a whole. By age 11, Type A had better visual–spatial skills than Type B, but the initial differences on verbal skills were not apparent. Despite these different developmental patterns, scores on the WRAT Reading and Spelling subtests did not differentiate these two subtypes. However, in addition to poor visual–spatial skills at each age point, Type B children had poorer Arithmetic scores than Type A children, whose scores were average relative to scores for the entire sample. Finally, the accelerated development of visual–spatial skills in Type A did not lead to better Reading and Spelling scores.

There was no subtype that showed more rapid development of verbal skills relative to visual–spatial skills. Type C was uniformly deficient on both skills at each age point. Children in this subtype had the lowest PPVT IQ scores and came from lower-SES backgrounds. In some respects, Type C resembled a slow-learner group that, from a developmental point of view, may be more similar to Types D and E than to the other subtypes of disabled learners (A and B). The differences among Types C, D, and E are primarily due to a severity dimension (i.e., profile elevation), not to ability patterns (i.e., profile shape). Type E showed slightly accelerated development of verbal and visual–spatial skills from ages 5 to 8, but tended to perform at higher levels than Type D at all ages. Both subtypes performed at higher levels than Type C.

The longitudinal results are also somewhat different from the subtypes apparent in the initial study (Satz & Morris, 1981). At age 11, Type C was similar to the mixed–global subtype from the initial study, while Type A resembled the general verbal subtype. Type B had a consistent visual–spatial deficiency over time, but the dissociation between verbal and spatial skills was less apparent at age 11 than for the visual–spatial subtype in the initial study. These differences point to the need for caution in extrapolating results from cross–sectional studies. However, the differences in results from these two studies can also be attributed to the use of normal and disabled learners and additional tests in the developmental study.

GENERAL CONCLUSIONS

The Florida Longitudinal Project was not designed for classification research. Nonetheless, the studies summarized in this chapter show that reliable subtypes can be identified with the methods applied to these data.

Perhaps the major contribution of these studies is the systematic application of multivariate classification techniques to neuropsychological data. The attempt to evaluate the internal validity of a subtype solution is fundamental to the application of multivariate techniques to these problems. These techniques may yield spurious results if their application is not carefully investigated in the manner described in this chapter (Morris *et al.*, 1981).

Some additional nonstatistical considerations are important for evaluating these cluster-analytic studies. First, the longitudinal nature of the project locked us into a set of variables that would not be viewed as ideal, given more recent developments in learning disabilities research. The absence of measures of memory, attention, and psycholinguistic skills is most apparent. Second, the sample was relatively homogeneous in terms of race, sex, and SES. Whether results will generalize to other samples requires additional research. Third, the design of the external validity studies did not permit sufficiently rigorous evaluations of emergent subtypes against external criteria. While we were fortunate to have data for the comparisons that were made, these studies were generally atheoretical. External validity studies should also generate *a priori* refutable hypotheses about subtype differences on external criteria (see Fletcher, Chapter 9, this volume). These types of studies will help illuminate the nature and validity of the subtypes.

These studies fully illustrate the value of multivariate quantitative approaches to the classification problem. Stable, reliable, and meaningful subtypes were clearly defined. However, some investigators have argued that clinical approaches to classification are more desirable than quantitative methods because of the limitations of most measures of children's abilities and the capriciousness of multivariate techniques (e.g., Kinsbourne, 1982). Unfortunately, the limitations of ability measures will also hinder a clinical approach. Problems with reliability and construct validity cannot be dealt with through thoughtful visual inspection. Furthermore, a clinician's judgment is no less capricious than a computer-based technique (Meehl, 1954). The tendency to view clinical and statistical approaches as representative of opposing points of view does not do justice to the true nature of both enterprises. The judicious use of multivariate techniques requires a clinical approach to the selection of variables and interpretation of results; otherwise, the data will not be fully explored. At the same time, the clinician's judgment must be carefully investigated, since belief and conviction are not particularly illuminating, given the amount of covariance in most data sets. The computer is better equipped than a clinician to deal with covariance, but results will be difficult to interpret without a careful conceptualization of the nature of the data and rational exploration of the results. The emphasis on methodology throughout this chapter has been designed to illustrate appropriate uses of multivariate techniques for classification research. Regardless of technique and theory, disabled learners are heterogeneous, and their performance patterns can be difficult to interpret. Clustering techniques, if appropriately applied, may be quite helpful in dealing with the multiple sources of covariance inherent in this research.

ACKNOWLEDGMENT

The contributions of Robin Morris to this program of research and his permission to describe his developmental study (pp. 55-60) are gratefully acknowledged.

REFERENCES

Beery, K., & Buktenica, N. A. *Developmental Test of Visual-Motor Integration*. Chicago: Follet Education Company, 1967.

Benton, A. L. Developmental dyslexia: Neurological aspects. In W. J. Friedlander (Ed.), *Advances in neurology* (Vol. 7). New York: Raven Press, 1975.

Blashfield, R. K. Propositions regarding the use of cluster analysis in clinical research. *Journal of Consulting and Clinical Psychology*, 1980, *3*, 456-459.

Boder, E. Developmental dyslexia: A diagnostic approach based on three atypical reading-spelling patterns. *Developmental Medicine and Child Neurology*, 1973, *15*, 663-687.

Carter, R. L., Morris, R., & Blashfield, R. K. *Clustering two-dimensional profiles: A comparative study*. Unpublished manuscript, 1983.

Cormack, R. M. A review of classification. *Journal of the Royal Statistical Society* (Series A), 1971, *134*, 321-367.

Critchley, M. *The dyslexic child*. Springfield, Ill.: Charles C Thomas, 1970.

Cronbach, L. J., & Gleser, G. C. Assessing similarity between profiles. *Psychological Bulletin*, 1953, *50*, 456-473.

Doehring, D. G. The tangled web of behavioral research on developmental dyslexia. In A. L. Benton & D. Pearl (Eds.), *Dyslexia: An appraisal of current knowledge*. New York: Oxford University Press, 1978.

Doehring, D. G., & Hoshko, I. M. Classification of reading problems by the Q-technique of factor analysis. *Cortex*, 1977, *13*, 281-294.

Doehring, D. G., Hoshko, I. M., & Bryans, B. N. Statistical classification of children with reading problems. *Journal of Clinical Neuropsychology*, 1979, *1*, 5-16.

Doehring, D. G., Trites, R. L., Patel, P. G., & Fiedorowicz, C. *Reading disabilities*. New York: Academic Press, 1981.

Everitt, B. *Cluster analysis*. London: Heinemann Educational Books, 1980.

Fisk, J. L., & Rourke, B. P. Identification of subtypes of learning disabilities at three age levels: A neuropsychological, multivariate approach. *Journal of Clinical Neuropsychology*, 1979, *1*, 289–310.

Fleiss, J. L., & Zubin, J. On the methods and theory of clustering. *Multivariate Behavioral Research*, 1969, *4*, 235–250.

Fletcher, J. M. Linguistic factors in reading acquisition: Evidence for decelopmental changes. In F. Pirozzolo & M. C. Wittrock (Eds.), *Neuropsychological and cognitive processes in reading*. New York: Academic Press, 1981.

Fletcher, J. M., & Satz, P. Developmental changes in the neuropsychological correlates of reading achievement: A six-year longitudinal follow-up. *Journal of Clinical Neuropsychology*, 1980, *2*, 23–37.

Fletcher, J. M., & Satz, P. Pre-school prediction of reading failure. In M. Levine & P. Satz (Eds.), *Middle childhood: Developmental variation and dysfunction between six and fourteen years*. New York: Appleton-Century-Crofts, 1984.

Fletcher, J. M., Satz, P., & Morris, R. The Florida Longitudinal Project: A review. In S. A. Mednick & M. A. Harway (Eds.), *U.S. longitudinal projects*. New York: Praeger, 1984.

Guertin, W., & Bailey, J. *Introduction to modern factor analysis*. Ann Arbor, Mich.: Edwards Brothers, 1970.

Jastak, J., Bijou, S. W., & Jastak, S. R. *The Wide Range Achievement Test*. Wilmington, Del.: Jastak Associates, 1965.

Johnston, C. *Learning disability subtypes: A cross-validation*. Doctoral dissertation in preparation, University of Florida, 1984.

Kinsbourne, M. The role of selective attention in reading disability. In R. N. Malatesha & P. G. Aaron (Eds.), *Reading disorders: Variety and treatments*. New York: Academic Press, 1982.

Lyon, R. Subgroups of LD readers: Clinical and empirical identification. In H. R. Myklebust (Ed.), *Progress in learning disabilities* (Vol. 5). New York: Grune & Stratton, 1982.

Mattis, S., French, J. H., & Rapin, I. Dyslexia in children and adults: Three independent neuropsychological syndromes. *Developmental Medicine and Child Neurology*, 1975, *119*, 121–127.

Meehl, P. *Clinical versus statistical prediction*. Minneapolis: University of Minnesota, 1954.

Milligan, G. W. A review of Monte Carlo tests of cluster analysis. *Multivariate Behavioral Research*, 1981, *16*, 379–407.

Morey, L. C. *Alcohol abuse: Patterns and subtypes*. Unpublished doctoral dissertation, University of Florida, 1981.

Morris, R. *The developmental classification of learning disabled children using cluster analysis*. Unpublished doctoral dissertation, University of Florida, 1982.

Morris, R., & Blashfield, R. *Monte Carlo comparative studies of Q-analysis and cluster analysis*. Unpublished manuscript, 1983.

Morris, R., Blashfield, R., & Satz, P. Neuropsychology and cluster analysis: Problems and pitfalls. *Journal of Clinical Neuropsychology*, 1981, *3*, 79–99.

Morris, R., Blashfield, R., & Satz, P. *Developmental classifications of learning disabled children*. Unpublished manuscript.

Overall, J. E., & Klett, C. J. *Applied multivariate analysis*. New York: McGraw-Hill, 1972.

Petrauskas, R., & Rourke, B. P. Identification of subgroups of retarded readers: A neuropsychological, multivariate approach. *Journal of Clinical Neuropsychology*, 1979, *1*, 17–37.

Rourke, B. P. Neuropsychological research in reading retardation. In A. L. Benton & D. Pearl (Eds.), *Dyslexia: An appraisal of current knowledge*. New York: Oxford University Press, 1978.

Rourke, B. P. Central processing deficiencies in children: Toward a developmental neuropsychological model. *Journal of Clinical Neuropsychology*, 1982, *4*, 1–18.

Rourke, B. P., & Adams, K. M. Quantitative approaches to the neuropsychological assessment of children. In R. E. Tarter & G. Goldstein (Eds.), *Advances in clinical neuropsychology* (Vol. 2). New York: Plenum, 1984.

Rourke, B. P., & Finlayson, M. A. J. Neuropsychological significance of variations in patterns of academic performance: Verbal and visual-spatial abilities. *Journal of Abnormal Child Psychology*, 1978, *6*, 121–133.

Rourke, B. P., & Strang, J. D. Neuropsychological significance of variations in patterns of academic performance: Motor, psychomotor, and tactile-perceptual abilities. *Journal of Pediatric Psychology*, 1978, *3*, 62–66.

Rutter, M. Emotional disorder and educational under-achievement. *Archives of Diseases in Childhood*, 1974, *49*, 249–256.

Satz, P., & Fletcher, J. M. Minimal brain dysfunctions: An appraisal of research concepts and methods. In H. Rie & E. Rie (Eds.), *Handbook of minimal brain dysfunctions*. New York: Wiley-Interscience, 1980.

Satz, P., Friel, J., & Rudegair, F. Some predictive antecedents of specific reading disability: A two-, three-, and four year follow-up. In J. T. Guthrie (Ed.), *Aspects of reading acquisition*. Baltimore: John Hopkins University Press, 1976.

Satz, P., & Morris, R. Learning disability subtypes: A review. In F. J. Pirozzolo & M. C. Wittrock (Eds.), *Neuropsychological and cognitive processes in reading*. New York: Academic Press, 1981.

Satz, P., Taylor, G., Friel, J., & Fletcher, J. M. Some developmental and predictive precursors of reading disabilities: A six-year follow-up. In A. L. Benton & D. Pearl (Eds.), *Dyslexia: An appraisal of current knowledge*. New York: Oxford University Press, 1978.

Schauer, C. A. *The developmental relationship between neuropsychological and achievement variables: A cluster analysis study*. Unpublished doctoral dissertation, University of Florida, 1979.

Skinner, H. A. Differentiating the contribution of elevation, scatter and shape in profile similarity. *Educational and Psychological Measurement*, 1978, *38*, 297–308.

Skinner, H. A. Toward the integration of classification theory and methods. *Journal of Abnormal Psychology*, 1981, *90*, 68–87.

Spreen, O., & Benton, A. L. *Spreen-Benton Language Examination Profile*. Iowa City: University of Iowa, 1969.

Taylor, H. G., & Fletcher, J. M. Biological foundations of "specific developmental disorders": Methods, finding, and future directions. *Journal of Clinical Child Psychology*, 1983, *12*, 46–65.

Taylor, H. G., Satz, P., & Friel, J. Developmental dyslexia in relation to other childhood reading disorders: Significance and clinical utility. *Reading Research Quarterly*, 1979, *15*, 84–101.

Vellutino, F. R. Toward an understanding of dyslexia: Psychological factors in specific reading disability. In A. L. Benton & D. Pearl (Eds.), *Dyslexia: An appraisal of current knowledge*. New York: Oxford University Press, 1978.

Wiggins, J. *Personality and prediction*. New York: Addison-Wesley, 1973.

Wishart, D. *CLUSTAN user manual* (3rd ed.). London: University of London, 1975.

4

Neuropsychological Subtypes
of Learning-Disabled Children
Who Exhibit the ACID Pattern
on the WISC

MICHAEL JOSCHKO
BYRON P. ROURKE

This chapter focuses on one approach to the problem of generating *reliable* and *valid* typologies in clinical neuropsychology. In particular, the study described herein involves the use of *cluster-analytic* methodology to identify reliable subtypes of learning-disabled children who exhibit a specific pattern on the Wechsler Intelligence Scale for Children (WISC) and the Wechsler Intelligence Scale for Children—Revised (WISC-R).

The WISC and the WISC-R (Wechsler, 1949, 1974) have long been used in identifying and evaluating learning disabilities in children. Some school administrators require that a child obtain a certain pattern of performance on the WISC or WISC-R before he/she can be "diagnosed" as learning-disabled and before remedial assistance can be provided. Administrative decisions such as this reflect the widespread notion that there are specific WISC/WISC-R profiles that reliably characterize learning-disabled children. What is immediately apparent from a review of the clinical and empirical literature dealing with the WISC/WISC-R profiles of learning-disabled children, however, is that no single pattern of

Michael Joschko. Department of Psychology, Queen Alexandra Hospital for Children, and University of Victoria, Victoria, British Columbia, Canada.

Byron P. Rourke. Department of Psychology, University of Windsor, and Department of Neuropsychology, Windsor Western Hospital Centre, Windsor, Ontario, Canada.

results is characteristic of all learning-disabled children. Rather, there are a number of different WISC/WISC-R profiles that have been found in studies of *groups* of learning-disabled children. This should come as no surprise, in light of the now widely accepted view that learning-disabled children are a heterogeneous group with respect to their academic difficulties and adaptive ability structures (Knights & Bakker, 1976; Rourke, 1978, 1983; Rourke & Strang, 1983; Satz & Morris, 1980).

According to Swartz (1974; cited in Ackerman, Dykman, & Peters, 1976; Dykman, Ackerman, & Oglesby, 1980; Petrauskas & Rourke, 1979), a pattern consisting of depressed scores on four WISC subtests, the ACID pattern (an acronym for Arithmetic, Coding, Information, and Digit Span), is characteristic of most samples of learning-disabled children. This view is also held by Lutey (1977). A review of the literature suggests that there is some truth to this assertion, but that this pattern is certainly not characteristic of all samples or subsamples of learning-disabled children.

The literature on learning-disabled children manifesting ACID profiles (e.g., Ackerman et al., 1976; Ackerman, Dykman, & Peters, 1977) suggests that a subtype of learning-disabled children with particularly poor prognosis for academic performance in reading, spelling, and arithmetic may be defined by serious early reading problems and depressed scores on the ACID subtests. Clinically, however, there would appear to be at least two definable subgroups of reading-disabled children who exhibit this pattern: (1) a group with particularly poor immediate auditory–verbal memory (sequencing) problems, and (2) a group with particularly poor visual-imagery abilities. Additional research is needed to cross-validate and to investigate further the characteristics of learning-disabled children exhibiting the ACID pattern. In this regard, there is already some empirical evidence available.

Huelsman (1970) and Rugel (1974) have provided extensive reviews of the WISC subtest score profiles obtained by disabled readers. The ACID pattern, although not recognized by these authors, is clearly evident upon reanalysis of the published data in 5 of the 20 studies reviewed by Huelsman (1970) and in 9 out of 25 studies reviewed by Rugel (1974). More recently, this pattern has been reported by the following: Ackerman et al. (1976, 1977), for a sample of learning-disabled boys; Dykman et al. (1980), for both a learning-disabled and a hyperactive sample; Milich and Loney (1979), for a sample of "hyperactive/minimal brain dysfunction" boys with academic deficits; and Petrauskas and Rourke (1979), for two subtypes of retarded readers.

Although the ACID pattern is frequently apparent in the *mean* WISC profiles of groups of learning-disabled children described in the literature, clinical experience and the literature in this area suggest (1) that the ACID pattern is not individually characteristic of the majority of learning-disabled children, and (2) that learning-disabled children who do exhibit the ACID pattern do not all have the same type of information-processing deficits. The literature reviews provided by Huelsman (1970) and Rugel (1974) lend support to this first point. The findings reported by Ackerman *et al.* (1976, 1977), Dykman *et al.* (1980), and Petrauskas and Rourke (1979) are consistent with the second point and provide the impetus for investigating the subtype structure of learning-disabled children who exhibit the ACID pattern.

The original research described in this chapter utilizes the differential-score approach as a method of analysis in the study of learning-disabled children (Rourke, 1975, 1981) in an attempt to determine the neuropsychological significance of the ACID pattern for a large group of learning-disabled children who *individually* demonstrate this pattern. The relationship of the ACID pattern to academic performance is also investigated. These goals are accomplished by the following means: (1) statistical generation of homogeneous subtypes of learning-disabled ACID children through cluster-analytic methodology; (2) comparisons, utilizing multivariate analyses of variance (MANOVAs), of the academic performances of the ACID subtypes to matched groups of learning-disabled children who did *not* exhibit the ACID pattern; and (3) interpretations of the neuropsychological and academic ability profiles associated with each of the subtypes.

Because the use of cluster analysis is not as straightforward as it might at first appear, the findings of this research are presented in a framework emphasizing a methodological description of the steps involved in applying cluster-analytic procedures to neuropsychological test data.

The advantages of automatic multidimensional classification procedures, such as cluster analysis, over clinical or visual classification procedures are well recognized and include the following: (1) the ability to deal with large multivariate data sets, and (2) the properties of objectivity and repeatability. As a result, cluster-analytic methodology is becoming increasingly popular in the behavioral sciences. However, many of the problems in the use of this methodology are often overlooked. Since Adams (see Chapter 2, this volume) and Fletcher and Satz (see Chapter 3, this volume) review these concerns, they are not discussed in detail here.

THE STUDY

METHOD

A total of 181 learning-disabled children who exhibited the ACID pattern and 181 learning-disabled controls who did *not* exhibit the ACID pattern were selected for study. The controls were individually matched to the children in the ACID group on age, WISC Full Scale IQ, sex, and handedness. There were no statistically significant differences between the groups on any of the matching variables. All subjects had received an extensive standardized battery of neuropsychological tests and were judged by at least two experienced clinical neuropsychologists to be exhibiting a central information-processing deficiency.

The criteria used to select the two groups were as follows:

1. Each subject obtained a WISC Full Scale IQ of 80 or greater.
2. Each subject obtained at least one Wide Range Achievement Test (WRAT; Jastak & Jastak, 1965) centile score of 30 or below.
3. No subject exhibited any defects in hearing or visual acuity (determined from the results of a puretone sweep hearing test; a questionnaire completed by the parents; and visual and auditory screening information, when available in a child's clinical file).
4. No subject had a history of medically documented cerebral trauma or neurological dysfunction.
5. All subjects spoke English as the primary language in their homes (determined from the parent questionnaire) and were enrolled in English-language schools.
6. No subject was believed to be culturally, environmentally, or educationally deprived (determined from the history documented in each child's clinical file).
7. No subject exhibited any primary emotional-behavioral disturbances (determined from the results of a neuropsychological evaluation and the history available in each child's clinical file).

The ACID group met the following additional WISC criteria, which were necessary to define a *clinically* meaningful ACID pattern:

1a. The subtest scaled scores on Arithmetic, Information, and Digit Span were less than those on Comprehension, Similarities, and Vocabulary, *or*

1b. Scores on at least two of the Arithmetic, Information, and Digit Span subtests were less than scores on the Comprehension, Similarities, and Vocabulary subtests, and the third subtest scaled score was equal to the lowest of the remaining verbal subtests.

2a. Coding was the lowest Performance subtest scaled score, *or*

2b. Coding was lower than all other Performance subtest scaled scores save one, and it was equal to that one.

At this point, it is important to emphasize that the criteria for subject selection were clinical and were chosen to exploit the differential-score approach. As such, the control group differed from the ACID group only in the *pattern* of their WISC subtest scores; that is, the control group, although clearly comprised of learning-disabled children, did not exhibit the ACID pattern.

The selection of tests and procedures used in this research was based upon the following criterion: The tests and procedures should be capable of reflecting a fairly broad spectrum of those abilities that are subserved by the human brain and that are expected to be impaired when its various systems are dysfunctional. For this reason, a number of measures of sensory–perceptual, motor, psychomotor, linguistic, and cognitive skills that have been shown to be sensitive to the functional integrity of cerebral hemispheres in children (Boll, 1974; Reitan, 1974; Rourke, 1981) were included.

Table 4-1 contains a list of the tests included in the neuropsychological test battery. For the most part, the tests and procedures were developed and standardized by Reitan (Reitan & Davison, 1974). Except where otherwise indicated, these measures are described in Reitan and Davison (1974) or Wechsler (1949). Those tests that were administered only to children between the ages of 5 to 8 years are followed by the designation "Younger." Those administered only to children within the age span of 9 to 15 years are followed by the designation "Older." In total, these tests provided 110 and 103 measures for the younger and older groups, respectively.

In order (1) to avoid artificially high correlations between variables because of positive correlations with age and (2) to express the many different variables in comparable units for ease of comparison between tests, all of the test scores for which the necessary data were available were

TABLE 4-1. Tests Included in Neuropsychological Test Battery

1. Tactile-perceptual and tactile-kinesthetic
   a. Reitan-Kløve Tactile-Perceptual and Tactile-Form Recognition Tests
       i. Tactile Imperception and Suppression
      ii. Finger Agnosia
     iii. Fingertip Number-Writing Recognition (Older)
          Fingertip Symbol-Writing Recognition (Younger)
      iv. Coin Recognition (Older)
          Tactile-Form Recognition (Younger)
   b. Tactual Performance Test

2. Visual-perceptual
   a. Reitan-Kløve Visual-Perceptual Test
   b. Constructional Dyspraxia Items, Halstead-Wepman Aphasia Screening Test
   c. WISC Picture Completion, Block Design, Object Assembly Subtests
   d. Color Form Test (Younger)
   e. Progressive Figures Test (Younger)
   f. Individual Performance Tests (Younger)
       i. Star Drawing
      ii. Concentric Squares Drawing

3. Auditory-perceptual and language-related
   a. Reitan-Kløve Auditory-Perceptual Test
   b. Seashore Rhythm Test
   c. Speech-Sounds Perception Test
   d. Auditory Closure Test (Kass, 1964)
   e. Sentence Memory Test (Benton, 1965)
   f. Verbal Fluency Test
   g. Peabody Picture Vocabulary Test (Dunn, 1965)
   h. Aphasoid Items, Aphasia Screening Test
   i. WISC Information, Comprehension, Similarities, Vocabulary subtests

4. Sequencing: Auditory and visual sequential perception, sequential motor responding
   a. WISC Coding, Digit Span, and Picture Arrangement subtests
   b. Trail Making Test for Children, Parts A and B (Older)
   c. Target Test
   d. Individual Performance Tests (Younger)
       i. Matching Figures
      ii. Matching V's
   e. Finger-Tapping Test
   f. Foot-Tapping Test (Knights & Moule, 1967)

5. Problem solving, concept formation, reasoning
   a. Halstead Category Test
   b. Matching Pictures Test (Younger)
   c. WISC Arithmetic subtest

6. Motor and psychomotor
   a. Reitan-Kløve Lateral Dominance Examination
   b. Dynamometer
   c. Kløve-Matthews Motor Steadiness Battery (Kløve & Matthews, 1963)
       i. Maze Coordination Test
      ii. Static Steadiness
     iii. Grooved Pegboard Test

7. Academic
   a. WRAT Reading, Spelling, and Arithmetic subtests (Jastak & Jastak, 1965)

Note. "Younger" denotes tests given only to children between the ages of 5 and 8 years.
"Older" tests are given only to children between the ages of 9 and 15 years.

transformed into T scores. Both the ACID and control subjects were divided into "younger" (6 years, 0 months to 8 years, 11 months; 54 males, 5 females) and "older" (9 years, 0 months to 14 years, 11 months; 117 males, 5 females) groups because of the differences in the test batteries administered to the two age groups and because it was expected that developmentally based differences in ability structures between younger and older learning-disabled children would be delineated. The two younger and older groups were then combined into "younger" and "older" data sets, which contained 63 and 54 neuropsychological measures, respectively.[1]

In order (1) to enhance the reliability and interpretability of the subtypes determined in later analyses, (2) to reduce redundancy in the variables used, and (3) to conserve computing resources, the initial analyses involved data reduction of the two age-based data sets through principal-components analysis (PCA) with orthogonal rotation to varimax criterion. For the younger data set, PCA reduced the 63 measures to 19 factors, which accounted for 76.3% of the variance. For the older data set, the 54 measures were reduced to 16 factors, which accounted for 68.1% of the variance.

Because "outliers"—unique individuals or disparate individuals resulting from measurement error—can affect most clustering procedures (Edelbrock, 1979; Everitt, 1974, Milligan, 1979), the scatter plots of the two age-based samples in the space of the first few principal components were examined for outliers. Four subjects in each group were determined to be outliers and were dropped, along with their matched controls, from further analyses.

CLUSTER ANALYSES AND INTERNAL VALIDATION
(RELIABILITY) PROCEDURES

The data for the older and the younger ACID groups were subjected separately to a number of different cluster analyses. In the interests of brevity from this point on, only the procedures applied to the younger

---

1. It should be noted that a number of neuropsychological measures were not included in the younger and older data sets because they were either composites of other measures used (i.e., summary scores), components of composite measures used (i.e., subtest scores), measures used to validate the subtypes obtained, measures used directly in the selections of the ACID subjects, or measures for which there were a high frequency of missing values or insufficient normative data available.

group are specifically described. It should be noted, however, that *identical* procedures were carried out with the older group.

Since different similarity measures can produce discrepant results even when the same data and clustering algorithms are used (Edelbrock, 1979; Mezzich, 1978), the choice of the similarity measure used in a cluster analysis demands careful consideration. Because it was believed that the *relative patterning* of the neuropsychological test scores, rather than differences in level of performance, would distinguish ACID subtypes, product–moment correlation was chosen as the measure of similarity between subjects. It is well recognized that distance measures, such as the popular squared Euclidean distance, are differentially sensitive to profile elevation and are inappropriate when profile shape (pattern) needs to be emphasized (Everitt, 1974; Fleiss & Zubin, 1969; Skinner, 1978).

Because a clustering algorithm will "find" clusters even in random data, and because different cluster-analytic algorithms using the same similarity measures can generate different groupings when applied to the same data set, it is important to demonstrate the "internal validity" (reliability) of a cluster solution. That is, it is important to demonstrate that the groupings determined are stable and that they actually exist in the data.

With this in mind, five different cluster analyses using correlation as a measure of similarity were carried out in order to ensure that the derived groupings were stable and replicable across different clustering techniques. This procedure is based on the premise that well-structured data will produce clusters that replicate well across different clustering methods that are applicable to a particular research problem (Everitt, 1974). Because homogeneous groups of subjects were expected, algorithms subject to "chaining" (Everitt, 1974) were excluded as possible clustering procedures.

Version 1C2 of the CLUSTAN (Wishart, 1975) computer software package was used to perform all cluster analyses utilized in this research, because of its versatility, reasonably detailed documentation, and increasing familiarity to researchers in the behavioral sciences.

Younger ACID Group

The choice of clustering algorithms in this research was based on their sensitivity to "group" structure and on the basis of previous research assessing the accuracy of different clustering algorithms (Edelbrock, 1974;

Mezzich, 1978). The five clustering procedures applied to the factor-score data matrix for the younger ACID group were as follows:

1. Group-average analysis (Sokal & Michener's [1958] unweighted pair–group method using arithmetic averages).
2. Centroid-sorting analysis (Sokal & Michener's [1958] unweighted pair–group centroid method).
3. Group-average analysis with iterative relocation.
4. Centroid-sorting analysis with iterative relocation.
5. Iterative relocation of a random partition of the data.

A problem common to all hierarchical agglomerative clustering methods, such as the group-average and centroid-sorting analyses, is in deciding at what stage in the procedure the clustering algorithm should stop generating more clusters (i.e., in deciding how many clusters represent the most appropriate solution). It has generally been suggested (Everitt, 1974; Wishart, 1975) that a significant "drop" or discontinuity in the clustering coefficient (a metric related to the amount of variance accounted for at each step of a clustering procedure) indicates that two dissimilar clusters have been combined to create a relatively heterogeneous cluster, and, therefore, that the preceding partition of the data represents the appropriate stopping point. Using this criterion, inspection of the plots of the cluster coefficients against the number of clusters for the group-average and centroid-sorting analyses and an evaluation of the cluster solutions at different levels in the hierarchy led to a decision to utilize the four-cluster classifications as the terminal solutions.

Since hierarchical clustering procedures do not allow for the re-allocation of subjects to correct for a poor initial grouping of the data, an iterative relocation procedure was applied to the classifications generated by the group-average and centroid-sorting analyses in order to assess the stability of the clusters derived by the hierarchical analyses, to increase homogeneity, and to decrease cluster overlap. To assess further the stability of the generated groupings, the iterative relocation method was also used to cluster a random initial classification of the factor-score data matrix. This allows for a comparison of solutions obtained from quite different starting points. If essentially the same solution is obtained, this can be taken as an indication that an acceptable solution has been reached (Wishart, 1975).

Comparisons of the classifications generated by the five different cluster analyses indicated that the closest agreement occurred between the centroid-sorting analysis with relocation and the relocation analysis of a random partition of the data (85% of the subjects were classified into the same clusters by both methods). Since essentially the same solution was obtained from quite different starting points, this was taken as evidence that an acceptable solution had been reached (Wishart, 1975). On the basis of these results, the cluster solution generated by centroid-sorting analysis with relocation was chosen to represent the underlying structure of the younger ACID group.

The agreement among the four-cluster solutions generated by five different cluster analyses described to this point is summarized in Table 4-2. The number of subjects correctly classified and the percentages of hits were calculated with the four-cluster solution produced by centroid-sorting analysis with iterative relocation as reference. Inspection of Table 4-2 reveals different concordance rates across the younger ACID clusters. Clusters 2 and 4 were well preserved over all cluster analyses, with mean percentages of hits of 88.16 and 89.58, respectively. These clusters would appear to constitute reliable subtypes. Clusters 1 and 3, on the other hand, were considerably less stable, with mean percentages of hits of 52.78 and 58.33, respectively. These clusters may represent artificial groupings forced on the data; therefore, these clusters are not described below in any detail.

TABLE 4-2. Concordance across Different Clustering Procedures for the Younger ACID Subtypes, with Cluster Solution Produced by Centroid-Sorting Analysis with Iterative Relocation as Reference

Cluster analysis procedure	Younger ACID clusters							
	Cluster 1		Cluster 2		Cluster 3		Cluster 4	
	Hits	(%)	Hits	(%)	Hits	(%)	Hits	(%)
CS-IR	9	(100)	19	(100)	15	(100)	12	(100)
AL-IR	6	(66.67)	16	(84.21)	15	(100)	11	(91.67)
IR (RANDOM)	8	(88.89)	16	(84.21)	8	(53.33)	11	(91.67)
AL	1	(11.11)	17	(89.41)	6	(40.00)	10	(83.33)
CS	4	(44.44)	18	(94.74)	6	(40.00)	11	(91.67)

Note. Abbreviations: CS-IR = centroid-sorting analysis with iterative relocation; AL-IR = group-average analysis with iterative relocation; IR (RANDOM) = iterative relocation from an initial random classification; AL = group-average analysis; CS = centroid-sorting analysis.

Note. Mean percentages of hits over methods AL-IR, IR (RANDOM), CS, and AL were as follows: Cluster 1, 52.78%; Cluster 2, 88.16%; Cluster 3, 58.33%; and Cluster 4, 89.58%.

Further evidence of the stability of Clusters 2 and 4 was obtained from inspection of the five- and three-cluster solutions. These clusters were well preserved at both of these levels in the hierarchical solution, while the less reliable groupings were not.

At this point, it should be noted that two reliable subtypes emerged when the results of five cluster-analytic techniques were analyzed. If only two cluster-analytic techniques had been used (i.e., centroid-sorting and group-average analyses), it would have been possible to conclude that four reliable subtypes had emerged (see Table 4-2). Therefore, it behooves the user of cluster-analytic methodology to attend most carefully to the evaluation of the reliability (referred to by some as "internal validity") of the derived classification.

The stability of the subtype structure was also assessed in the face of changes to the set of clustering variables. Correlation similarity matrices were calculated for data sets consisting of the T scores of the variables with the two highest loadings on each factor and a data set consisting of a subset of the original 19 principal-component factor scores. These data matrices were then subjected to centroid-sorting analysis with relocation. The groupings generated by these analyses were consistent with the previous results: Clusters 2 and 4 were relatively well preserved in both cluster solutions.

The final step in assessing the stability of the classifications generated in this investigation was to cluster-anayze the combined sample of ACID and control subjects. The results of this analysis indicated that Clusters 2 and 4 remained well preserved even when other subjects were added to the data matrices.

Older ACID Group

The series of analyses described above was also applied to the older ACID group. Table 4-3 contains the number of subjects correctly classified and the percentages of hits over the different cluster analyses; identical groupings were produced by the centroid-sorting and group-average analyses with iterative relocation. Therefore, calculations were performed arbitrarily with the four-cluster solution produced by centroid sorting with iterative relocation as reference in order to maintain consistency with the procedures applied to the younger ACID group. Inspection of Table 4-3 reveals different concordance rates across the older ACID clusters. Clusters 1 and 2, which were well preserved over all cluster analyses,

TABLE 4-3. Concordance across Different Clustering Procedures for the Older ACID Subtypes, with Cluster Solution Produced by Centroid-Sorting Analysis with Iterative Relocation as Reference

Cluster analysis procedure	Older ACID clusters							
	Cluster 1		Cluster 2		Cluster 3		Cluster 4	
	Hits	(%)	Hits	(%)	Hits	(%)	Hits	(%)
CS-IR	41	(100)	34	(100)	21	(100)	22	(100)
AL-IR	41	(100)	34	(100)	21	(100)	22	(100)
IR (RANDOM)	32	(78.05)	21	(61.76)	13	(61.90)	3	(13.64)
CS	31	(75.61)	33	(97.06)	12	(57.14)	6	(27.27)
AL	33	(80.49)	22	(64.71)	12	(57.14)	17	(77.27)

Note. Abbreviations: CS-IR = centroid-sorting analysis with iterative relocation; AL-IR = group-average analysis with iterative relocation; IR (RANDOM) = iterative relocation from an initial random classification; CS = centroid-sorting analysis; AL = group-average analysis.

Note. Mean percentages of hits over methods AL-IR, IR (RANDOM), CS, and AL were as follows: Cluster 1, 83.54%; Cluster 2, 80.88%; Cluster 3, 69.04%; and Cluster 4, 54.54%.

would appear to constitute reliable subtypes. Clusters 3 and 4, however, were considerably less stable and may represent artificial groupings forced on the data; therefore, these clusters are not described below in any detail.

Clusters 1 and 2 were well preserved by five- and three-cluster solutions. These clusters also had the highest concordance rates when the four-cluster solutions produced by centroid sorting with relocation for three different sets of clustering variables were compared. The results stemming from the cluster analysis of the combined sample of older ACID and control subjects were not as clear-cut as those obtained with the younger data set. This may be due to the generally larger standard deviations of the variables in the older data set. Nonetheless, Cluster 1 was well preserved in the combined analysis, and this provides some further evidence of the stability of the derived classification of the older ACID group; Cluster 2, however, was the least well preserved of the four older ACID clusters.

PREDICTIVE (EXTERNAL) VALIDITY OF THE TAXONOMY

The aforementioned procedures indicate that the same clusters consistently appeared in these data, but this only demonstrates the internal validity or reliability of the derived classification. The external validity and clinical meaningfulness of the subtypes generated in this research are discussed in this section.

A number of authors (e.g., Blashfield, 1980; Fletcher, Chapter 9, this volume; Satz & Morris, 1980) have stressed that the external validity of a cluster solution should be assessed by means of variables that are independent of those used in the cluster analysis. That is, groups deter-mined from a cluster analysis should differ with respect to variables not used in the actual classification. In this regard, a series of MANOVAs, analyses of variance (ANOVAs), and Newman–Keuls tests were used to assess the validity of the subtypes generated in this research by comparing ACID clusters to their matched controls and by evaluating intercluster differences on the subtests of the WRAT. These analyses indicated that the ACID group obtained significantly poorer WRAT Reading and Arithmetic scores than did their matched controls at the younger ages and poorer Arithmetic scores at the older ages. No significant intercluster differences, however, were found. Further work with these data will be necessary to determine whether there are qualitative intercluster dif-ferences in academic performance.

The aforementioned validation procedures utilized one of the two principal types of external validity commonly employed in subtype analyses—that is, differences on other (e.g., academic) tasks. The evalu-ation of differences in response to treatment represents another com-monly employed procedure for external validation. Although the ACID subtypes identified do not differ on academic tasks, they may differ in response to remedial treatment. That is, they may be deficient on aca-demic tasks for quite different reasons, and they might make gains on academic tasks for much different reasons. There is some evidence in support of this hypothesis for the ACID subtypes derived in this in-vestigation.

Although the ACID subtypes generated in this research do not differ significantly in terms of *level* of academic performance, the plots of the factor-score profiles for each of the reliable subtypes indicate that they have *qualitatively different* ability profiles, which may have practical implications with respect to the habilitation and education of learning-disabled children who exhibit the ACID pattern. When the mean neuro-psychological test profiles were plotted for each of the reliable subtypes, some clinically meaningful patterns emerged.

The distinguishing features of the reliable subtypes at each of the two age levels are summarized in Table 4-4 and are discussed below. In order to simplify comparisons among the subtypes, the neuropsychological

TABLE 4-4. Performance Characteristics of Reliable ACID Subtypes

Neuropsychological measures	ACID subtypes			
	Younger Subtype 2	Younger Subtype 4	Older Subtype 1	Older Subtype 2
Tactile–perceptual	Poor	Average	Average	Poor
Visual–perceptual	Poor	Average	Average	Average
Auditory–perceptual and language-related	Poor	Poor	Poor	Poor
Sequencing	Average	Poor	Poor	Average
Concept formation and reasoning	Average	Average	Average	Average
Motor	Poor	Average	Average	Poor
Academic	Poor	Poor	Poor	Poor

Note. "Poor" indicates a tendency for poorer test performances in comparison to the norms for the test. "Average" indicates test performances generally within one standard deviation of the normative mean.

measures are grouped rationally into seven areas: tactile–perceptual; visual–perceptual; auditory–perceptual and language-related; sequential analysis and sequential motor responding; concept formation and reasoning; motor; and academic (see Table 4-1).

Younger ACID Subtype 2 was characterized by poor performances with the right hand relative to the left hand on a number of measures in the tactile–perceptual category. The poorest performance in this area was on a test involving the perception of symbols written on the fingertips. In comparison to Younger ACID Subtype 4, Subtype 2 exhibited a pattern of outstandingly poor performances on four tests (Color Form Test, Progressive Figures Test, Star Drawing, and Concentric Square Drawing) in the visual–perceptual category. It should be noted, however, that other tests in the visual–perceptual category (i.e., WISC Block Design, Object Assembly, and Picture Completion) were performed normally or in an above-average manner. With the exception of performances well below the mean on tests involving auditory–visual matching (Speech-Sounds Perception Test), sentence memory (Sentence Memory Test), and verbal fluency (Verbal Fluency Test), performances on tests in the auditory–perceptual and language-related category were within one standard deviation of the mean. Likewise, the performances of Subtype 2 subjects on the measures in the sequencing and concept-formation categories were generally within one standard deviation of the mean. Within the motor category, Subtype 2 exhibited an outstanding deficiency in kinetic steadiness ability with the left upper extremity (Maze Coordination Test).

Subtype 2 exhibited the highest Full Scale and Performance IQs and the largest Verbal–Performance IQ discrepancy (10.58 IQ points favoring the Performance scale) of any of the younger ACID clusters. Their WRAT Spelling subtest scores were somewhat poorer than their Reading and Arithmetic scores.

In general, there is some similarity between the pattern of neuropsychological strengths and weaknesses exhibited by Subtype 2 and the neuropsychological pattern exhibited by adults with well-documented lesions that are confined to the temporal and adjacent posterior regions of the left cerebral hemisphere (Luria, 1973). With respect to the underlying neuropsychological deficit affecting academic performance, a clinical interpretation of their group profile suggests that Subtype 2 children may be experiencing a predominant deficiency in the "revisualization" of symbols. This would seem to be reflected in the poor performances of this subtype on the Fingertip Symbol-Writing Recognition Test, the WRAT Spelling subtest, the Speech-Sounds Perception Test, the WISC Coding subtest, and, possibly, the WISC Arithmetic and Digit Span subtests and the Target Test. Further investigations, including a qualitative analysis of the spelling and reading errors evidenced by Subtype 2 children, will be necessary to test this hypothesis.

Similar problems in revisualization have been described by Johnson and Myklebust (1967) in their classic text. This ACID subtype may be similar to Boder's (1971) "dyseidetic dyslexia" group and to a subtype of reading-problem children described by Doehring and Hoshko (1977) who exhibited poor auditory–visual matching.

Younger ACID Subtype 4 was distinguished from the other younger ACID clusters by a pattern of good performance in the tactile–perceptual category, together with consistently poorer performances on tests in the sequencing category. With the exception of an outstandingly poor performance on the Concentric Squares Drawing test, Subtype 4 performed well on tests in the visual–perceptual category. As was the case for Subtype 2 children, the performance of Subtype 4 subjects was quite poor on the Speech-Sounds Perception Test and the Sentence Memory Test, while their performances were within one standard deviation of the mean on most of the other auditory–perceptual and language-related measures. The performances of Subtype 4 subjects on the measures in the concept-formation and motor categories were generally within one standard deviation of the mean.

Compared to the other younger ACID clusters, Subtype 4 exhibited the lowest WISC Verbal and Full Scale IQs. A Verbal–Performance IQ discrepancy of 7.24 IQ points in favor of the Performance scale characterized Subtype 4. This subtype also exhibited the lowest Peabody Picture Vocabulary Test IQ and the poorest performance on a test involving sustained attention, fine auditory discrimination, and auditory sequencing (the Seashore Rhythm Test). Their WRAT Reading and Spelling subtest scores were somewhat poorer than were their Arithmetic scores.

In summary, the mean profile of Subtype 4 reflected deficits in auditory, visual–spatial, and motoric sequential processing. This may be the limiting feature responsible for the academic difficulties of this group. Whether immediate auditory–verbal and visual–spatial memory problems per se are also present or whether the apparent mnemonic deficiency is a reflection of a "sequencing" deficit is moot. Qualitative analyses of the Digit Span and Sentence Memory performance of these subjects could be expected to shed some light on this issue. In any case, various authors (reviewed by Rourke, 1978) have postulated that sequencing deficits may account for reading disorders in some children. In particular, Denckla (1977) and Mattis (1978) have described small groups of learning-disabled children with isolated sequencing deficits who bear a striking resemblance to Subtype 4. Petrauskas and Rourke (1979) have also described a subtype of 7- and 8-year-old retarded readers who, as a group, exhibited the ACID pattern and "sequencing" difficulties.

In view of the sequencing deficiencies exhibited by Subtype 4 and the overall profile of neuropsychological strengths and weaknesses exhibited by this group, it would seem reasonable to hypothesize that some of the abilities ordinarily thought to be subserved by the temporo-parietal region of the left cerebral hemisphere are compromised in this Younger ACID subtype.

The distinguishing characteristics of Older ACID Subtype 1 are a pattern of normal performances (within one standard deviation of the mean) on the measures in the tactile–perceptual category; deficient performances on two symbolic sequencing and visual scanning tasks (Trail Making Test for Children, Parts A and B); and outstandingly slow performances bilaterally on a measure of kinetic steadiness (Maze Coordination Test). This subtype also exhibited the highest WISC Full Scale IQ and the smallest Verbal–Performance IQ discrepancy (9.22 IQ points in favor of the Performance scale) of the older ACID clusters. The WRAT Spelling and Arithmetic scores of Older ACID Subtype 1 subjects were somewhat poorer than were their Reading scores.

Older ACID Subtype 1 bears some resemblance to Younger ACID Subtype 4 and may represent an "older version" of this younger subtype.

Clearly, however, a longitudinal investigation is needed to test this hypothesis.

Older ACID Subtype 2 exhibited the largest WISC Verbal–Performance IQ discrepancy (11.76 IQ points in favor of the Performance scale) of the four older ACID clusters. As a group, the children classified into Older ACID Subtype 2 exhibited a pattern of mildly impaired performances on all three of the WRAT subtests.

The distinguishing features of the neuropsychological test performances of Older ACID Subtype 2 are as follows: (1) poor performances bilaterally on a number of tactile–perceptual measures involving the "mental imaging" of numbers (Fingertip Number-Writing Recognition) and objects (Coin Recognition, Tactual Performance Test, Location Component) and (2) outstandingly poor kinetic steadiness abilities bilaterally (Maze Coordination Test). This pattern of tactile–perceptual and kinetic steadiness deficiencies, together with deficiencies in certain auditory–perceptual (Speech-Sounds Perception Test) and language-related (Sentence Memory Test, Verbal Fluency Test) skills, is similar to neuropsychological profiles seen commonly in clinical practice; it raises the possibility that some of the abilities normally thought to be subserved primarily by the temporal and adjacent posterior cortical regions of the left cerebral hemisphere (Luria, 1973) may be compromised. As such, this pattern of neuropsychological strengths and weaknesses bears *some* resemblance to that of Younger ACID Subtype 2. A longitudinal tracking of Younger ACID Subtype 2 children, however, will be necessary to determine whether Older ACID Subtype 2 represents an older "version" of this younger ACID subtype.

CONCLUSIONS AND IMPLICATIONS

The purpose of this chapter has been to demonstrate the application of cluster-analytic procedures to the problem of determining reliable and meaningful subtypes of children who exhibit central processing deficiencies. The results of the study described in this chapter indicate that, at each of the two age levels studied, there are at least two reliable subtypes of learning-disabled children who individually exhibit the ACID pattern. This is consistent with clinical experience and the available literature, which suggests that children who exhibit the ACID pattern are a heterogeneous population with respect to their adaptive ability structures. These findings have obvious implications for school psychologists and others who might tend to base remedial recommendations on a unitary view of the ACID pattern as, say, a measure of "freedom from distractibility." Furthermore, although there is some evidence to indicate that the ACID subtypes found in the older age group exhibit information-processing deficiencies similar to those exhibited by the younger ACID subtypes, it is not possible to determine whether the older subtypes actually represent older versions of the younger subtypes. A longitudinal study would be necessary to address this issue.

The identification of reliable subtypes of children who exhibit the ACID pattern is consistent with the results of previous investigations (Doehring & Hoshko, 1977; Doehring, Hoshko, & Bryans, 1979; Fisk & Rourke, 1979; Petrauskas & Rourke, 1979), which have indicated that learning-disabled children are a heterogeneous group and that reliable subtypes can be determined through the use of automatic multivariate classification procedures. With respect to the ACID pattern, the issue now is to determine the predictive validity and clinical meaningfulness of the classification.

The similarities of the ACID subtypes identified in the present study to other specific groups of learning-disabled children described in the literature (e.g., the similarity of Younger ACID Subtype 4 to groups of children described by Denckla, 1977, and Mattis, 1978) are encouraging vis-à-vis the consensual validity of the ACID subtypes generated in this research. Further in-depth qualitative analyses of the information-processing deficiencies exhibited by these subtypes, however, is necessary to confirm these similarities. We are now undertaking such qualitative analyses, including analyses of types of spelling errors (see Sweeney & Rourke, 1978, and Chapter 7, this volume).

Qualitative analyses could also be expected to lead to an evaluation of the appropriateness of specific remedial techniques for certain "types" of learning-disabled children. For example, one might expect that Younger ACID Subtype 4 and Older ACID Subtype 1 would benefit from specific training and drill in the various dimensions of visual and auditory sequentialization (Gaddes, 1981; Johnson & Myklebust, 1967). Such a remedial approach would train a child to recall the temporal or spatial order of sequentially presented stimuli. An approach that also allows for the progression of stimuli from nonverbal auditory or visual patterns, followed by syllables or letters within words and then by words in a sentence, could be expected to be most effective and to have the broadest range of application. Because the sequencing deficiencies of these children might affect their ability to profit from a phonics-based approach to reading and spelling, whole-word, multisensory strategies might be more appropriate until the sequencing deficiencies are remediated. The relative emphasis on remediation within the visual or auditory modalities, however, would have to be based on a careful clinical analysis of the individual child's particular adaptive strengths and weaknesses. Since it is possible that children with these sequencing deficiencies differ with respect to the extent that the sequencing problem contributes to difficulties in auditory comprehension or reading, the specific emphasis of the remedial approaches used would be expected to require some modifications among children.

The remediation of the revisualization deficiencies of Younger ACID Subtype 2 and Older ACID Subtype 2 also requires careful clinical analysis of the nature of their deficiencies and the academic abilities affected. In general, however, specific training and drill in the revisualization of letters and words through the use of a tactile- and kinesthetic-perceptual approach (e.g., the multisensory methods of Fernald, 1943) and the visual-memory strategies of Johnson and Myklebust (1967) might be appropriate remedial techniques for these children. Intensive drill in phonics through a phonetic-visual approach that stresses visual-auditory associations might help to circumvent the effects of revisualization deficiencies on the reading and spelling performances of these children. Likewise, verbal mediation strategies might be effective in circumventing any problems in arithmetic due to these deficiencies.

At this juncture, it must be emphasized that remediation for the individual child *must* be based on an evaluation of that child's specific pattern of strengths and weaknesses, and not solely on the basis of inferences made from group data. Failure to attend to this principle may, in part, contribute to the current confusion in the literature and within school systems regarding the efficiency and effectiveness of various remedial approaches for learning-disabled children (Rourke, Bakker, Fisk, & Strang, 1983).

Although the ACID subtypes determined in the research described in this chapter are similar to other subtypes of learning-disabled children described in the literature, none of the ACID subtypes bear any close resemblance to other groups of children described in the literature who exhibit the "ACID" pattern. At first glance, the failure to find reliable ACID subtypes similar to groups of ACID-pattern children described in the literature is perplexing. There is at least one major difference, however, between the subjects used in the present research and those used in previous investigations that may account for this phenomenon. All of the ACID subjects utilized in the present research *individually* exhibited the ACID pattern. There is little evidence to indicate that the ACID groups described in previous investigations consisted of such well-defined ACID-pattern children; in most cases, it would seem that group means rather than individual profiles served to define the ACID groups (e.g., see Ackerman *et al.*, 1976, 1977).

The dissimilarities between the ACID subtypes identified in this investigation and children who as a group exhibit the ACID pattern would seem to highlight some important clinical considerations. There are clear pitfalls inherent in attributing clinical utility to profiles based on mean scores, which may not be representative of individual children constituting the group. Previous conclusions based on such group profiles (e.g., that the ACID pattern per se portends a particularly poor prognosis for academic performance in reading, spelling, and arithmetic, as measured by the WRAT; see Ackerman *et al.*, 1976) must be viewed with some caution. The results of the cross-sectional research described in this chapter would not support this conclusion vis-à-vis learning-disabled children in general. Although the older ACID group obtained lower WRAT Arithmetic scores than did a group of matched learning-disabled controls who did not evidence the ACID pattern, the two groups were not differentiated significantly in terms of their levels of reading or spelling performances. Clearly, a longitudinal follow-up of younger ACID children will be necessary to determine whether the ACID pattern is predictive of exceptionally poor academic prognosis.

Not only do the ACID subtypes described herein differ from the controls on some WRAT subtests, but there is evidence that the ACID subtypes have ability profiles that differ qualitatively from the subgroups of matched learning-disabled controls. At first blush, this would seem to be further evidence in favor of the hypothesis that the ACID subtypes define a clinically meaningful classification of learning-disabled children. However, because the control groups were not subjected to cluster-analytic procedures, their subgroup ability profiles cannot be considered to represent more than the mean profiles of a heterogeneous group of learning-disabled children. Therefore, the differences between the ability profiles of the ACID subtypes and the control subgroups is only evidence in favor of the *internal* validity (reliability) of the ACID subtype structure. Further analyses of the subtype structure of the control groups will be necessary to determine whether and to what extent ACID subtypes differ in their ability profiles (i.e., information-processing deficiencies) from other subtypes of learning-disabled children.

The investigation described in this chapter represents an attempt to cluster a group of learning-disabled children who individually exhibited a specific, clinically meaningful pattern on the WISC. Although samples of learning-disabled children commonly exhibit the ACID pattern as a group, only a small proportion of learning-disabled children would seem to exhibit this pattern on an individual basis. For example, of the large number of children (3500) contained in the data base utilized in the present study, fewer than 6% exhibited the ACID pattern (there would have been more if the criteria had been looser). It is noteworthy that two distinct and reliable subtypes, with little in common, emerged when only a very small percentage of a population of learning-disabled children was subjected to subtyping. This would seem to indicate that finer levels of subtype analyses can be quite heuristic. Rather than limiting subtype analyses to broad-band classifications of learning-disabled or reading-disabled children in general, the approach used in this investigation demonstrates the value of subtyping children with more circumscribed characteristics. Del Dotto and Rourke (Chapter 5, this volume), Sweeney and Rourke (Chapter 7, this volume), and Strang and Rourke (Chapter 8, this volume) provide other examples of subtype analyses at these finer levels.

Cluster analysis, as a classification tool, is frequently valued because of its objectivity and repeatability. However, lest the reader be left with the impression that the methodology described in this chapter represents an entirely objective approach to the classification of learning-disabled children, the following methodological considerations are offered. The determination of the ACID pattern based on the *relative* pattern of WISC subtest scores clearly limits the generalizability of the classification discussed in this chapter. A different subtype structure might eventuate if the ACID pattern were determined on the basis of a certain minimum difference (e.g., the standard error of measurement, or the "abnormality of the difference"; see Piotrowski, 1978) between the ACID subtests and the remaining WISC scales.

A number of issues related to the cluster analyses may also affect the generalizability of the ACID classification. The choice of the clustering variables, similarity coefficient, clustering algorithms, and terminal cluster solutions, although defensible on rational grounds, all basically involved subjective decisions on the part of Joschko. Clearly, other choices that may have affected the derived subtype structure were possible. Therefore, the subtype structure of ACID children described above needs to be confirmed empirically before it is accepted as valid. In this regard, cross-validation and the application of further external validation procedures are necessary to establish firmly the predictive validity of the taxonomy generated by the cluster analyses in this research.

ACKNOWLEDGMENTS

The research described in this chapter formed the basis of a doctoral dissertation completed by Joschko at the University of Windsor. The initial phases of this research were supported by a Research Studentship from the Ontario Mental Health Foundation. The support of Mr. N. John Scholten, Director of the Sarnia–Lambton Centre for Children and Youth, and the assistance of Mrs. Barb Metcalfe and Mrs. Gwen Paquette are gratefully acknowledged.

REFERENCES

Ackerman, P. T., Dykman, R. A., & Peters, J. E. Hierarchical factor patterns on the WISC as related to areas of learning deficit. *Perceptual and Motor Skills*, 1976, *42*, 583–615.

Ackerman, P. T., Dykman, R. A., & Peters, J. E. Learning-disabled boys as adolescents: Cognitive factors and achievement. *Journal of the American Academy of Child Psychiatry*, 1977, *16*, 296–313.

Benton, A. L. *Sentence Memory Test*. Iowa City, Iowa: Author, 1965.

Blashfield, R. K. Propositions regarding the use of cluster analysis in clinical research. *Journal of Consulting and Clinical Psychology*, 1980, *48*, 456–459.

Boder, E. Developmental dyslexia: Prevailing diagnostic concepts and a new diagnostic approach. In H. R. Myklebust (Eds.), *Progress in learning disabilities* (Vol. 2). New York: Grune & Stratton, 1971.

Boll, T. J. Behavioral correlates of cerebral damage in children aged 9 through 14. In R. M. Reitan & L. A. Davison (Eds.), *Clinical neuropsychology: Current status and applications*. Washington, D.C.: V. H. Winston & Sons, 1974.

Denckla, M. B. Minimal brain dysfunction and dyslexia: Beyond diagnosis by exclusion. In M. E. Blaw, I. Rapin, & M. Kinsbourne (Eds.), *Child neurology*. New York: Spectrum, 1977.

Doehring, D. G., & Hoshko, I. M. Classification of reading problems by the Q-technique of factor analysis. *Cortex*, 1977, *13*, 281–294.

Doehring, D. G., Hoshko, I. M., & Bryans, B. N. Statistical classification of children with reading problems. *Journal of Clinical Neuropsychology*, 1979, *1*, 5–16.

Dunn, L. M. *Expanded manual for the Peabody Picture Vocabulary Test*. Minneapolis: American Guidance Service, 1965.

Dykman, R. A., Ackerman, P. T., & Oglesby, D. M. Correlates of problem solving in hyperactive, learning disabled, and control boys. *Journal of Learning Disabilities*, 1980, *13*, 309–318.

Edelbrock, C. Mixture model tests of hierarchical clustering algorithms: The problem of classifying everybody. *Multivariate Behavioral Research*, 1979, *14*, 367-384.

Everitt, B. *Cluster analysis.* London: Heinemann Educational Books, 1974.

Fernald, G. M. *Remedial techniques in basic school subjects.* New York: McGraw-Hill, 1943.

Fisk, J. L., & Rourke, B. P. Identification of subtypes of learning disabled children at three age levels: A neuropsychological, multivariate approach. *Journal of Clinical Neuropsychology*, 1979, *1*, 289-310.

Fleiss, J. L., & Zubin, J. On the methods and theory of clustering. *Multivariate Behavioral Research*, 1969, *4*, 235-250.

Gaddes, W. H. An examination of the validity of neuropsychological knowledge in educational diagnosis and remediation. In G. W. Hynd & J. E. Obrzut (Eds.), *Neuropsychological assessment and the school-age child.* Toronto: Grune & Stratton, 1981.

Huelsman, C. B. The WISC subtest syndrome for disabled readers. *Perceptual and Motor Skills*, 1970, *30*, 535-550.

Jastak, J. F., & Jastak, S. R. *The Wide Range Achievement Test.* Wilmington, Del.: Guidance Associates, 1965.

Johnson, D., & Myklebust, H. *Learning disabilities: Educational principles and practices.* New York: Grune & Stratton, 1967.

Kass, C. E. Auditory Closure Test. In J. J. Olson & J. L. Olson (Eds.), *Validity studies on the Illinois Test of Psycholinguistic Abilities.* Madison, Wisc.: Photo Press, 1964.

Kløve, H. Clinical neuropsychology. In F. M. Forster (Ed.), *The medical clinics of North America.* New York: Saunders, 1963.

Knights, R. M., & Bakker, D. J. *The neuropsychology of learning disorders: Theoretical approaches.* Baltimore: University Park Press, 1976.

Knights, R. M., & Moule, A. D. Normative and reliability data on finger and foot tapping in children. *Perceptual and Motor Skills*, 1967, *25*, 717-720.

Luria, A. R. *The working brain.* Harmondsworth, England: Penguin Books, 1973.

Lutey, C. *Individual intelligence testing: A manual and sourcebook* (2nd ed.). Greeley, Colo.: Carol L. Lutey Publishing, 1977.

Mattis, S. Dyslexia syndromes: A working hypothesis that works. In A. L. Benton & D. Pearl (Eds.), *Dyslexia: An appraisal of current knowledge.* New York: Oxford University Press, 1978.

Mezzich, J. E. Evaluating clustering methods for psychiatric diagnosis. *Biological Psychiatry*, 1978, *13*, 265-281.

Milich, R. S., & Loney, J. The factor composition of the WISC for hyperkinetic/MBD males. *Journal of Learning Disabilities*, 1979, *12*, 491-495.

Milligan, G. W. An examination of the effect of error perturbation of constructed data on fifteen clustering algorithms (Doctoral dissertation, The Ohio State University, 1978). *Dissertation Abstracts International*, 1979, *39*, 4010B-4011B. (University Microfilms No. 7902188)

Petrauskas, R. J., & Rourke, B. P. Identification of subtypes of retarded readers: A neuropsychological, multivariate approach. *Journal of Clinical Neuropsychology*, 1979, *1*, 17-37.

Piotrowski, R. J. Abnormality of subtest score differences on the WISC-R. *Journal of Consulting and Clinical Psychology*, 1978, *46*, 569-570.

Reitan, R. M. Psychological effects of cerebral lesions in children of early school age. In R. M. Reitan & L. A. Davison (Eds.), *Clinical neuropsychology: Current status and applications.* Washington, D.C.: V. H. Winston & Sons, 1974.

Reitan, R. M., & Davison, L. A. (Eds.). *Clinical neuropsychology: Current status and applications.* Washington, D.C.: V. H. Winston & Sons, 1974.

Rourke, B. P. Brain–behavior relationships in children with learning disabilities: A research program. *American Psychologist*, 1975, *30*, 911–920.

Rourke, B. P. Neuropsychological research in reading retardation: A review. In A. L. Benton & D. Pearl (Eds.), *Dyslexia: An appraisal of current knowledge.* New York: Oxford University Press, 1978.

Rourke, B. P. Neuropsychological assessment of children with learning disabilities. In S. B. Filskov & T. J. Boll (Eds.), *Handbook of clinical neuropsychology.* New York: Wiley-Interscience, 1981.

Rourke, B. P. Reading and spelling disabilities: A developmental neuropsychological perspective. In U. Kirk (Ed.), *Neuropsychology of language, reading, and spelling.* New York: Academic Press, 1983.

Rourke, B. P., Bakker, D. J., Fisk, J. L., & Strang, J. D. *Child neuropsychology: An introduction to theory, research, and clinical practice.* New York: Guilford Press, 1983.

Rourke, B. P., & Strang, J. D. Subtypes of reading and arithmetical disabilities: A neuropsychological analysis. In M. Rutter (Ed.), *Developmental neuropsychiatry.* New York. Guilford Press, 1983.

Rugel, R. P. WISC subtest scores of disabled readers: A review with respect to Bannatyne's recategorization. *Journal of Learning Disabilities*, 1974, *7*, 48–55.

Satz, P., & Morris, R. Learning disability subtypes: A review. In F. J. Pirozzolo & M. C. Wittrock (Eds.), *Neuropsychological and cognitive processes in reading.* New York: Academic Press, 1980.

Skinner, H. A. Differentiating the contribution of elevation, scatter, and shape in profile similarity. *Educational and Psychological Measurement*, 1978, *38*, 297–308.

Sokal, R. R., & Michener, C. D. A statistical method for evaluating systematic relationships. *University of Kansas Science Bulletin*, 1958, *38*, 1409–1438.

Swartz, G. A. *The language-learning system.* New York: Simon & Schuster, 1974.

Sweeney, J. E., & Rourke, B. P. Neuropsychological significance of phonetically accurate and phonetically inaccurate spelling errors in younger and older retarded spellers. *Brain and Language*, 1978, *6*, 212–225.

Wechsler, D. *Manual for the Wechsler Intelligence Scale for Children.* New York: Psychological Corporation, 1949.

Wechsler, D. *Manual for the Wechsler Intelligence Scale for Children—Revised.* New York: Psychological Corporation, 1974.

Wishart, D. *CLUSTAN user manual* (3rd ed.). London: Computer Centre, University of London, 1975.

5

Subtypes of Left-Handed Learning-Disabled Children

JEREL E. DEL DOTTO
BYRON P. ROURKE

This chapter discusses the results from a study that was conducted with two specific purposes in mind. First, an attempt was made to isolate systematically and to report on the adaptive similarities and dissimilarities between subtypes of left- and right-handed learning-disabled children. Toward this end, multivariate quantitative taxonomic procedures were applied to the scores collected from a battery of neuropsychological measures. A systematic study of the typology of cognitive strengths and weaknesses associated with learning diabilities in these two particular groups of children evolved from the burgeoning evidence, suggesting that handedness and the organization of higher cognitive abilities are, to some extent, correlated with each other. Indeed, data collected from studies aimed at identifying different patterns of cortical organization and the extent of cerebral specialization in relation to handedness have led to the widely accepted view that patterns of hemispheric specialization vary more among sinistrals than among dextrals.

The second aim of the investigation was to offer some evidence to show that similar subtypes could be generated in a reliable fashion through the application of different numerical taxonomy or classification techniques. The fact that learning-disabled children may constitute a

Jerel E. Del Dotto. Division of Neuropsychology, Henry Ford Hospital, Detroit, Michigan, USA.

Byron P. Rourke. Department of Psychology, University of Windsor, and Department of Neuropsychology, Windsor Western Hospital Centre, Windsor, Ontario, Canada.

heterogeneous population in regard to their adaptive ability structure has been the focus of attention by several investigators, who have employed both clinical inferential methods (Boder, 1973; Mattis, 1978; Mattis, French, & Rapin, 1975) and more elaborate and sophisticated multi-variate classification procedures (Doehring & Hoshko, 1977; Doehring, Hoshko, & Bryans, 1979; Fisk & Rourke, 1979; Petrauskas & Rourke, 1979). With respect to the latter approach, both Q-type factor analysis and cluster-analytic techniques have been shown to isolate subgroups of children with learning disabilities in a fairly reliable fashion. Undoubtedly, the detection of a reliable taxonomy of learning disabilities could offer potentially useful information in regard to the remedial management of such children. However, up to this point in the "subtyping" literature, research efforts have focused almost exclusively on the elucidation of adaptive skill deficiencies associated with academic retardation in the *right-handed* learning-disabled child. To the best of our knowledge, no systematic study of the typology of cognitive impairment associated with learning disabilities in the *left-handed* child appears within the literature. We present, therefore, the findings from a study that compared the ways in which the performance measurements collected on an equal number of sinistral and dextral learning-disabled children were classified statistically by several multivariate procedures.

Even a cursory review of the large amount of handedness literature that has accumulated over the years eventuates in the impression that left-handers differ from right-handers on a host of performance measures. For example, several studies have reported, as a function of handedness, differences in language disturbance following unilateral lesions of either hemisphere (Ettlinger, Jackson, & Zangwill, 1956; Goodglass & Quadfasel, 1954; Hardyck & Petrinovich, 1977; Hecaen & de Ajuriaguerra, 1964; Hecaen & Sauguet, 1971; Hicks & Kinsbourne, 1978; Humphrey & Zangwill, 1951; Satz, 1979, 1980), and differences in the degree and extent of recovery from various aphasic conditions (Gloning, 1977; Gloning, Gloning, Haub, & Quatember, 1969; Gloning & Quatember, 1966; Subirana, 1964, 1969; Zangwill, 1964).

In addition to the information gathered by lesion-produced deficits, a number of studies utilizing an approach of dichotically presenting verbal information to normal, neurologically intact subjects have demonstrated smaller recall difference scores between the two ears for the left-handed individual, as compared to the usual right-ear advantage exhibited by a right-handed person (Bryden, 1965; Curry & Rutherford, 1967; Geffen & Taub, 1979; Lishman & McMeekan, 1977; Satz, Achenbach, Pattisball, & Fennell, 1965). Similarly, studies employing visual half-field preference measures have demonstrated that sinistrals differ from dextrals in the perception of tachistoscopically presented verbal information by exhibiting either a greater overall recognition in the left visual field, a right-visual-field superiority that is less marked, or no consistent visual-field differences (Beaumont & Dimond, 1973; Bradshaw, Gates, & Nettleton, 1977; Bryden, 1965; Hines & Satz, 1974; McKeever & Gill, 1972). Some researchers have even posited that, in addition to language processes, other cognitive abilities may be organized differently within the cerebral hemipsheres of sinistrals. Thus, there have been several published reports demonstrating the following: that the left-handed show performance decrements on a variety of visual–perceptual tasks (Flick, 1966; Hicks & Beveridge, 1978; Johnson & Harley, 1980; Levy, 1969; McGlone & Davidson, 1973; Miller, 1971; Nebes, 1971; Silverman, Adevai, & McGough, 1966); that left-handers as a group tend to be more "field-dependent" than right-handed individuals (Dawson, 1977a, 1977b; Oltman & Capobianco, 1967); and that left-handers differ from right-handers on tasks involving somatic pressure sensitivity (Weinstein & Sersen, 1961) and on tasks involving the execution of certain hand and finger movements (Kimura, 1973; Whilke & Sheeley, 1979).

It has also been suggested by several authors that, for left-handers in particular, hemispheric specialization patterns may be influenced by such factors as an individual's handwriting posture (Gregory & Paul, 1980; Levy, 1973; Levy & Reid, 1976, 1978), his/her intensity or degree of left-handedness (Dee, 1971; Hecaen & Sauguet, 1971; Knox & Boone, 1970; Lishman & McMeekan, 1977; Newcombe & Ratcliff, 1973; Satz, Achenbach, & Fennell, 1967; Searleman, 1978; Shankweiler & Studdert-Kennedy, 1975), and whether or not he/she has any biological family members who are left-handed (Andrews, 1977; Annett, 1973, 1974; Bradshaw & Taylor, 1979; Briggs & Nebes, 1976; Bryden, 1975; Geffen & Taub, 1979; Hecaen & Sauguet, 1971; Lishman & McMeekan, 1977; McKeever & Van Deventer, 1977; Newcombe & Ratcliff, 1973; Piazza, 1980; Schmuller & Goodman, 1979; Varney & Benton, 1975; Zurif & Bryden, 1969). While these studies have generated conflicting results, a pattern emerges that suggests that it is either the left-hander who exhibits a normal writing posture, or the left-hander who demonstrates an unadulterated tendency toward sinistral hand preference, or the left-hander who tends to report a family history of sinistrality who is most likely to exhibit a type of cerebral organization that is different from that seen in the right-handed individual.

The notion that left-handedness may be related to learning deficits in general, and reading disability in particular, is certainly not a recent one. Ever since Orton (1937) suggested that the lack of consistent laterality preference reflected some degree of mixed cerebral dominance, which then resulted in some type of learning disability, researchers have been interested in the relationship among patterns of lateral preference, cerebral dominance, and learning difficulties. For example, several reports have suggested that children who present with difficulties in learning to read are often found to be more poorly lateralized; that is, they exhibit a much higher incidence of mixed hand dominance, or they are noted to demonstrate a higher incidence of left-handedness among the group members (Annett & Turner, 1974; Ayres, 1972; Bryden, 1970; Gordon, 1921; Harris, 1957; Hecaen & de Ajuriaguerra, 1964; Shearer, 1968). This latter finding has led many to speculate that sinistrality may be a manifestation of brain pathology, especially when one views it in the context of a clinical population (Annett, 1964; Bakan, 1971, 1977; Gur, 1977; Harris, 1980; Satz, 1972, 1973; Satz, Baymur, & van der Vlugt, 1979). When researchers have examined the interrelationships among hand, foot, eye, and ear laterality measures, the findings have tended to bolster the notion that children with specific learning problems exhibit different information-processing deficits as a function of congruent or incongruent laterality patterns (Berman, 1971; Dean, Schwartz, & Smith, 1981; McBurney & Dunn, 1976; Porac, Coren, & Duncan, 1980; Swanson, Kinsbourne, & Horn, 1980). Performance differences observed between children who exhibit a mixed and children who exhibit a consistent laterality preference are then interpreted as indicating the presence of differences in brain organization between the two groups.

Perhaps one of the most convincing investigations aimed at examining the relationship among lateral preference, hemispheric specialization, and academic-related difficulties was conducted recently by Schevill (1980). Interested in examining the effect of handedness on tactual–perceptual functioning within children who exhibit reading difficulties, Schevill looked for disparities between reading-disabled dextrals and sinistrals in the ability to store and transfer tactile skin-writing images bilaterally. The results from this study suggested the following: (1) that left-handers may tend to use a greater degree of dominant- (i.e., verbal-)hemisphere bias in processing tactile–verbal sorts of information, and (2) that left-handed children may partially disregard the nondominant spatial function and may utilize a dominant bias for both spatial and verbal processing. These findings, however, stand in marked contrast to several reports that have failed to identify any appreciable disparities in verbal and nonverbal abilities between left- and right-handed reading-impaired children (Annett & Turner, 1974; Fagin-Dubin, 1974; Wussler & Barclay, 1970).

It would appear that the effects of handedness on cortical organization are controversial and that the issue is far from being resolved. Given this state of affairs, the need for further investigation into the relation between adaptive ability structure and preferred handedness appeared to be especially warranted. Moreover, while researchers have made considerable progress in their attempts to identify how patterns vary for cerebral organization as a function of handedness by using a number of different clinical research methods (e.g., lesion-produced deficits, right–left perceptual asymmetries), we felt that multivariate taxonomic methods offered a viable and useful alternative approach to investigating this problem, especially since we were predominantly interested in isolating and defining subgroups of left- and right-handed learning-disabled children.

Because of the exploratory nature of the current study, the formulation of specific hypotheses appeared rather difficult. However, we felt that certain expectations could be advanced on the basis of some of the previously cited research. First, there was reason to expect that the number and type of cognitive deficits associated with learning disability in the left-handed child may well be different from those seen in the right-handed child. Secondly, if variables such as familial handedness or intensity of handedness are influential factors in regard to variation in cognitive organization (i.e., hemispheric specialization), then it would be expected that the derived subgroups would exhibit membership compositions reflective of their influence. Finally, in regard to the issue of the subtyping of learning-disabled children, it was expected that the subgroups generated by means of one multivariate statistical procedure should be able to be detected through the application of several other classification methods as well.

METHOD

SUBJECTS

A total of 322 children were drawn from a population pool of over 3500 individuals who were referred to a large urban children's clinic for comprehensive neuropsychological evaluation. Initially, 161 left-handers were selected, and then a comparable group of 161 right-handers was chosen. The criteria for the study sample were as follows: All children had to be between the chronological ages of 108–179 months; exhibit a Wechsler Intelligence Scale for Children (WISC) Full Scale IQ within the range of 85–115; and be free of sensory acuity defects, primary socioemotional disturbance, or evidence of compromised environmental influences.

As part of the assessment procedure, the subjects were administered the Harris Tests of Lateral Dominance (Harris, 1947). Included in this inventory are a series of questions regarding preferred hand usage for the following seven different manual tasks: throwing a ball, hammering a nail, cutting with a knife, turning a door knob, using a scissors, using an eraser, and writing one's name. All subjects were initially classified as right- or left-handed on the basis of choice of writing hand, such that they formed two groups of 161 subjects each. Left-handers were comprised of 136 males and 25 females, whereas there were 134 male and 27 female right-handers. Moreover, of the total of 161 left-handed writers, 86 were found to employ their left hand on all seven of the Harris Inventory items (i.e., were pure-dominant), whereas 75 reported a tendency to use their right hand on one or more of the remaining questionnaire items (i.e., were mixed-dominant). Right-handed writers, on the other hand, were composed almost entirely ($n = 151$) of pure-dominant individuals (i.e., reported the use of their right hand for all of the inventory items).

Left- and right-handed groups were closely matched with respect to mean age (11.45 years vs. 11.28 years), and a breakdown of familial handedness history revealed that 65 left- and 64 right-handed children reported the presence of left-handedness within the family (with "presence" defined as at least one immediate biological family member—that is, mother, father, sibling—being left-handed), whereas 75 sinistrals and 92 dextrals reported the absence of sinistrality tendencies among family members. Information pertaining to the handedness of family members was derived from a questionnaire that the parents were requested to complete.

TEST MEASURES

Included among the tests that comprised the comprehensive neuropsychological test battery were 42 measures presumably thought to represent various neuropsychological adaptive skill areas as outlined by Reitan (1974). These skill areas included the following: (1) tactile–perceptual and tactile–kinesthetic abilities; (2) visual–motor, visual–perceptual, and visual–spatial skills; (3) sequential processing abilities; (4) auditory–perceptual and language-related abilities; (5) simple motor and psychomotor skills; and (6) conceptual reasoning and nonverbal problem-solving capabilities. Fairly complete discriptions of the test measures used in this study can be obtained elsewhere (Benton, 1965; Dunn, 1965; Kass, 1964; Reitan, 1969; Reitan & Davison, 1974; Rourke, Bakker, Fisk, & Strang, 1983; Wechsler, 1949).

Of the 42 dependent measures, 21 were selected for data analysis. These test measures are listed in Table 5-1 and represent the same ones used by Fisk and Rourke (1979) in their study of right-handed learning-disabled children.

TABLE 5-1. List of Dependent Test Measures

Test measures	Abbreviation
1. Tactile Finger Recognition—Right Hand	FAGNR
2. Fingertip Number Writing—Right Hand	FTWR
3. Tactual Performance Test—Dominant Hand	TPTDT
4. Tactual Performance Test—Nondominant Hand	TPTNDT
5. WISC Picture Completion subtest	PICCOM
6. WISC Block Design subtest	BLKDES
7. WISC Object Assembly subtest	OBJASS
8. Target Test	TARGET
9. WISC Arithmetic subtest	ARITH
10. WISC Digit Span subtest	DIGITS
11. WISC Coding subtest	CODING
12. WISC Information subtest	INFO
13. WISC Comprehension subtest	COMP
14. Speech-Sounds Perception	SSPER
15. Auditory Closure	AUDCLO
16. Finger Oscillation—Right Hand	TAPR
17. Finger Oscillation—Left Hand	TAPL
18. Grooved Pegboard—Right Hand	PEGSRT
19. Grooved Pegboard—Left Hand	PEGSLT
20. Category Test	CATTOT
21. Trail Making Test, Part B	TRSBT

PROCEDURE

Q-Type Factor Analysis

To facilitate comparisons between and among the many different test measures, raw scores collected on each of the dependent measures were first converted to *T* scores. Each handedness-based sample was then subjected to *Q*-type factor analysis independently. As a basic input to the factor analysis, *T* scores were transposed, and product–moment correlation coefficients were calculated between each pair of subjects within the target sample. Next, factor analysis was applied to the correlational matrix, using an iterated principal-axis solution (communality estimates based on 1.00 in the diagonals initially). To achieve simpler, more meaningful factor patterns, the initial extracted factors that yielded eigenvalues greater than or equal to the ratio of number of subjects/ number of variables were then retained and rotated orthogonally to varimax criterion (SAS PROC FACTOR, method = Prinit; Helwıg & Council, 1979).

In the factor analysis, children were assigned to each subtype in terms of the factor for which they showed the highest single factor loading above .50. For each subtype, *T*-score means for the variables used in the factor analysis were calculated, and these values were then plotted. Analyses of the similarities and differences between factor solutions generated for the left- and right-handed samples were conducted through visual inspection of the factor profiles, and by means of Pearson product–moment correlational analysis between each plot separately.

Cluster-Analytic Classification Procedures

To confirm the existence of subtypes that had been identified by *Q*-type factor analysis, cluster analyses of the same data sets were performed. The number and variety of cluster-analytic techniques is overwhelming, and there are numerous methodological considerations that surround the use of the techniques. For example, Blashfield (1980) and Morris, Blashfield, and Satz (1981) point out that the choice of clustering method, similarity measure, computer program, and procedure for estimating the number of clusters in the data must be clearly defined. Moreover, adequate evidence of a cluster solution's validity should be provided as well (e.g., replicating a solution across different cluster-analytic methods or across a different collection of variables). Space limitations, however, preclude any detailed discussion on each of these considerations. What follows, therefore, is brief descriptive information in regard to each issue (the reader is referred to Blashfield, 1980, and Morris *et al.*, 1981, for a more complete discussion).

To begin with, since one objective of this study was to compare classifications derived from different taxonomic procedures, a decision was made to apply cluster analysis to the same 21 *T*-score measures collected on the same target populations used in the initial factor analysis.

Second, since it was felt that the similarity of profile shapes, rather than how far apart the profiles were, was more important in identifying different subtypes of left-handed learning-disabled children, the product–moment correlation coefficient was selected as the measure of similarity between subjects.

Third, to lessen the possibility of accepting misleading solutions, two clustering methods were chosen to analyze the data in the present study. Because the hierarchical agglomerative techniques have been accepted as the clustering methods of choice in a number of investigations, a decision was made to adopt two of these techniques, group average or average linkage (CLUSTAN, version IC2, procedure = Hierarchy, method = Group Average; Wishart, 1978), and centroid sorting (CLUSTAN, version IC2, procedure = Centroid; Wishart, 1978).

Fourth, to clarify further the cluster solutions derived by means of the two hierarchical methods, an iterative relocation procedure was applied to both. Each initial clustering solution was reexamined to see whether any of the classified subjects should be reallocated to another group. Moreover, since it is often difficult to find a "global optimum" solution when clustering very large populations (e.g., where $n > 150$), different "starting configurations" (i.e., shape difference, random classification arrays) were utilized in the "relocate" step.

Fifth, a persistent problem in cluster analysis is the difficulty of deciding on the correct number of groups to consider for a given set of data. Two commonly used methods or indicators for the number of clusters present in the data include an examination of the dendrogram or mapping of the data, and an analysis of the clustering coefficients. Both of these methods were employed in the present study.

Finally, to determine the stability and usefulness of the clustering solutions, a split-sample validation design was employed: The 161 children were randomly divided into two subsamples, and each half was clustered independently. Membership assignment in the partitioned samples was checked against the cluster solutions derived for the sample as a whole. Also, solutions derived from the different clustering techniques were compared.

The solutions derived from the cluster analyses were then compared against the subtypes generated by *Q*-type factor analysis. This was accomplished in three ways. First, *T*-score means for the variables used to define a cluster were calculated. These values were then plotted to enable visual inspection of the similarity between intercluster profiles, and between *Q*-type and cluster-analytic profiles. Secondly, Pearson product–moment correlational analyses were calculated between each plot separately. Finally, the results of the cluster analyses were evaluated and interpreted with reference to the classification obtained in the *Q*-type analysis (i.e., the number of subjects from each of the *Q*-type subtypes who were not classified together by a given method of cluster analysis).

Figure 5-1 presents an illustration of the steps involved in the Q-type factor-analytic and cluster-analytic procedures.

Subtype Analyses of Left-Handedness

The last step in the treatment of the data was to compare subtype composition across the variables of intensity of left-handedness and familial handedness tendencies. This was accomplished through the application of a series of chi-square goodness-of-fit tests. An examination of intensity of left-handedness involved inspection of two parameters:

1. Hand preference—the consistency or degree to which an individual reported the use of his/her left hand on a series of questionnaire items regarding hand preference; in the case of the Harris inventory, individuals who reported a tendency to engage the left hand on all seven manual tasks were considered to be "pure" left handers, whereas individuals who exhibited any deviation from a consistent sinistral tendency for the preference items (e.g., a person who wrote his/her name with the left hand but threw a ball with the right) were considered to be of "mixed" preference.

2. Hand proficiency—the consistency of hand usage across two behavioral tasks: one involving simple motor speed, as measured by the rapid tapping of a key with the index finger (i.e., Finger Oscillation Task), and a second involving fine eye–hand coordination, as measured by the placement of steel pegs into slots or holes varying in directional orienta-

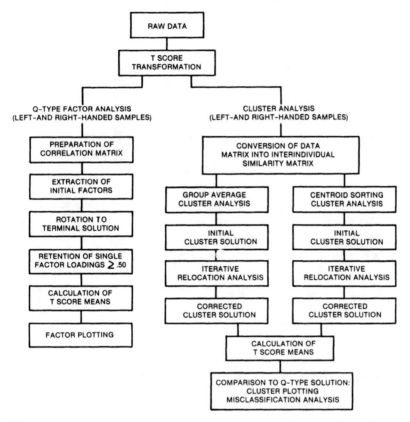

FIG. 5-1. Illustration of the steps involved in the *Q*-type and cluster-analytic classification procedures.

tion (i.e., Grooved Pegboard Test). For this parameter, individuals were identified as being "congruous" left-handers if they wrote with the left hand and also exhibited a higher level of performance with the left hand relative to the right hand on both the Grooved Pegboard and Finger Oscillation Tasks; as "incongruous" left-handers if they wrote with the left hand but exhibited a higher level of performance with the right hand on both behavioral measures; and as "mixed-proficient" left-handers if they wrote with the left hand but exhibited a mixed proficiency pattern on the two behavioral tasks (i.e., left-handed performance superior to right-handed performance on one task, and vice versa).

RESULTS

Q-Type Factor Analysis Solutions

The results of the *Q*-type factor analyses applied to the scores of the two handedness samples independently are presented in Table 5-2. The eigenvalue limitation used to terminate factoring was 7.66 for both handedness samples. This value yielded seven factors for each of the factor analyses, which accounted for 96.9% and 97.5% of the common variance for the left- and right-handed samples, respectively.

The breakdown of factor loadings is shown in Table 5-3. Only individuals with a high positive loading ($\geq .50$) on one factor were considered in the determination of subtypes. This criterion accounted for 68% of the left-handed and 72% of the right-handed samples.

Visual inspection of the plots of the *T*-score means of the variables used in the factor-analytic procedures for each left- and right-handed *Q*-analysis factor revealed that the first three factors of the sinistral sample exhibited almost identical profile characteristics to the first three factors of the dextral sample. Pearson product–moment correlations based on comparisons between mean *T* scores for all variables between all possible pairs of subtypes revealed that the correlation between Factor 1 of the left-handers and Factor 2 of the right-handers was .94. Left-handed Factor 2 and right-handed Factor 1, as well as left-handed Factor 3 and right-handed Factor 3, correlated at a .84 level. These values are indicative of the high degree of similarity between the pattern of mean *T* scores for these factors. The three factors from each handedness sample accounted for a total of 78% of the left-handed and 55% of the right-handed children.

TABLE 5-2. Factor Analysis Solutions for Sinistral and Dextral Samples

Data	Factors						
	1	2	3	4	5	6	7
Sinistrals							
Eigenvalues	33.399	22.619	16.102	15.471	11.361	9.052	8.273
Variance	0.276	0.187	0.133	0.128	0.094	0.075	0.068
Cumulative variance	0.276	0.462	0.595	0.723	0.816	0.891	0.959
Dextrals							
Eigenvalues	34.926	24.756	17.648	12.538	11.010	10.232	8.386
Variance	0.285	0.202	0.144	0.102	0.090	0.083	0.068
Cumulative variance	0.285	0.487	0.631	0.733	0.083	0.906	0.975

TABLE 5-3. Number of Classified (Single-Factor Loadings ≥ .50), Multiple Loadings, and Unclassified Subjects for Sinistral and Dextral Samples

	Sample	
Loadings	Sinistrals	Dextrals
Single loadings		
1	41	20
2	26	26
3	19	18
4	9	11
5	6	18
6	4	8
7	5	15
Total	110	116
% of sample	68%	72%
Multiple loadings		
Total	15	20
% of sample	9%	12%
Unclassified		
Total	36	25
% of sample	23%	16%

LEFT-HANDED CLUSTER SOLUTIONS

The hierarchical trees (dendrograms) obtained by applying the group-average and centroid-sorting techniques to the sinistral data set indicated clearly that the data were structured and contained several clusters. Both inspection of the dendrograms and analyses of the plots of the clustering coefficients favored a four-cluster terminal solution for each method. Subsequent iterative relocation analyses of the four-cluster solutions from the group-average and centroid-sorting analyses indicated that only 7% and 9% of the subjects, respectively, were actually placed in a different cluster. Moreover, the results of the relocation analyses were replicated perfectly from different starting classifications.

Group membership distributions for the four-cluster relocation solutions can be ascertained from Table 5-4. The number of subjects classified into eight clusters down to two are provided in Table 5-4 in order to view the incorporation of clusters during the fusion process. It also allows for the detection and removal of "outliers" (defined as unique individuals within the sample or viewed as resulting from measurement errors) from

TABLE 5-4. Number of Left-Handed Children in Each Cluster for 8, 7, 6, 5, 4, 3, and 2 Relocation Cluster Results

Cluster analysis method	Clusters						
	8	7	6	5	4	3	2
Group average							
1	45	45	45	48	49	64	72
2	20	20	22	20	26	31	89
3	14	14	14	47	51	66	
4	11	24	28	28	35		
5	38	39	39	18			
6	7	10	13				
7	24	9					
8	2						
Centroid sorting							
1	34	38	38	48	51	66	72
2	14	15	15	16	35	64	89
3	19	29	30	30	49	31	
4	46	46	46	49	26		
5	14	14	18	18			
6	14	14	14				
7	5	5					
8	15						

the data. In the current study, no children were removed from the analyses. As indicated in Table 5-4, the group-average and centroid-sorting relocation methods generated identical four-cluster solutions.

Visual inspection of the mean T-score plots indicated that there was a high degree of visual similarity between the four cluster profiles and four of the sinistral and three of the dextral profiles generated from the factor analyses. Pearson product–moment correlations based on comparisons between mean T scores for all variables between all possible pairs of left- and right-handed Q-analysis factors and left-handed cluster groups revealed that the correlation values between the four sinistral clusters and the first four left-handed factors were .94 and above. These correlation values attest to the near-perfect match between performance patterns generated from the Q-type factor analysis and performance patterns derived from the cluster-analytic methods following the application of both procedures to the same sample of left-handed children. Comparisons between sinistral Clusters 1, 3, and 4 and the first three dextral factors revealed very high correlation values of .81 and above between these pairs of T-score plots as well.

Misclassification analysis was the last method used to compare the cluster-analytic and factor-analytic solutions derived from the left-handed data set. Table 5-5 shows the number of children from each of the Q-type factors who were not classified together by a given method of cluster analysis. As can be seen from Table 5-5, all of the children classified together by Q-type factor analysis were also classified together by cluster analysis. In other words, on the basis of subtype membership, the classification solutions generated from the two different multivariate taxonomic methods were in perfect agreement with each other.

Taken together, the visual-similarity findings between cluster and factor profiles, correlation values between clusters and factors, and the results of the misclassification analyses seemed to support the notion that there were four distinct subtypes of left-handers within the data set, three of which were highly similar to three subtypes of age-equivalent right-handers that had been derived by means of Q-type factor analysis.

RELIABILITY AND CROSS-VALIDATION OF LEFT-HANDED CLUSTERS

With respect to reliability, the identical assignment of subjects into clusters between the group-average and centroid-sorting relocation methods at the four-cluster solution level tends to support the presence of well-defined clusters within the data.

Second, the results of the split-sample study indicated that the group-average and centroid-sorting relocation methods generated identical four-cluster solutions in the case of both subsample analyses. Moreover, misclassification analyses revealed that, between the two subsamples, only 16% of the subjects changed from their original clusters, leaving 84% of the subjects who clustered together in both procedures.

Finally, gross visual inspection of the plots of the mean T scores for each variable for each subsample cluster revealed, for the most part, a

TABLE 5-5. Number of Left-Handed Children from Each of the Q-Type Factors Misclassified by Cluster-Analytic Methods

Cluster analysis method	Number of clusters	Q-type factors				Total misclassification $(n = 95)$
		1 $(n = 41)$	2 $(n = 26)$	3 $(n = 19)$	4 $(n = 9)$	
Group average	4	0	0	0	0	0
Centroid sorting	4	0	0	0	0	0

high degree of similarity between profile characteristics of the standard and split-sample clusters.

RIGHT-HANDED CLUSTER SOLUTIONS

The hierarchical trees summarizing cluster solutions obtained by applying the group-average and the centroid-sorting techniques to the dextral data set clearly showed clusters in this data set as well. From an analysis of the changes in cluster coefficients, and from inspections of the clustering coefficient plots, a seven-cluster solution appeared to be plausible.

Iterative relocation analysis of the seven-cluster group-average solution resulted in 17% of the subjects being placed in a different cluster, while 38% of the children were reallocated to a different cluster for the seven-cluster centroid-sorting results.

When the relocation procedure was repeated using a different starting configuration, the results indicated that there was a 95% conformity rate between solutions derived from the different starting points.

Membership distributions for the seven-cluster relocation solutions can be ascertained from Table 5-6. For the right-handed sample, no children were removed from the analyses. As can be seen in Table 5-6, cluster sizes between the group-average and centroid-sorting relocation methods were very similar.

Visual inspection of the plots of the T-score means of the variables used in the cluster analysis for each centroid-sorting and group-average cluster indicated that there was a high degree of similarity between group-average and centroid-sorting relocation cluster profiles. Moreover, Pearson product–moment correlations between six of the cluster plots were at the .97 level and above. Since intercorrelations were so high between the two solutions, only the group-average relocation results were compared against the left- and right-handed profiles derived from factor analysis.

Intercorrelation values between all factors and clusters reported up to this point indicated the following: Cluster 2 of the group-average relocation solution for the dextral sample correlated highest with Factor 2 from the dextral sample ($r = .99$), with Factor 1 from the sinistral sample ($r = .93$), and with Cluster 1 from the sinistral sample ($r = .92$). These values would suggest that the patterns of mean scores for these profiles were quite similar. Cluster 3 of the group-average relocation solution for the dextral sample correlated highest with both Factor 5 ($r = .86$) and

TABLE 5-6. Number of Right-Handed Children in Each Cluster for 8, 7, 6, 5, 4, 3, and 2 Relocation Cluster Results

Cluster analysis method	Clusters						
	8	7	6	5	4	3	2
Group average							
1	19	24	31	31	64	43	109
2	29	30	32	36	40	47	52
3	37	41	43	46	30	71	
4	18	21	21	24	27		
5	20	12	10	24			
6	9	10	24				
7	9	23					
8	20						
Centroid sorting							
1	31	30	32	36	40	44	52
2	23	40	43	46	63	44	109
3	18	22	21	24	29	73	
4	20	22	24	31	29		
5	12	15	31	24			
6	9	9	10				
7	25	23					
8	23						

Factor 1 ($r = .83$) from the dextral sample, with Factor 2 from the sinistral sample ($r = .80$), and with Cluster 3 from the sinistral sample ($r = .83$), indicating a high degree of similarity in the pattern of scores for these profiles. Cluster 4 of the group-average solution for the dextral sample correlated highest with Factor 3 from the dextral sample ($r = .92$), with Factor 3 from the sinistral sample ($r = .92$), and with Cluster 4 from the sinistral sample ($r = .91$). These values would indicate that the patterns of mean T scores for these profiles were quite similar as well. The profiles of performances associated with these factors and clusters, as well as the correlation coefficients between factors and clusters, are seen as evidence that validates the existence of three highly similar subtypes of left- and right-handed learning-disabled children.

The following intercorrelation values were obtained for the remaining dextral group-average relocation clusters. Cluster 1 from this sample correlated highest with Cluster 2 from the sinistral sample ($r = .79$) and with Factor 4 from the sinistral sample ($r = .76$). The similarities in these profiles may represent another similar subtype of left- and right-handed children. Cluster 6 from the group-average relocation solution for the dextral sample correlated highest with Factor 6 from the dextral sample ($r = .75$) and with Factor 5 from the sinistral sample ($r = .67$). Again, these profiles may represent another similar subtype of sinistral and dextral children, despite the fact that Factor 5 from the left-handed sample included a total of only six children. Cluster 7 from the group-average relocation solution for the dextral sample correlated at a level of .68 with both Factor 7 from the dextral sample and Factor 7 from the sinistral sample. Finally, there was a high correlation ($r = .92$) between Cluster 5 from the group-average relocation solution and Factor 4 from the dextral sample, suggesting that these profiles may represent a separate right-handed subtype.

The results of a misclassification analysis used to compare the cluster-analytic and factor-analytic solutions derived from the right-handed data set are summarized in Table 5-7. A total of 35 children (30% of the total sample) classified together by Q-type factor analysis were not classified together by the group-average method of cluster analysis, leaving 81 subjects (70% of the data set) that were classified into the same groups. Agreement between the centroid-sorting method and the Q-type analysis was slightly lower, with a total of 40 subjects (35% of the sample) misclassified, and 76 of the children (65% of the data set) classified together.

RELIABILITY AND CROSS-VALIDATION OF RIGHT-HANDED CLUSTERS

With respect to reliability, comparison of the group-average and centroid-sorting relocation procedures revealed almost perfect membership agreement between the two methods. More specifically, the results showed that fewer than 5% of the subjects were placed into a different cluster for the seven-cluster solution.

Second, the split-sample analyses produced, in the case of both subsamples, highly similar seven-cluster solutions between the group-average and centroid-sorting results following iterative partitioning of both. Moreover, misclassification analyses revealed that, in total, fewer than 30% of the subjects were changed from their original clusters, using any of the clustering methods.

Finally, visual inspection of the graphic illustrations of the mean T scores for each variable for the clusters derived in split-sample analyses 1 and 2 revealed, in most cases, a high degree of similarity between profile characteristics of the solutions derived from split-sample analyses 1 and 2 and the results obtained from clustering the entire sample together.

TABLE 5-7. Number of Right-Handed Children from Each of the Q-Type Factors Misclassified by Cluster-Analytic Methods

Cluster analysis method	Number of clusters	Q-type factors							Total misclassifications ($n = 116$)
		1 ($n = 20$)	2 ($n = 26$)	3 ($n = 18$)	4 ($n = 11$)	5 ($n = 18$)	6 ($n = 8$)	7 ($n = 15$)	
Group average	7	7	3	6	3	4	4	8	35
Centroid sorting	7	10	3	7	4	2	5	9	40

CHI-SQUARE ANALYSES

Finally, the results of a series of chi-square analyses indicated that the derived subtypes could not be differentiated from one another on the basis of hand preference (i.e., Harris Inventory responses), hand proficiency (i.e., performances on skilled motor tasks, such as Finger Tapping and Grooved Pegboard), or familial handedness composition. That is to say, there were no particular subtypes that exhibited either an unusually large or small number of congruent, incongruent, or mixed-proficient left-handers, pure or mixed-preference left-handers, or subjects with predominantly sinistral or dextral family members.

DISCUSSION

The principal findings from this study suggested, first and foremost, that left- and right-handed learning-disabled children exhibit several similar patterns (i.e., subtypes) of neuropsychological abilities and deficits, and, secondarily, that subtypes generated by means of one multivariate statistical procedure can be reliably detected through the application of several other classification methods as well. In this section, a more detailed and comprehensive discussion of these findings is preceded by comments on some methodological considerations of the study. Next, characteristics of the subtypes are identified and described, and comparisons are then made to other subtypes reported in the literature. Within this context, there is some discussion regarding the reliability and stability of the isolated subtypes. Then, the implications of the findings as they relate to the issue of handedness are addressed, including their apparent relevance for assessment and intervention. Finally, directions for future research are provided.

METHODOLOGICAL CONSIDERATIONS

First, the present investigation compared the adaptive ability profiles of independent groups of left- and right-handed subjects who were selected from a *clinical* rather than from a *normal* population of school-age children. As such, conclusions in regard to the relation between handedness and neuropsychological ability structure are apt to be most appropriate and meaningful to that population of children referred to clinics for learning difficulties. Investigation of a normal sample of school-age children may be expected to eventuate in quite different sets of conclusions.

Second, other clinically affected samples—for example, those exhibiting psychometric intelligence values outside the range utilized within this investigation (i.e., below a WISC Full Scale IQ of 85)—may demonstrate very different patterns of cognitive abilities and deficits as a function of preferred handedness. The findings from this study, therefore, are by no means intended to reflect a general typology of cognitive strengths and weaknesses associated with lateral hand preference patterns per se. Rather, they should be viewed and interpreted within the context of the limitations imposed by sampling considerations.

As mentioned earlier, a number of methodological issues surround the use of cluster analysis. For example, there is always the problem of deciding how many variables are appropriate for study. To minimize test redundancy and to maximize cluster interpretability, one usually seeks to reduce the number of input variables. This is often accomplished by means of principal-components analysis. However, this procedure was not followed in the present study. Instead, 21 variables that had been utilized in past subtyping research efforts (Fisk & Rourke, 1979) were chosen as dependent measures for the current investigation. *T*-score matrices of these variables were then analyzed by the different clustering algorithms. According to Everitt (1974), similar classifications should emerge from the use of either the first few principal-component scores or the complete set of data, provided the data are well structured. On the other hand, widely divergent solutions may be derived when the groups are not as clearly defined within the data set. In the present study, applying clustering algorithms to the raw data may have produced solutions quite different from those that would have been obtained had factor scores been used as input to the clustering method.

Since we were interested in elucidating the similarities and differences between left- and right-handed learning-disabled children in adaptive ability profile *patterns*, correlation was selected as the measure of interindividual similarity. Distance measures are felt to be a more appropriate metric when one is interested in the similarity of the average profile *levels*. That is, two profiles could exhibit very similar patterns of performance, but could be quite far apart in level of performance. These quite different ways of defining similarity between subjects may result in rather different, yet clinically meaningful, conclusions. This being the case, one may wish to reanalyze the data using distance measures.

It is not uncommon in clustering problems to find that a single set of scores analyzed by several different techniques may result in entirely different solutions or groupings of the data. Despite the fact that several clustering algorithms were utilized in the present study, other types of group structure may have emerged through the application of different clustering techniques. There is certainly no reason to believe that the results derived from the clustering algorithms utilized in the present investigation are the only types of structure present in the data.

As pointed out earlier, a persistent problem in cluster analysis is the difficulty in deciding the correct number of groups to consider for a given set of data. In this investigation, a review of both mappings of the data and clustering coefficient results provided some notion of the number of clusters suitable for representation of the data matrices. However, inspection of these two sets of results did not always provide an unequivocal answer to this question. In fact, in several cases, a range of clustering solutions appeared to be quite plausible. It is clear that a host of interpretations or judgments could have eventuated in regard to the subtype structure existing within the data had an examination been made of other partitioning results.

Finally, the Q-type solutions generated in this study were validated by the clustering results, and these findings, in turn, were validated through the application of a split-sample procedure to the data set. However, to bolster the existence of "real" subtypes within the data, several alternative ways of validating the clustering results derived in this study should be carried out (e.g., altering the input data matrix through the omission or deletion of variables, or demonstrating that clusters have predictive value with respect to variables not included in the original clustering procedure).

One final note on this issue: The ultimate test of a factor or clustering solution's validity would seem to lie in its usefulness and meaningfulness from a clinical point of view. In this connection, questions such as the following are relevant: Are the characteristics of the derived subgroups interpretable? Are they reasonably consonant with those that one would expect to find within the data? These questions are answered in the next section, where the features and characteristics of the derived subtypes are outlined.

DESCRIPTION OF SUBTYPES

The profiles of test performance associated with derived factors and clusters, the correlation values between clusters and factors, and the results of the misclassification analyses were interpreted to define three highly similar and reliable subtypes of left- and right-handed learning-disabled children. In addition, four other interpretable but less well-defined subtypes emerged. In this section, subtype composites are described, and comparisons are made to other subtypes reported in the literature.

Subtype I

Subtype I was composed of children who constituted Factor 1 ($n = 41$) and Cluster 1 ($n = 49$) from the left-handed sample, and Factor 2 ($n = 26$), group-average Cluster 2 ($n = 30$), and centroid-sorting Cluster 1 ($n = 30$) from the right-handed sample. A graphic illustration of this subtype is depicted in Figure 5-2. Since the factor and cluster intercorrelations were so remarkably high within this group (i.e., $r = .92$ or above), a composite

FIG. 5-2. Profile of Subtype 1. (For key to abbreviations of test measures, see Table 5-1.)

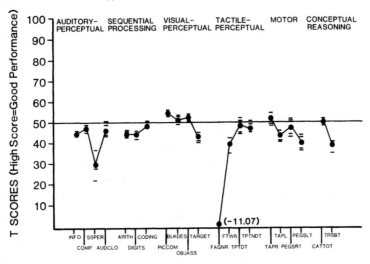

of all mean *T*-score profiles for all the factors and clusters represented in this subtype is presented in Figure 5-2. The dashes on this figure as well as on the two subsequent figures represent the various independent factor and cluster *T*-score means for each variable.

Children in this group exhibited the following profile characteristics:

1. Poor performances on several auditory–linguistic and sequential-processing types of tasks, involving phoneme–grapheme matching, sound blending, general fund of information, "mental" numerical reasoning, and immediate recall for sequences of digits.
2. Roughly normal performances on a task intended to determine understanding of social conventionality and social judgment (as assessed through a person's verbal reports), and on an associative-learning task involving speed and accuracy of symbolic transcription.
3. Age-appropriate or better performances on tasks intended to assess appreciation for visual–spatial relationships, and involving visual–perceptual skill participation.
4. Well-developed motor manipulatory and tactually guided problem-solving ability, as well as adequate nonverbal reasoning skills with visually or spatially presented stimuli.
5. Some difficulties in remembering sequences of visual stimuli and in performing visual-sequencing types of tasks involving symbolic shifting.
6. Haptic deficiencies involving mild right-sided finger dysgraphesthesia and marked right-sided finger agnosia.
7. Normally developed simple motor speed and fine finger dexterity with the right hand, but reduced motoric celerity and manipulative dexterity with the upper left extremity.

In sum, Subtype I children were distinguished by the presence of a normally developed visual information-processing system, rather good nonverbal problem-solving capabilities, some mild auditory information-processing deficits, and pronouncd haptic deficiencies, especially tactile finger localization. Moreover, Subtype I children exhibited a mean WISC Performance IQ that exceeded their mean Verbal IQ, and mean WRAT Reading, Spelling and Arithmetic scores that were all below the 30th centile.

The test profile for Subtype I is strikingly similar to Subtype A of the Fisk and Rourke (1979) study, exhibiting almost identical profile characteristics. Subtype A in that investigation was derived from a *Q*-type multivariate analysis conducted on a sample of 264 right-handed learning-disabled children. Subtype I also bears some relation to a group of children in the Satz, Friel, and Rudegair (1974) study and to Type 2 of the Petrauskas and Rourke (1979) study. In all of these instances, problems in tactile finger localization was a prominent feature in the pattern of abilities and deficits exhibited by the learning-disabled children.

Subtype II

Subtype II was composed of children who constituted Factor 2 ($n = 26$) and Cluster 3 ($n = 51$) from the left-handed sample, and Factor 1 ($n = 20$), group-average Cluster 3 ($n = 41$), and centroid-sorting Cluster 2 ($n = 40$) from the right-handed sample. Figure 5-3 is a graphic representation of Subtype II. Again, this figure represents a composite of all mean *T*-score profiles constituting this subtype.

The Subtype II profile was characterized by the following:

1. Clear impairment on some auditory–verbal and psycholinguistic tasks involving the associating of sounds and symbols, assessing of general knowledge (as is normally acquired through everyday

FIG. 5-3. Profile of Subtype II. (For key to abbreviations of test measures, see Table 5-1.)

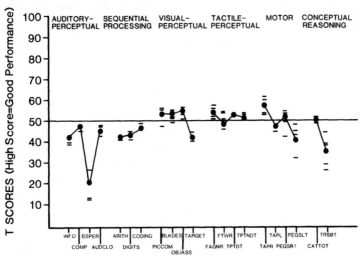

activities), "mental" numerical reasoning, and mnestic skill participation (e.g., immediate memory for series of numbers), as well as some mild difficulty in blending sounds to form words.

2. Relatively better but slightly depressed performances on a test intended to assess understanding of social conventionality and social judgment, and on a task requiring the associating of symbols to their appropriate numerical counterparts.
3. Well-developed visual–perceptual and spatial visualization abilities.
4. Some difficulty in reproducing graphically sequences of visual stimuli and in negotiating visual–spatial arrays on the basis of numerical and alphabetical sequences.
5. Age-appropriate tactile– and kinesthetic–perceptual skills, including well-developed nonverbal tactually guided problem-solving abilities.
6. Adequate performance on a task involving inductive and deductive reasoning with visually or spatially presented stimuli.
7. Normally developed simple motor speed bilaterally, and fine manipulative dexterity with the right hand, but deficits in fine finger dexterity with the left hand.

In sum, Subtype II children manifested well-developed visual and tactile information-processing systems, appeared to be good problem-solving strategists, and presented with reasonably well-developed simple and more complex psychomotor skills. Conversely, they exhibited clear weaknesses in their ability to process information of an auditory–verbal nature and demonstrated some deficiencies in verbal coding or verbal labeling. Children in this group were also seen to exhibit the largest mean WISC low Verbal–high Performance IQ discrepancy, and mean WRAT Reading, Spelling and Arithmetic subtest performances were all well below the 30th centile.

These children bear a striking resemblance to Subtype B of the Fisk and Rourke (1979) study, and to Type 1 of the Petrauskas and Rourke (1979) study. In both of these instances, problems in processing information of an auditory–verbal nature were a cardinal feature in the pattern of abilities and deficits exhibited by the learning-disabled children. Subtype II is also most similar to the language disorder groups of Kinsbourne and Warrington (1963) and Mattis *et al.* (1975), and to the sound–symbol integration deficiency group (i.e., dysphonetic dyslexia) of Boder (1973).

Subtype III

Included in Subtype III were children who constituted Factor 3 ($n = 19$) and Cluster 4 ($n = 35$) from the left-handed sample, and Factor 3 ($n = 18$), group-average Cluster 4 ($n = 21$), and centroid-sorting Cluster 4 ($n = 22$) from the right-handed sample. Once again, the test profile for this group is plotted in terms of a composite of all mean *T*-score patterns in Figure 5-4.

Visual inspection of the profile for Subtype III children revealed the following characteristics:

1. Some auditory–verbal processing weaknesses, involving a limited acquisition of general information, deficient sound–symbol matching skills, poor sound-blending abilities, and somewhat under-developed "mental" numerical reasoning skills. Immediate recall for short bursts of nonredundant auditory–verbal information (e.g., sequences of digits) was mildly impaired, as were understanding of social conventionality and social judgment. An associative-learning task involving speed and accuracy of symbolic transcription was performed in an age-appropriate manner.

2. Normally developed visual–perceptual, perceptual–organizational, and visual–spatial skills.

FIG 5-4. Profile of Subtype III. (For key to abbreviations of test measures, see Table 5-1.)

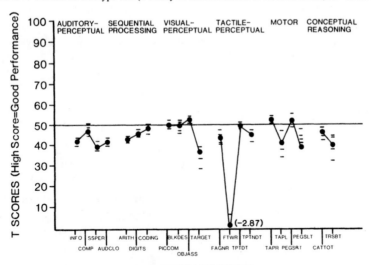

TEST MEASURES

3. Poor performance on one visual–spatial sequential-memory task.
4. Mild finger agnosia and pronounced finger dysgraphesthesia with the upper right extremity; average and below-average tactually guided problem-solving capabilities with the dominant and non-dominant hands, respectively.
5. Normally developed simple motor speed and speeded eye-hand coordination with the right hand, but clearly impaired skills within these areas with the left hand.
6. Slightly impoverished capabilities of nonverbal reasoning, and clear difficulties in performing visual-sequencing tasks involving symbolic shifting.

Children in this group exhibited reasonably well-developed visual information-processing skills, normally developed simple motor skills, and normal motor manipulatory problem-solving abilities with the upper right extremity. On the other hand, children in this subtype could be described as having some poor auditory–verbal and psycholinguistic skills, mild right-sided finger recognition deficits, and pronounced haptic deficiencies involving the detection of numbers written on the fingertips of the right hand. For Subtype III children, mean WISC Performance IQ exceeded Verbal IQ, and mean WRAT Reading, Spelling and Arithmetic subtest scores were all below the 30th centile ranking.

The adaptive profile that characterized the Subtype III children was quite similar to that of Subtype C of the Fisk and Rourke (1979) study. In fact, Subtype III children exhibited the highest mean age (12.59) of all of the groups, a finding consonant with the fact that Subtype C emerged only in the two oldest age-based samples (i.e., 11–12 years and 13–14 years) of the Fisk and Rourke investigation. These children exhibited problems primarily in the ability to detect numbers written on the fingertips of the right hand.

The three groups of children described above appeared to be the most reliable subtypes, having been generated across all possible factor and clustering procedures. They accounted for 71% of the total sample of 322 children, 84% of the left-handed sample, and 58% of the right-handed sample. Four other less reliable (in the sense of having been only partially replicated) subtypes of learning-disabled children emerged. A brief description of each of these is provided below.

Subtype IV

Subtype IV was composed of Factor 4 ($n = 9$) and Cluster 2 ($n = 26$) from the left-handed sample, and group-average Cluster 1 ($n = 24$) and centroid-sorting Cluster 7 ($n = 23$) from the right-handed sample.

Visual inspection of the profile for Subtype IV children revealed the following cardinal features:

1. A slight reduction in general fund of information, and mild deficiencies in phoneme–grapheme matching skills.
2. A well-developed understanding of social conventionality, and exceptionally good sound-blending skills.
3. Mildly impaired arithmetic reasoning, auditory–verbal amnestic skills, and symbolic transcribing capabilities.
4. Relatively good visual information-processing skills; mildly impaired performances on immediate memory for visual sequences, and on a visual-sequencing task requiring the ability to shift "mental" set.
5. Normally developed right-hand tactile finger localization and dominant-hand tactually guided problem-solving skills; mild right-sided finger dysgraphesthesia, and weak tactually guided behavior with the nondominant extremity.
6. Adequate nonverbal reasoning abilities; average and mildly deficient simple motor speeds with the right and left hands, respectively; and bilateral deficits in fine finger dexterity, somewhat more pronounced with the left hand.

The distinguishing features of Subtype IV children were their deficiencies in fine eye–hand coordination under speeded conditions. Children in this group were more apt to exhibit a very small WISC Verbal–Performance IQ discrepancy, or, in some cases, a higher Verbal–lower Performance pattern. Reading performance on the WRAT was more likely to exceed the 30th centile, while both Spelling and Arithmetic subtest scores were below this value.

Subtype V

Included in Subtype V were children who constituted Factor 5 ($n = 6$) from the left-handed sample, and Factor 6 ($n = 8$), group-average Cluster

6 ($n = 10$), and centroid-sorting Cluster 6 ($n = 9$) from the right-handed sample. However, intercorrelations between left-handers and right-handers within this group were rather low, whereas comparisons among the dextral sample yielded higher, more reliable intercorrelations. Thus, it would appear that this subtype may constitute an independent right-handed subtype.

Examiniation of all mean *T*-score patterns for this group suggested that Subtype V children were characterized by the following:

1. Inconsistent performance on auditory–linguistic tasks involving understanding of social conventionality, phoneme–grapheme matching, and sound blending, together with consistent depression of both general fund of information and arithmetic reasoning. Performances on immediate recall for digits and on an associate-learning task involving speed and accuracy of symbolic transcription were roughly age-appropriate.
2. Normally developed visual– and tactile–perceptual information-processing skills.
3. Good nonverbal problem-solving skills, as well as the ability to moderate performances when the task required conceptual shifting.
4. Mildly and moderately deficient simple motor speed with the right and left hands, respectively; average and mildly impaired fine manipulative skills with the dominant and nondominant hands, respectively.

These subjects also exhibited a fairly low Verbal–high Performance IQ discrepancy on the WISC. While their WRAT subtest performance patterns were somewhat inconsistent, there was a trend for Reading to be somewhat higher than either Spelling or Arithmetic.

Subtype VI

Subtype VI contained childen who constituted sinistral Factor 7 ($n = 5$), dextral Factor 7 ($n = 15$), dextral group-average Cluster 7 ($n = 23$), and dextral centroid-sorting Cluster 3 ($n = 22$).

While there was some degree of visual similarity between factor and cluster plots within this group, most intercorrelation values were rather low. This would suggest that this subtype is the most unreliable. Briefly, however, with the exception of some inconsistency among performances within the auditory–linguistic and sequential-processing realms, most neuropsychological adaptive skill areas yielded age-appropriate or better levels of performance. A low Verbal–high Performance IQ discrepancy of fairly large magnitude on the WISC was exhibited by these children as well.

Subtype VII

The final group, Subtype VII, was composed of children who constituted Factor 4 ($n = 11$) and group-average Cluster 5 ($n = 12$) from the right-handed sample. Subtype VII would appear to represent another independent right-handed subtype, despite the fact that it did not emerge when the centroid-sorting clustering procedure was applied.

Inspection of the profile for Subtype VII children revealed the following:

1. Some mild auditory–perceptual deficiencies involving a reduced store of general information, underdeveloped sound-blending skills, and a somewhat limited understanding of social conventionality.
2. "Mental" numerical reasoning skills and auditory–verbal mnestic abilities that were roughly normal, but mildly deficient performance on the Coding subtest of the WISC.
3. Well-developed visual and haptic information-processing skills; good nonverbal reasoning capabilities; inconsistent performances on visual-sequencing tasks requiring symbolic shifting.
4. Normally developed simple motor speed and speeded fine eye–hand coordination with the upper right extremity, but clearly deficient performances with the left hand within these same areas.
5. Pronounced difficulties in immediate memory for sequences of visual stimuli.

The distinguishing feature of Subtype VII children centered around deficiencies on the Target Test, a finding that may be reflective of a compromised ability in these children to apply verbal-coding or verbal-labeling strategies efficiently. This group exhibited a minimal Verbal–Performance IQ discrepancy on the WISC. It should also be noted that this subtype obtained mean WRAT Arithmetic scores that were below the 30th centile level, while both Reading and Spelling scores were above this value. A summary of the profile characteristics for Subtypes IV, V, VI, and VII is provided in Table 5-8.

TABLE 5-8. Profile Characteristics for Subtypes IV, V, VI, and VII

Test measure[a]	Subtype			
	IV	V	VI	VII
INFO	(−)	(−)	−	(−)
COMP			(−)	
SSPER	(−)			(+)
AUDCLO	(+)	+	−	
ARITH	(−)	(−)	(−)	
DIGITS	(−)			
CODING	(−)			(−)
PICCOM				(−)
BLKDES		(+)		
OBJASS		(+)	(+)	
TARGET	−			−−
FAGNR		(+)		
FTWR	(−)		(+)	
TPTDT		(+)		
TPTNDT	(−)			
TAPR		(−)	+	(+)
TAPL	−	−	(−)	−
PEGSRT	−−	(+)	+	
PEGSLT	−−−	(−)		−
CATTOT				
TRSBT	−	(−)		

Note. Key: Blank = average performance; (−) = ½ standard deviation below average; − = 1 standard deviation below average; (+) = ½ standard deviation above average; + = 1 standard deviation above average.

[a] For key to abbreviations of test measures, see Table 5-1.

EVALUATION OF EXPECTATIONS

Our first hypothesis suggested that different patterns of adaptive strengths and weaknesses may emerge in left- and right-handed learning-disabled children as a function of differences in specific patterns of cerebral organization that have been hypothesized to exist between the handedness groups. This expectation was clearly not supported. In fact, the sorts of adaptive deficiencies exhibited by the group of left-handed learning-disabled children were found to be remarkably similar to the types of neuropsychological skill deficiencies seen in a comparable group of right-handed age-mates included in the investigation, as well as to several other dextral learning-disabled subtypes reported in the literature.

That there were no disparities associated with sinistrality in regard to adaptive ability structure may be reflective of the problems in identification or the difficulty in constructing a workable definition of sinistrality. In the current study, name-writing hand was chosen as an initial index of hand dominance. Left-handers identified on this basis were then examined more closely to determine their demonstrated hand proficiency on two skilled manual dexterity tasks: simple motor speed and speeded fine eye–hand coordination. Neither one of these considerations appeared to influence the patterns of performance seen within the population of children assessed. Perhaps different methods of handedness determination (or classification) would reveal measurable differences between dextral and sinistral learning-disabled children (Roszkowski, Snelbecker, & Sacks, 1981). In addition, a closer examination of hand, foot, and eye dominance may eventuate in findings that are consistent with ability differences as a function of lateral preference patterns (Dean *et al.*, 1981).

Our second and third hypotheses dealt with two different issues, one focusing on the importance of an individual's familial handedness history and one focusing on the significance of degree or intensity of an individual's left-handedness. Both of these factors have been posited as possessing predictive value in terms of being able to distinguish between sinistrals with different patterns of hemispheric specialization. In the present study, we felt that, if these particular variables were related to cerebral laterality, then the multivariate classification methods should generate subtypes whose members report mostly sinistral or mostly dextral biological relatives, and/or subtypes that exhibit a membership composition reflective of different measurable variations in consistency and degree of hand usage across a variety of manipulative and behavioral tasks. Neither of these expectations was supported by the data. That is to say, the results of a series of chi-square nonparametric analyses indicated that the derived subtypes could not be distinguished from one another on the basis of hand preference, hand proficiency, or familial handedness composition.

In regard to the familial sinistrality findings, there were at least two problems in obtaining an accurate assessment of familial handedness tendencies. First, since this study tended to regard familial sinistrality as positive if at least one parent or sibling was left-handed, a large number of "false positives" could have been reported. For instance, 60% of the left- and 65% of the right-handed subjects were considered to have a history of left-handedness within the family, based on a single-sibling criterion. However, included within these percentages were several very young siblings (i.e., under 3 years of age) who had been reported by parents as exhibiting a left-sided preference, despite the likelihood that hand dominance had not yet been clearly established in these children. Gesell and Ames (1947), for example, reported the presence of considerable bilaterality in regard to handedness within the age range of 2.5–3.5 years. The second problem was pointed out by Bishop (1980), who suggested that family size may be an important factor to consider when assessing familial sinistrality. According to Bishop, the *a priori* probability that an individual will have a sinistral relative increases with the number of relatives he/she has. This being the case, adopting a single-parent or single-sibling criterion could possibly confound the effects of familial sinistrality and family size.

Finally, it has been demonstrated rather convincingly that subtypes generated by means of one multivariate statistical procedure can be detected reliably through the application of several other classification methods as well. Indeed, Q-type factor-analytic and cluster-analytic solutions were in perfect agreement for the left-handed sample of children, while solutions remained fairly well defined across taxonomic procedures for the right-handed data set. These findings, together with the success Doehring *et al.* (1979) have experienced in their application of multiple classification methods, confirm the usefulness and suitability of these instruments for providing a reliable taxonomy of learning disabilities.

IMPLICATIONS

Several conclusions or generalizations can be drawn from the results of this study.

1. Left- and right-handed learning-disabled children would appear to exhibit very similar adaptive ability profiles. The classification analyses suggested the presence of at least three highly similar subtypes of learning-disabled children within two age-equivalent handedness-based samples. In turn, the subtypes were found to bear a striking resemblance to other dextral subtypes reported in the research literature (Boder, 1973; Fisk & Rourke, 1979; Mattis *et al.*, 1975; Petrauskas & Rourke, 1979). These findings support the notion that learning-disabled children constitute a heterogeneous group in regard to their adaptive structures (Benton, 1975; Rourke, 1978, 1983a, 1983b; Vernon, 1977). Furthermore, it would appear that handedness per se may not be an especially important consideration in the search for subtypes of learning-disabled children. This finding would appear to be in agreement with several studies that have reported the absence of any significant ability differences between left- and right-handed reading-disabled children (Annett & Turner, 1974; Fagin-Dubin, 1974; Wussler & Barclay, 1970), but it seems to be at odds with other studies that have reported the existence of information-processing differences between the handedness groups (Dean *et al.*, 1981; Schevill, 1980).

2. To aid in subtype interpretability, the independent factor and cluster graphs that illustrated Subtype I, Subtype II, and Subtype III individually were combined, and an overall mean *T*-score illustration was provided for each group. However, it was interesting to note that closer visual inspection of the independent factor and cluster profiles within each group revealed one feature that distinguished sinistral and dextral children. In all cases, dextrals exhibited a clearly better right-hand than left-hand performance on the two psychomotor tasks (i.e., Finger Tapping and Grooved Pegboard), whereas sinistrals were found to demonstrate a smaller between-hand discrepancy. Most of the difference between the two handedness groups on this dimension occurred within the right-handed performances, where dextrals were clearly more proficient. Left-handed performances were usually quite similar between the two samples. The differences seen on tasks of a motoric nature could suggest one of two alternative states of affairs. First, within the group of left-handers, the left-handed performances on skilled motor tasks may be reflecting some "shift" in handedness as a consequence of having sustained some degree of left-hemispheric dysfunction. This would imply that the sinistral tendencies seen in these children are a manifestation of brain pathology, a view expounded upon by a number of investigators (Annett, 1964; Bakan, 1971, 1977; Satz, 1972, 1973). However, this possibility seems rather remote, since there was little evidence to suggest that left-handers in this study encountered any particular difficulties with the right hand that would have caused them to engage the use of their left hand as the dominant extremity (e.g., Finger Tapping and Grooved Pegboard scores were usually within an age-appropriate range with the right hand). A

second, more parsimonious, possibility is that the motor performances within the ability repertoires of both handedness groups represent the results of social conditioning and practice (Collins, 1970, 1975). That is, perhaps sinistrals exhibit a smaller between-hand discrepancy because they are natural left-handers who have been actively taught to use the right hand as a result of social and cultural influences. The same social conditioning in natural right-handers, of course, would result in a larger difference score between the upper extremities.

3. The findings of this investigation, together with the results of handedness studies of lesion-produced deficits and of right–left auditory and visual perceptual asymmetries, certainly invite further study into the relation among handedness, adaptive ability structure, and performance on visual half-field, dichotic-listening, or dichotic-monitoring tasks.

4. Related to paragraph 3 above, an obvious research direction to pursue would be to obtain some further information on the possible neurological determinants underlying the different subtype structures. Neurophysiological investigations involving visual or auditory evoked potentials would be especially helpful in this regard (see Fletcher, Chapter 9, this volume; Lovrich & Stamm, 1983).

5. An *internal* validation method (e.g., split-sample replication) was employed in the present study to determine the stability and usefulness of the clustering solutions. As an alternative, it would be of interest to see whether one subtype could be distinguished from other subtypes on a variety of measures and attributes that were not included in the initial classification process (i.e., externally validating the derived solutions). For example, subtype differences across such variables as academic achievement level (WRAT Reading, Spelling, and Arithmetic), presence of learning problems among other family members, prevalence and/or type of birth complication, or birth order could be assessed through the application of parametric (analysis of variance, multivariate analysis of variance) or nonparametric (chi-square) statistical methods.

6. The clarification and differentiation of the quality of cognitive impairment associated with learning difficulties has obvious implications for remedial management. Since one important therapeutic objective is to promote academic remedial programs tailored to the individual's specific cognitive strengths and weaknesses, identification of the "patterning" of deficits in adaptive skills becomes especially important. Indeed, clinical experience has suggested that a remedial management intervention that fails to "fit" the adaptive ability makeup of the child can, in effect, be

counterproductive in respect to the acquisition of basic academic-related skills, with consequent (often negative) impact on personality development. Specific instances of these assertions are contained in other chapters within this volume (see especially Ozols & Rourke, Chapter 13, and Strang & Rourke, Chapter 14).

7. Finally, there has been a persistent tendency to attribute a variety of behavioral deficits to sinistrality. Researchers continue to argue for an association between deficits and left-handedness, despite the burgeoning amount of evidence to disclaim any significant link between cognitive deficiency and handedness. It would seem likely that the tendency to believe that sinistrality is a sign of possible deficit pervades much of clinical practice with learning-disabled children, and other types of abnormal children as well. The results of the current investigation would suggest that left-handedness, more often than not, should be viewed as a "red herring," not worthy of the pathognomic importance attributed to it.

REFERENCES

Andrews, R. J. Aspects of language lateralization correlated with familial handedness. *Neuropsychologia*, 1977, *15*, 769–778.

Annett, M. A model of the inheritance of handedness and cerebral dominance. *Nature*, 1964, *204*, 59–60.

Annett, M. Handedness in families. *Annals of Human Genetics*, 1973, *37*, 93–105.

Annett, M. Handedness in the children of two left handed parents. *British Journal of Psychology*, 1974, *65*, 129–131.

Annett, M., & Turner, A. Laterality and the growth of intellectual abilities. *British Journal of Educational Psychology*, 1974, *44*, 37–46.

Ayres, A. J. Types of sensory integrative dysfunction among disabled learners. *American Journal of Occupational Therapy*, 1972, *26*, 13–18.

Bakan, P. Handedness and birth order. *Nature*, 1971, *229*, 195.

Bakan, P. Left handedness and birth order revisited. *Neuropsychologia*, 1977, *15*, 837–839.

Beaumont, J. G., & Dimond, S. J. Transfer between the cerebral hemispheres in human learning. *Acta Psychologia*, 1973, *37*, 87–91.

Benton, A. L. *Sentence Memory Test.* Iowa City, Iowa: Author, 1965.

Benton, A. L. Development dyslexia: Neurological aspects. In W. J. Friedlander (Ed.), *Advances in neurology* (Vol. 7). New York: Raven Press, 1975.

Berman, A. The problem of assessing cerebral dominance and its relationship to intelligence. *Cortex*, 1971, *7*, 372–386.

Bishop, D. V. M. Measuring familial sinistrality. *Cortex*, 1980, *16*, 311–313.

Blashfield, R. K. Propositions regarding the use of cluster analysis in clinical research. *Journal of Consulting and Clinical Psychology*, 1980, *48*, 455–459.

Boder, E. Developmental dyslexia: A diagnostic approach based on three atypical reading-spelling patterns. *Developmental Medicine and Child Neurology*, 1973, *15*, 663–687.

Bradshaw, J. L., Gates, A., & Nettleton, N. C. Bihemispheric involvement in lexical decisions: Handedness and a possible sex difference. *Neuropsychologia*, 1977, *15*, 277–286.

Bradshaw, J. L., & Taylor, M. J. A word-naming deficit in nonfamilial sinistrals? Laterality effects of vocal responses to tachistoscopically presented letter strings. *Neuropsychologia*, 1979, *17*, 21–32.

Briggs, G. G., & Nebes, R. D. The effects of handedness, family history and sex on the performance of a dichotic listening task. *Neuropsychologia*, 1976, *14*, 129–133.

Bryden, M. P. Tachistoscopic recognition, handedness and cerebral dominance. *Neuropsychologia*, 1965, *3*, 1–8.

Bryden, M. P. Laterality effects in dichotic listening: Relations with handedness and reading ability in children. *Neuropsychologia*, 1970, *8*, 443–450.

Bryden, M. P. Speech lateralization in families: A preliminary study using dichotic listening. *Brain and Language*, 1975, *2*, 201–211.

Collins, R. L. The sound of one paw clapping: An inquiry into the origin of left-handedness. In G. Lindzey & D. D. Thiessen (Eds.), *Contribution to behavior*-genetic analysis—the mouse as a prototype. New York: Meredity Corporation, 1970.

Collins, R. L. When left-handed mice live in right-handed worlds. *Science*, 1975, *187*, 181–184.

Curry, F. K. W., & Rutherford, D. R. Recognition and recall of dichotically presented verbal stimuli by right- and left-handed persons. *Neuropsychologia*, 1967, *5*, 119–126.

Dawson, J. L. M. Alaskan Eskimo hand, eye, auditory dominance and cognitive style. *Psychologia*, 1977, *20*, 121–135. (a)

Dawson, J. L. M. An anthropological perspective on the evolution and lateralization of the brain. *Annals of the New York Academy of Science*, 1977, *299*, 424–447. (b)

Dean, R. S., Schwartz, N. H., & Smith, L. S. Lateral preference patterns as a discriminator of learning difficulties. *Journal of Consulting and Clinical Psychology*, 1981, *49*, 227–235.

Dee, H. L. Auditory asymmetry and strength of manual preference. *Cortex*, 1971, *7*, 236–245.

Doehring, D. G., & Hoshko, I. M. Classification of reading problems by the Q-technique of factor analysis. *Cortex*, 1977, *13*, 281–294.

Doehring, D. G., Hoshko, I. M., & Bryans, B. N. Statistical classification of children with reading problems. *Journal of Clinical Neuropsychology*, 1979, *1*, 5–16.

Dunn, L. M. *Expanded manual for the Peabody Picture Vocabulary Test*. Minneapolis: American Guidance Service, 1965.

Ettlinger, G., Jackson, C. V., & Zangwill, O. L. Cerebral dominance in sinistrals. *Brain*, 1956, *79*, 569–588.

Everitt, B. *Cluster analysis*. London: Heinemann Educational Books, 1974.

Fagin-Dubin, L. Lateral dominance and development of cerebral specialization. *Cortex*, 1974, *10*, 69–74.

Fisk, J. L., & Rourke, B. P. Identification of subtypes of learning-disabled children at three age levels: A neuropsychological, multivariate approach. *Journal of Clinical Neuropsychology*, 1979, *1*, 289–310.

Flick, G. L. Sinistrality revised: A perceptual–motor approach. *Child Development*, 1966, *37*, 613–622.

Geffen, G., & Taub, E. Preferred hand and familial sinistrality in dichotic monitoring. *Neuropsychologia*, 1979, *17*, 527–531.

Gesell, A., & Ames, L. B. The development of handedness. *Journal of Genetic Psychology*, 1947, *70*, 155–175.

Gloning, K. Handedness and aphasia. *Neuropsychologia*, 1977, *15*, 355–358.

Gloning, I., Gloning, K., Haub, G., & Quatember, R. Comparison of verbal behavior in right-handed and non-right-handed patients with anatomically verified lesion of one hemisphere. *Cortex*, 1969, *5*, 43–52.

Gloning, K., & Quatember, R. Statistical evidence of neuropsychological syndromes in left-handed and ambidextrous patients. *Cortex*, 1966, *2*, 484–488.

Goodglass, H., & Quadfasel, F. A. Language laterality in left-handed aphasics. *Brain*, 1954, *77*, 521–568.

Gordon, H. Left-handedness and mirror writing, especially among defective children. *Brain*, 1921, *43*, 313–368.

Gregory, R., & Paul, J. The effects of handedness and writing posture on neuropsychological test results. *Neuropsychologia*, 1980, *18*, 231–235.

Gur, R. E. Motoric laterality in schizophrenia: A possible concomitant of left hemispheric dysfunction. *Archives of General Psychiatry*, 1977, *34*, 33–37.

Hardyck, C., & Petrinovich, L. F. Left-handedness. *Psychological Bulletin*, 1977, *84*, 385–404.

Harris, A. J. *Harris Tests of Lateral Dominance: Manual of directions for administration and interpretation*. New York: Psychological Corporation, 1947.

Harris, A. J. Lateral dominance, directional confusion and reading disability. *Journal of Psychology*, 1957, *44*, 283–394.

Harris, L. J. Left-handedness: Early theories, facts and fancies. In J. Herron (Ed.), *Neuropsychology of left-handedness*. New York: Academic Press, 1980.

Hecaen, H., & de Ajuriaguerra, J. *Left-handedness: Manual superiority and cerebral dominance*. New York: Grune & Stratton, 1964.

Hecaen, H., & Sauguet, J. Cerebral dominance in left-handed subjects. *Cortex*, 1971, *7*, 19–48.

Helwig, J. T., & Council, K. A. (Eds.). *SAS Users Guide, 1979 Edition*. Cary, N.C.: SAS Institute Inc., 1979.

Hicks, R. A., & Beveridge, R. Handedness and intelligence. *Cortex*, 1978, *14*, 304–307.

Hicks, R. E., & Kinsbourne, M. Human handedness. In M. Kinsbourne (Ed.), *Asymmetrical function of the brain*. Cambridge, England: Cambridge University Press, 1978.

Hines, D., & Satz, P. Cross-modal asymmetries in perception related to asymmetry in cerebral functions. *Neuropsychologia*, 1974, *12*, 239–247.

Humphrey, M. E., & Zangwill, O. L. Dysphasia in left-handed patients with unilateral brain lesions. *Journal of Neurology, Neurosurgery and Psychiatry*, 1951, *15*, 184–193.

Johnson, O., & Harley, C. Handedness and sex differences in cognitive tests of brain laterality. *Cortex*, 1980, *16*, 73–82.

Kass, C. E. Auditory Closure Test. In J. J. Olsen & J. L. Olsen (Eds.), *Validity studies on the Illinois Test of Psycholinguistic Abilities*. Madison Wisc.: Photo Press, 1964.

Kimura, D. Manual activity during speaking: II. Left-handers. *Neuropsychologia*, 1973, *11*, 51–55.

Kinsbourne, M., & Warrington, E. K. Developmental factors in reading and writing backwardness. *British Journal of Psychology*, 1963, *54*, 145–156.

Knox, A. W., & Boone, D. R. Auditory laterality and tested handedness. *Cortex*, 1970, *6*, 164–173.

Levy, J. Possible basis for the evolution of lateral specialization of the human brain. *Nature*, 1969, *244*, 614–615.

Levy, J. Lateral specialization of the human brain. Behavioral manifestations and possible evolutionary basis. In J. Kiger (Ed.), *The biology of behavior*. Corvallis: Oregon State University Press, 1973.

Levy, J., & Reid, M. Variations in writing posture and cerebral organization. *Science*, 1976, *194*, 337–339.

Levy, J., & Reid, M. Variations in cerebral organization as a function of handedness, hand posture in writing and sex. *Journal of Experimental Psychology*, 1978, *107*, 119–144.

Lishman, W. A., & McMeekan, E. R. L. Handedness in relation to direction and degree of cerebral dominance for language. *Cortex*, 1977, *13*, 30–43.

Lovrich, D., & Stamm, J. S. Event-related potential and behavioral correlates of attention in reading retardation. *Journal of Clinical Neuropsychology*, 1983, *5*, 13–37.

Mattis, S. Dyslexia syndromes: A working hypothesis that works. In A. L. Benton & D. Pearls (Eds.), *Dyslexia: An appraisal of current knowledge*. London: Oxford University Press, 1978.

Mattis, S., French, J. H., & Rapin, I. Dyslexia in children and young adults: Three independent neuropsychological syndromes. *Developmental Medicine and Child Neurology*, 1975, *17*, 150–163.

McBurney, A. K., & Dunn, H. C. Handedness, footedness, eyedness: A prospective study with special reference to the development of speech and language skills. In R. M. Knights & D. J. Bakker (Eds.), *Neuropsychology of learning disorders: Theoretical approaches*. Baltimore: University Park Press, 1976.

McGlone, J., & Davidson, W. The relation between cerebral speech laterality and spatial ability with special reference to sex and hand preference. *Neuropsychologica*, 1973, *11*, 105–113.

McKeever, W. F., & Gill, K. M. Visual half-field differences in masking effects for sequential letter stimuli in the right- and left-handed. *Neuropsychologia*, 1972, *10*, 111–117.

McKeever, W. F., & Van Deventer, A. D. Familial sinistrality and degree of left-handedness. *British Journal of Psychology*, 1977, *68*, 469–471.

Miller, E. Handedness and the pattern of human ability. *British Journal of Psychology*, 1971, *62*, 111–112.

Morris, R., Blashfield, R., & Satz, P. Neuropsychology and cluster analysis: Potentials and problems. *Journal of Clinical Neuropsychology*, 1981, *3*, 79–99.

Nebes, R. D. Handedness and the perception of part–whole relationships. *Cortex*, 1971, *7*, 350–356.

Newcombe, F., & Ratcliff, G. Handedness, speech lateralization and ability. *Neuropsychologia*, 1973, *11*, 399–407.

Oltman, P. K., & Capobianco, F. Field dependence and eye dominance. *Perceptual and Motor Skills*, 1967, *25*, 645–646.

Orton, S. T. *Reading, writing and speech problems in children*. New York: Norton, 1937.

Petrauskas, R. J., & Rourke, B. P. Identification of subtypes of retarded readers: A neuropsychological multivariate approach. *Journal of Clinical Neuropsychology*, 1979, *1*, 17–37.

Piazza, D. M. The influence of sex and handedness in the hemispheric specialization of verbal and non-verbal tasks. *Neuropsychologia*, 1980, *18*, 163–176.

Porac, C., Coren, S., & Duncan, P. Lateral preference in retardates: Relationships between hand, eye, foot and ear preference. *Journal of Clinical Neuropsychology*, 1980, *2*, 173–188.

Reitan, R. M. *Manual for administration of neuropsychological test batteries for adults and children*. Seattle, Wash.: Author, 1969.

Reitan, R. M. Psychological effects of cerebral lesions in children of early school age. In R. M. Reitan & L. A. Davison (Eds.), *Clinical neuropsychology: Current status and applications*. New York: Wiley, 1974.

Reitan, R. M., & Davison, L. A. (Eds.). *Clinical neuropsychology: Current status and applications.* New York: Wiley, 1974.

Roszkowski, M. J., Snelbecker, G. E., & Sacks, R. Children's, adolescents' and adults' reports of hand preference: Homogeneity and discriminating power of selected tasks. *Journal of Clinical Neuropsychology,* 1981, *3,* 199–213.

Rourke, B. P. Reading, spelling, arithmetic disabilities: A neuropsychologic perspective. In H. R. Myklebust (Ed.), *Progress in learning disabilities* (Vol. 4). New York: Grune & Stratton, 1978.

Rourke, B. P. Outstanding issues in research on learning disabilities. In M. Rutter (Ed.), *Developmental neuropsychiatry.* New York: Guilford Press, 1983. (a)

Rourke, B. P. Reading and spelling disabilities: A developmental neuropsychological perspective. In U. Kirk (Ed.), *Neuropsychology of language, reading and spelling.* New York: Academic Press, 1983. (b)

Rourke, B. P., Bakker, D. J., Fisk, J. L., & Strang, J. D. *Child neuropsychology: An introduction to theory, research, and clinical practice.* New York: Guilford Press, 1983.

Satz, P. Pathological left-handedness: An explanatory model. *Cortex,* 1972, *8,* 121–135.

Satz, P. Left-handedness and early brain insult: An explanation., *Neuropsychologia,* 1973, *11,* 115–117.

Satz, P. A test of some models of hemispheric speech organization in the left- and right-handed. *Science,* 1979, *203,* 1131–1133.

Satz, P. Incidence of aphasia in left-handers: A test of some hypothetical models of cerebral organization. In J. Herron (Ed.), *Neuropsychology of left-handedness.* New York: Academic Press, 1980.

Satz, P., Achenbach, K., & Fennell, E. Correlations between assessed manual laterality and predicted speech laterality in a normal population. *Neuropsychologia,* 1967, *5,* 295–310.

Satz, p., Achenbach, K., Pattisball, E., & Fennell, E. Order of report, ear asymmetry and handedness in dichotic listening. *Cortex,* 1965, *1,* 377–396.

Satz, P., Baymur, L., & van der Vlugt, H. Pathological handedness: Cross-cultural tests of a model. *Neuropsychologia,* 1979, *17,* 77–81.

Satz, P., Friel, J., & Rudegair, F. Differential changes in the acquisition of developmental skills in children who later become dyslexic: A three-year follow-up. In D. Stein, J. Rosen, & N. Butters (Eds.), *Plasticity and recovery of function in the central nervous system.* New York: Academic Press, 1974.

Schevill, H. S. Tactile learning, handedness and reading disability. In J. Herron (Ed.), *Neuropsychology of left-handedness.* New York: Academic Press, 1980.

Schmuller, J., & Goodman, R. Bilateral tachistoscopic perception, handedness and laterality. *Brain and Language,* 1979, *8,* 81–91.

Searleman, A. Subject variables as predictors of cerebral organization for language: Evidence from dichotic listening. *Dissertation Abstracts International,* 1978, *39*(6-B), 3027–3028.

Shankweiler, D., & Studdert-Kennedy, D. A continuum of lateralization for speech perception. *Brain and Language,* 1975, *2,* 212–225.

Shearer, E. Physical skills and reading backwardness. *Educational Research,* 1968, *10,* 197–206.

Silverman, A. J., Adevai, G., & McGough, E. Some relationships between handedness and perception. *Journal of Psychomatic Research,* 1966, *10,* 151–158.

Subirana, A. The relationship between handedness and language function. *International Journal of Neurology,* 1964, *4,* 215–234.

Subirana, A. Handedness and cerebral dominance. In P. J. Vinken & G. W. Bruyn (Eds.),

Handbook of clinical neurology: Disorders of speech, perception and symbolic behavior (Vol. 4). Amsterdam: North-Holland, 1969.

Swanson, J. M., Kinsbourne, M., & Horn, J. M. Cognitive deficit and left-handedness: A cautionary note. In J. Herron (Ed.), *Neuropsychology of left-handedness*. New York: Academic Press, 1980.

Varney, N. R. & Benton, A. L. Tactile perception of direction in relation to handedness and familial handedness. *Neuropsychologia*, 1975, *13*, 449–454.

Vernon, M. D. Varieties of deficiency in the reading process. *Harvard Educational Review*, 1977, *47*, 396–410.

Wechsler, D. *Wechsler Intelligence Scale for Children*. New York: Psychological Corporation, 1949.

Weinstein, S., & Sersen, E. A. Tactual sensitivity as a function of handedness and laterality. *Journal of Comparative and Physiological Psychology*, 1961, *54*, 665–669.

Whilke, J. T., & Sheeley, E. M. Muscular or directional preferences in finger movement as a function of handedness. *Cortex*, 1979, *15*, 561–569.

Wishart, D. *CLUSTAN IC Release 2 User Manual*. London: University College, University of London, 1978.

Wussler, M., & Barclay, A. Cerebral dominance, psycholinguistic skills and reading disability. *Perceptual and Motor Skills*, 1970, *31*, 419–425.

Zangwill, O. L. The current status of cerebral dominance. *Research Publications Association for Research in Nervous and Mental Disease*, 1964, *42*, 103–118.

Zurif, E. B., & Bryden, M. P. Familial handedness and left–right differences in auditory and visual perception. *Neuropsychologia*, 1969, *7*, 179–187.

III

Reading, Spelling, and Arithmetic Disability Subtypes

6

Reading Disability Subtypes: Interaction of Reading and Nonreading Deficits

DONALD G. DOEHRING

RESULTS OF THE RESEARCH TO DATE

In this chapter, I describe our research on reading disability subtypes in relation to other subtype research, and then suggest the possible usefulness of alternative research strategies. After completing a large-scale study in which I compared a group of disabled readers to a group of normal readers on a wide range of nonreading skills (Doehring, 1968), I became aware of the need for a more thorough analysis of the patterns of reading skill deficits in disabled readers, and for the study of individual differences in these patterns. In a subsequent study, my colleagues and I did carry out detailed assessments of reading skills in disabled readers. We found that the determination of individual differences by the inspection of individual profiles of reading skill deficits was difficult and scientifically inadequate (Doehring, 1976). A study by Aram and Nation (1975) suggested that Q-type factor analysis might provide an objective means of classifying disabled readers into subtypes. We identified several subtypes by this procedure (Doehring & Hoshko, 1977), and subsequently confirmed them by cluster analysis (Doehring, Hoshko, & Bryans, 1979).

This first statistical classification study was successful as far as it went. However, reading disabilities have traditionally been defined in

Donald G. Doehring. School of Human Communication Disorders, McGill University, Montreal, Quebec, Canada.

terms of deficient nonreading skills that presumably "cause" the reading problems. We next undertook to classify disabled readers on the basis of language and neuropsychological deficits as well as reading deficits (Doehring, Trites, Patel, & Fiedorowicz, 1981). As a group, the 88 subjects were deficient on all 31 of our reading measures, being most deficient in the oral reading of nonsense syllables and least deficient in the visual matching of letters and words. However, there was a large overlap on all reading measures between the reading-disabled sample and normal readers of the same ages. Statistical classification of the reading measures revealed essentially the same three subtypes that had been most clearly identified in the first study. The largest subtype (38% of the sample of 88 subjects) contained disabled readers who were particularly poor in the oral reading of letters, nonsense syllables, and words, relative to their silent reading skills. Members of the second subtype (25% of the sample) were relatively slow and inaccurate in associating printed and spoken letters, syllables, and words; and the third subtype (19% of the sample) was characterized by poor oral and silent reading of orthographically regular letter sequences in syllables and words, relative to the reading of single letters. Only 16 subjects (18% of the sample), many of whom had relatively mild reading problems (we included a number of siblings of disabled readers in order to compare familial patterns of reading and nonreading deficits), were unclassified.

We were quite satisfied that the three subtypes derived from the 31 reading measures were stable and reliable. Not only had the same subtypes been found in the earlier study (Doehring & Hoshko, 1977), but we also found the same three subtypes when we subdivided the present sample into three age-matched samples and three samples of different ages (8–10, 11–13.5, and 13.6–27); when we selected a subsample by more stringent criteria of reading disability; when we added eight measures of reading-related skills to the battery of reading measures; when we retested a subsample of 18 subjects; when the subjects were classified by cluster analysis; and when we inspected the individual profiles of reading deficits. Both the factor loadings on the Q-type factor analysis and the individual profiles indicated that the subtypes were not homogeneous and independent. Only a few subjects showed the idealized profile defined by the factor scores derived from the Q-type factor analysis, with 26% of the subjects having relatively high loadings on two or more of the three factors that defined the reading disability subtypes. A number of other analyses of the reading measures were also carried out, including intercorrelations among the reading measures, *R*-type factor analyses of the reading measures, and correlations between the reading measures and standardized measures of reading achievement, details of which are given elsewhere (Doehring *et al.*, 1981).

We next classified the subjects on the basis of 22 language measures and 37 measures from a battery of neuropsychological tests. If each of the three patterns of reading skill deficits were related to a particular pattern of deficits on the language and/or neuropsychological measures, we should have found language and neuropsychological subtypes that contained the same subjects as the reading subtypes. This would have permitted us to speculate about cause-and-effect relationships between the reading and nonreading deficits. Although the results were interesting and suggestive, classifications of the language and the neuropsychological measures by the *Q*-technique did not reveal such a simple correspondence between reading and nonreading deficits. The results are summarized below, with complete details given in Doehring *et al.* (1981).

As a group, the subjects did quite poorly on the language tests, particularly on phonemic, morphophonemic, syntactic, and serial-naming measures, but with considerable overlap between disabled readers and normal readers on all measures. However, *Q*-type factor analyses of the language measures revealed two subtypes containing only 58% of the subjects, mainly differentiated by their ability to repeat strings of spoken words. To gain further insight into the relationship between reading and language deficits, we next carried out *Q*-type factor analyses that included the 39 measures of reading and reading-related skills and the 22 language measures. Only three of the five factors that were found had reading–language profiles that could be interpreted. These three subtypes identified only 65% of the subjects. Our very provisional interpretation of the reading–language subtypes was that some disabled readers with oral reading disability tended to be very poor in repeating word strings, while others with oral reading disability tended to be very poor in naming colors and pictures; and disabled readers with sound–letter association problems and letter-sequence problems tended to be relatively good in repeating word strings and relatively poor in naming days and months.

On the 37 neuropsychological measures, the 88 subjects as a group showed the usual deficiency on Wechsler Intelligence Scale for Children (WISC) Verbal subtests, and tended to be at or above the average of other neuropsychology clinic patients of the same age on the remaining tests, the lowest scores occurring in finger agnosia, finger-tapping speed, and strength of grip. *Q*-type factor analyses of the 37 neuropsychological measures failed to reveal interpretable factors, perhaps because there were still differences in the scoring scales of the various measures even after all scores had been standardized. However, a *Q*-type factor analysis of the 12 WISC subtests alone did give some confirmation of short-term memory problems in a small subgroup of subjects with oral reading disability who had particularly low scores on the Digit Span subtest. Because of differences in test norms (the reading and language measures were scored in terms of centiles based on samples of normal readers of different ages, whereas all neuropsychological tests were scored relative to normal controls or clinic samples of the same age), *Q*-type factor analyses of combined reading and neuropsychological measures, and of combined reading, language, and neuropsychological measures, could not be carried out.

Although *Q*-type factor analyses of the language and neuropsychological measures did not reveal nonreading disability subtypes that corresponded exactly to the reading disability subtypes, it was still possible that some other form of analysis might reveal a more definite relationship between reading and nonreading deficits. Inspection of the average language scores for the three reading disability subtypes and discriminant analyses of the language measures for the three reading disability subtypes did not provide any new information. However, additional analyses of neuropsychological measures did provide some suggestions of differences among the three reading disability subtypes on the neuropsychological measures. Discriminant analyses of various subsets of neuropsychological measures suggested that there might be characteristic patterns of neuropsychological deficits associated with each type of reading disability. Subjects with oral reading problems tended to be generally least impaired; those with sound–letter association problems tended to be most impaired, particularly in verbal skills and finger-tapping speed; and those with letter-sequence problems tended to perform poorly on Progressive Matrices and on a measure of finger agnosia. When the average subtype profiles on the neuropsychological tests were clinically evaluated, there was no clear indication of cerebral dysfunction in oral reading problems, some indication of left-hemisphere dysfunction in letter–sound association problems, and some suggestion of posterior cerebral dysfunction—particularly in the right hemisphere—in letter-sequence problems. Blind clinical evaluations of individual neuropsychological profiles did not, however, reveal any consistent indication of lateralized cerebral dysfunction for any subtype, except for a larger proportion of possible bilateral posterior dysfunction in subjects with letter-sequence problems. Details of other analyses—including *R*-type factor analyses of the language and neuro-psychological measures; correlations among the reading, language, and neuropsychological measures; and correlations of the language and neuro-psychological measures with standardized measures of reading achievement —are given elsewhere (Doehring *et al.*, 1981).

The results of the language and neuropsychological measures did not go as far as we would have liked in showing what types of nonreading deficits are associated with each pattern of reading deficit). There was just enough information to formulate a provisional interpretation. When we put the results of all the different analyses of reading and nonreading measures together and stretched our collective imaginations to the fullest, some tentative hypotheses regarding the possible interactions of reading and nonreading deficits in disabled readers emerged. Some patterns of reading deficits may be associated with more than one pattern of non-reading deficit, and some patterns of nonreading deficits may be asso-ciated with more than one pattern reading deficit. Disabled readers with oral reading problems may be subdivided into as many as three different subtypes of nonreading deficit, involving difficulties in naming, in auditory-verbal short-term memory, and in motor planning or co-ordination, respectively. These disabled readers generally show the least indication of cerebral dysfunction. Disabled readers with problems in rapidly associating letters and sounds tend to be most likely to have cerebral dysfunction, with their particular deficiency on verbal tests sug-gesting possible left-hemisphere involvement. However, we found no direct connection between these reading problems and more generalized deficits in intermodal association, probably because our nonreading measures did not include sufficiently direct tests of such deficits. There was no direct indication of nonreading sequencing problems in disabled readers with letter-sequence problems, perhaps because of a lack of appropriate tests, but there was some suggestion of a visual-perceptual or conceptual deficit that might be associated with posterior bilateral cere-bral dysfunction.

Why did we not find a more clear-cut relationship between reading and nonreading deficits? There may actually be none, but it seems more likely that we did not succeed in demonstrating relationships that do exist. The sampling of both reading and nonreading skills could have been inadequate; perhaps there were too many measures of some types of skill and too few or no measures of other relevant skills. The sample of subjects may not have been representative of the population of disabled readers, which is very difficult to define (Doehring, 1978). Some of our tests may not have adequately sampled the abilities that they purported to measure, or there may have been too many tests involving more than one kind of ability.

Although the study did replicate the subtypes of reading deficits found earlier and contributed a wealth of additional information about the interrelationships among reading and nonreading skills in disabled readers, it did not yield a satisfactory description of the reading and nonreading deficits associated with different types of reading disability. Such a description still remains to be determined. We have to be content with the provisional conclusions derived from this study, which is the only one to date in which disabled readers were classified either objectively or subjectively according to a systematic assessment of both reading and nonreading deficits.

One interesting outcome of the use of several different test batteries was the variety of possible strategies for data analysis that could be applied. Because we wanted to replicate the subtypes found in the earlier study (Doehring & Hoshko, 1977), we chose first to classify subjects according to reading skill deficits by Q-type factor analysis. Then we evaluated patterns of nonreading deficits with reference to the three reading disability subtypes based on patterns of reading deficits. This was done through separate Q-type factor analyses of nonreading tests, through analysis of the profiles of nonreading deficit associated with each pattern of reading deficit, and through determination by discriminant analyses of the nonreading skills that best differentiated the three patterns of reading deficits. Other investigators may choose to use different strategies to investigate the interactions of reading and nonreading deficits. For example, it might be reasonable in some instances first to classify subjects on the basis of patterns of nonreading deficits, and then to determine whether the resulting subtypes differ in patterns of reading deficit. The ideal strategy, of course, would be to have a single battery of reading and nonreading tests that would yield replicable subtypes, based on patterns of combined reading and nonreading deficit.

COMPARISONS WITH OTHER RESEARCH RESULTS

At this stage of knowledge, it is not surprising that our results do not completely agree with those of other investigators. As stated above, the most obvious reasons are differences in tests, in subject populations, and in methods of analysis. There was, however, considerable concordance with both single- and multiple-syndrome explanations of reading disabilities. With regard to overall trends in our sample of disabled readers, the severe deficit on the language tests could be interpreted as supporting Vellutino's (1979) postulation of a language deficit in disabled readers, and the particularly severe phonemic and morphophonemic deficits could be interpreted as supporting the growing number of explanations (cf. Frith, 1981) of reading disability as involving a phonemic deficit.

With regard to the subtypes we tentatively identified, others have reported disorders of the same type, either as unitary disorders or as subtypes. These include deficits in naming (Denckla, 1979; Mattis, 1978; Wolf, 1981), short-term memory (Denckla, 1979; Farnham-Diggory & Gregg, 1975; Jorm, 1979, Torgeson, 1978–1979), oral–motor deficits (Denckla, 1979; Mattis, 1978; Myklebust, 1978), and letter-sequence problems (Bakker & Schroots, 1981; Denckla, 1979; Venezky & Massaro, 1979). Although other writers (Benton, 1975; Myklebust, 1978) have speculated about the possible existence of a subtype involving difficulty in rapid intersensory association, no other direct empirical evidence of this subtype has come to our notice.

We did not find an unequivocal visual-perception subtype, perhaps because the relative rarity of this type of reading disability (Boder, 1973; Mattis, 1978) might reduce the possibility of its identification by statistical classification procedures. It is possible, however, that our letter-sequence subtype involves some kind of visual-perception problem. More puzzling was the failure to find a specific pattern of reading skill deficits strongly associated with phonemic deficits, as postulated by a growing number of writers. Our language battery included what we thought were five good measures of phonemic segmentation skills, four of which were highly loaded on one factor of an *R*-type factor analysis. Further study is needed with additional measures related to phonemic processing to determine whether there is a subtype or subtypes particularly deficient in phonemic skills. There should also be attempts to determine more about the nature of the deficiency—whether the basic problem is difficulty in discriminating rapid changes in the acoustic speech signal (Tallal & Stark, 1981), bringing phonemic segments into conscious awareness (Fox & Routh, 1980; Liberman & Shankweiler, 1979; Mattingly, 1980), the use of phonological codes in short-term memory (Jorm, 1979), or knowledge of the articulatory gestures associated with phonemes (Frith, 1981; Snowling, 1981). Additional measures of reading skills might provide more insight into the role of phonemic deficits.

I will not compare our results with those of other statistical classification studies, since those studies are discussed more fully elsewhere in this volume. As far as we know, no other statistical classifications have been based upon reading skills or combined reading and nonreading skills.

SUGGESTIONS FOR FURTHER RESEARCH

Several suggestions can be offered regarding future research of this type. The choice of subjects is very important in research involving multivariate correlational analyses. In studies where statistical classifications are based on reading and nonreading skills, it is probably best first to classify samples of subjects who meet the usual criteria of severe reading disability into subtypes, and then to test broader samples of poor readers to see whether the same subtypes are found (Mattis, 1978; Satz & Morris, 1980). There is a definite need for an integrated battery of tests of reading and nonreading skills in which skills are differentiated by systematically varying the operations of a basic test paradigm, such as that used by Tallal, Stark, Kallman, and Mellits (1981), rather than batteries of tests with such diverse operations that unambiguous operational definitions of skills are not possible. It is essential that the integrated test battery be derived from a single theoretical model encompassing the reading and nonreading skills that may be involved in reading disabilities, in contrast to the loosely integrated constructs of attention, perception, memory, cognition, and language from which present tests are derived. The successful construction of a comprehensive, theoretically based battery of reading and nonreading tests would be a major contribution to research on reading disability. We have made a small beginning in this direction, using an approach based on standard information theory (Doehring, Backman, & Waters, 1983), but an entirely different approach to the assessment of human abilities may be needed.

In thinking about factors that could have contributed to our subtypes, it became inescapable that theories of reading disabilities must take the possible role of experience into consideration (cf. Fischer, 1980). Although definitions of reading disabilities that require normal educational opportunity and adequate sociocultural background are intended to control for experience, there is no way to rule out completely the possible influence of experiential differences on patterns of reading and nonreading deficits.

One way to study the influence of experience on certain skills is to give intensive training in the deficient skills. In doctoral research now being carried out, Christina Fiedorowicz has trained deficient reading skills in disabled readers and has compared patterns of reading skill deficits before and after training. We hope to determine the extent to which deficits can be eliminated by training, and how much transfer of training there is from trained skills to nontrained skills and to the reading of connected discourse. This research should give us more insight into the effects of experience on the observed patterns of reading skill deficits in disabled readers, and also into the possibility of eliminating these deficits through intensive context-free drill. We are particularly interested in testing the hypothesis that some or all reading disabilities involve the lack of rapid, automatic operations at some point in the reading process (LaBerge & Samuels, 1974), and we want to determine whether intensive context-free training will lead to automaticity and thus facilitate the rapid reading of connected discourse.

The importance of this new direction of research with respect to advances in the analysis of learning disabilities is that the intensive training of individual children would appear to rule out the possibility of assessing the large samples of subjects that are needed for statistical classification. For the immediate future, we plan to analyze the reading and nonreading deficits in disabled readers by intensive individual assessment and training procedures, as described below.

CURRENT RESEARCH PLANS

The first step in our current research was to design a provisional model of reading from which experimental measures for assessment and training could be derived. After reviewing other models of reading and reading disability, Joan Backman, Gloria Waters, and I formulated the model shown in Figure 6-1. This model is similar to other recent models, but more detailed with respect to those aspects of reading that may be involved in different types of reading disabilities. The severe reading disabilities that we first propose to study involve difficulties in reading letters, letter patterns, or words. For example, problems in visual perception could result from deficits in brief sensory storage, visual feature extraction, visual letter recognition, letter-pattern recognition, or word recognition; letter–sound association problems could occur at the level of

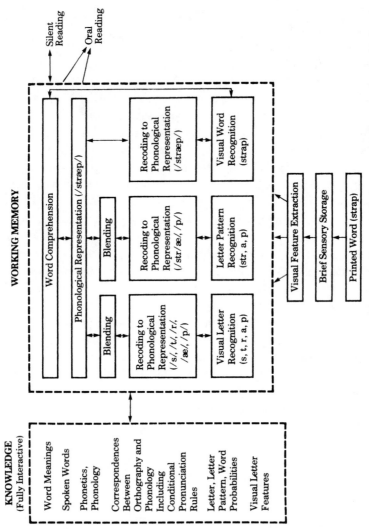

FIG. 6-1. A provisional model of letter, letter-pattern, and word reading for use in research on reading disabilities. (From D. G. Doehring, J. Backman, & G. Waters, Theoretical models of reading disabilities: Past, present and future. *Topics in Learning and Learning Disabilities*, 1983, 3, 84–94. Copyright 1983 by Aspen Systems Corporation. Reprinted by permission.)

recoding to phonological presentation; and letter-sequence problems could occur at the level of letter-pattern recognition or blending. Further details of the operation of the model and its application to reading disabilities are given elsewhere (Doehring, *et al.*, 1983).

Although the model is quite complex already, more detailed descriptions of present components and additional descriptions of new components will be needed in the future. Within the present model, we may need more detailed descriptions of recoding mechanisms and knowledge in order to specify different types of sound–letter correspondence that may be associated with different subtypes of reading disability. More complete descriptions of phonetic and phonological perception may be needed to describe preliminary stages of auditory analysis that could be involved in deficits of phonological recoding. It will also be necessary to elaborate the output stages to permit precise description of the processes involved in naming and articulation; and at some point we will need to go beyond the level of word perception and include descriptions of higher-level syntactic and semantic processes. For the moment, however, we are using the processes defined by the reading model in Figure 6-1.

We will begin by presenting letters, letter patterns, and words in printed and spoken form, and by assessing the speed and accuracy of visual identification, phonological recoding, and oral reading to determine which aspects of reading are most deficient. Then we will directly train the most deficient skills to determine how such experience alters the pattern of reading skill deficits. Once we have satisfactorily delineated areas of intractable reading skill deficits, we will expand the model to describe classes of deficient nonreading skills that might be associated with the reading deficits, and we will devise procedures for testing and training these skills. After the patterns of nonreading deficits have been reliably determined in this manner, the models of reading and nonreading skills, the procedures for assessing and training these skills, and the description of the type of reading disability can be successively modified until we achieve an integrated theoretical description of the individual's reading disability in terms of an operational description of the reading and nonreading deficiencies.

We have only begun the very first stages of this research. In a sense, it is diametrically opposed to our previous approach to investigating reading disabilities. Individuals are studied intensively over a period of time, as opposed to a single assessment of a large group of subjects. We will use some form of longitudinal single-subject research design (Denenberg,

1979; Hersen & Barlow, 1976). One potential advantage of this approach is that it may facilitate the discovery of cause-and-effect relationships among reading and nonreading deficits. Another potential advantage is that the testing and training procedures are much closer to the procedures used in practical diagnosis and treatment than are the procedures used in cross-sectional research. This may enable us to attack directly the notorious gap between research and practice, and to make more direct use of the insights of experienced clinicians in modifying our models, testing–training procedures, and final descriptions of reading disabilities. What we do not know at this stage is how much time it will take to accumulate a sufficient number of individual cases to arrive at comprehensive descriptions of different types of reading disabilities.

At this point in our lengthy, laborious efforts to discover the salient characteristics of reading disabilities, we need to make the best guess possible as to the most fruitful research approaches. Although it may be technically impossible to determine adequately all relevant interactions by conventional group studies (Cronbach, 1975; Denenberg, 1979), joint interpretation of individual and group studies could suggest useful directions for further research. What must be avoided at all costs is the spurious feeling that we are approaching the final answer. Whatever the best path may be, a great deal more hard work in designing, carrying out, and interpreting research will be needed before we reach a satisfactory understanding of these complex phenomena.

ACKNOWLEDGMENTS

The statistical classification research described herein was carried out with the collaboration of Irene Hoshko, Ronald L. Trites, P. G. Patel, and Christina A. M. Fiedorowicz, and financed by Grants 604-7-858 and 605-1326-44 from the National Health Research and Development Program of Canada and Grant MA-1652 from the Medical Research Council of Canada. Ms. Fiedorowicz's research on the training of deficient reading skills was financed by Grant 81-48 from The Hospital for Sick Children Foundation, Toronto, Ontario, Canada.

REFERENCES

Aram, D. M., & Nation, J. E. Patterns of language behavior in children with developmental language disorders. *Journal of Speech and Hearing Research*, 1975, *18*, 229–241.
Bakker, D. J., & Schroots, H. J. Temporal order in normal and disturbed reading. In G. T.

Pavlidis & T. R. Miles (Eds.), *Dyslexia: Experimental research and educational implications.* London: Wiley, 1981.

Benton, A. L. Developmental dyslexia: Neurological aspects. In W. J. Friedlander (Ed.), *Advances in neurology* (Vol. 7). New York: Raven Press, 1975.

Boder, E. Developmental dyslexia: A diagnostic approach based on three atypical reading patterns. *Developmental Medicine and Child Neurology,* 1973, *15,* 663–687.

Cronbach, L. J. Beyond the two disciplines of scientific psychology. *American Psychologist,* 1975, *30,* 116–127.

Denckla, M. B. Childhood learning disabilities. In K. M. Heilman & E. Valenstein (Eds.), *Clinical neuropsychology.* New York: Oxford University Press, 1979.

Denenberg, V. H. Dilemmas and designs for developmental research. In C. L. Ludlow & M. E. Doran-Quine (Eds.), *The neurological bases of language disorders in children: Methods and directions for research* (NINCDS Monograph No. 2, U.S. DHEW Publication No. (NIH) 79-440). Washington, D.C.: U.S. Government Printing Office, 1979.

Doehring, D. G. *Patterns of impairment in specific reading disability.* Bloomington: Indiana University Press, 1968.

Doehring, D. G. Evaluation of two models of reading disability. In R. M. Knights & D. J. Bakker (Eds.), *The neuropsychology of learning disorders: Theoretical approaches.* Baltimore: University Park Press, 1976.

Doehring, D. G. The tangled web of behavioral research on developmental dyslexia. In A. L. Benton & D. Pearl (Eds.), *Dyslexia: An appraisal of current knowledge.* New York: Oxford University Press, 1978.

Doehring, D. G., Backman, J., & Waters, G. Theoretical models of reading disabilities: Past, present and future. *Topics in Learning and Learning Disabilities,* 1983, *3,* 84–94.

Doehring, D. G., & Hoshko, I. M. Classification of reading problems by the Q technique of factor analysis. *Cortex,* 1977, *13,* 281–294.

Doehring, D. G., Hoshko, I. M., & Bryans, B. N. Statistical classification of children with reading problems. *Journal of Clinical Neuropsychology,* 1979, *1,* 5–16.

Doehring, D. G., Trites, R. L., Patel, P. G., & Fiedorowicz, C. A. M. *Reading disabilities: The interaction of reading, language, and neuropsychological deficits.* New York: Academic Press, 1981.

Farnham-Diggory, S., & Gregg, L. Short-term memory function in young readers. *Journal of Experimental Child Psychology,* 1975, *19,* 279–298.

Fischer, K. W. A theory of cognitive development: The control and construction of hierarchies of skills. *Psychological Review,* 1980, *7,* 477–531.

Fox, B., & Routh, D. K. Phonemic analysis and severe reading disability in children. *Journal of Psycholinguistic Research,* 1980, *9,* 115–119.

Frith, U. Experimental approaches to developmental dyslexia. *Psychological Research,* 1981, *43,* 97–109.

Hersen, M., & Barlow, D. H. *Single case experimental designs: Strategies for studying behavioral change.* New York: Pergamon Press, 1976.

Jorm, A. F. The nature of the reading deficit in developmental dyslexia. *Cognition,* 1979, *7,* 429–433.

LaBerge, D., & Samuels, S. J. Toward a theory of automatic information processing. *Cognitive Psychology,* 1974, *6,* 293–323.

Liberman, I. Y., & Shankweiler, D. Speech, the alphabet, and teaching to read. In L. B. Resnick & P. A. Weaver (Eds.), *Theory and practice of early reading* (Vol. 2). Hillsdale, N.J.: Erlbaum, 1979.

Mattingly, I. G. *Reading, linguistic awareness, and language acquisition* (Haskins Laboratories Status Report on Speech Research SR-61). New Haven, Conn.: Haskins Laboratories, 1980.

Mattis, S. Dyslexia syndromes: A working hypothesis that works. In A. L. Benton & D. Pearl (Eds.), *Dyslexia: An appraisal of current knowledge*. New York: Oxford University Press, 1978.

Myklebust, H. R. Toward a science of dyslexiology. In H. R.Myklebust (Ed.), *Progress in learning disabilities* (Vol. 4). New York: Grune & Stratton, 1978.

Satz, P., & Morris, R. Learning disability subtypes: A review. In F. J. Pirozzolo & M. C. Wittrock (Eds.), *Neuropsychological and cognitive processes in reading*. New York: Academic Press, 1980

Snowling, M. J. Phonemic deficits in developmental dyslexia. *Psychological Research*, 1981, *43*, 219–234.

Tallal, P., & Stark, R. Speech acoustic-cue discrimination abilities of normally developing and language impaired children. *Journal of the Acoustical Society of America*, 1981, *69*, 568–579.

Tallal, P., Stark, R., Kallman, C., & Mellits, D. A reexamination of some nonverbal perceptual abilities of language-impaired and normal children. *Journal of Speech and Hearing Research*, 1981, *24*, 351–357.

Torgeson, J. K. Performance of reading disabled children on serial memory tasks. *Reading Research Quarterly*, 1978–1979, *14*, 57–87.

Vellutino, F. R. *Dyslexia: Theory and research*. Cambridge, Mass.: MIT Press, 1979.

Venezky, R. L., & Massaro, D. W. The role of orthographic regularity in word recognition. In L. B. Resnick & P. A. Weaver (Eds.), *Theory and practice of early reading* (Vol. 1). Hillsdale, N.J.: Erlbaum, 1979.

Wolf, M. The word retrieval process and reading in children and aphasics. In K. Nelson (Ed.), *Children's language* (Vol. 3). New York: Gardner Press, 1981.

7

Spelling Disability Subtypes

JAMES E. SWEENEY
BYRON P. ROURKE

The ability to spell is usually discussed in the context of the development of reading skills, especially in educational circles. This situation may have developed not only because learning to read has some educational priority, but also because little has been known regarding those skills crucial to the development of spelling ability itself. Up to this point in time, knowledge about the adaptive significance of spelling performance has been extremely limited. The determination of clear relationships between the graphic representations of words and cognitive processes is an exciting possibility. The analysis of the manner in which the spoken word is graphically represented may very well be an important avenue through which meaningful hypotheses regarding cognitive processes can be tested.

Studies of spelling disorders (e.g., Bannatyne & Wichiarojote, 1969; Newton, 1961; Russell, 1955) have produced somewhat ambiguous, inconsistent, and sometimes contradictory findings. Since learning how to spell may involve the interaction of many subskills that may vary in salience at different stages of the development of this skill, the utilization of a "level-of-performance" approach (i.e., comparison of normal and deficient spellers on one or many dependent variables) in such studies may be inadequate. Only relatively recently have researchers begun to recognize this possibility. This has led to the consideration that qualitatively distinct deficits in processing capabilities may prompt the develop-

James E. Sweeney, District of Parry Sound Child and Family Centre, Parry Sound, Ontario, Canada.

Byron P. Rourke. Department of Psychology, University of Windsor, and Department of Neuropsychology, Windsor Western Hospital Centre, Windsor, Ontario, Canada.

ment of very different unsuccessful spelling strategies, and that these may, in turn, eventuate in similar levels of spelling retardation. Some progress has been made in isolating such strategies by classifying errors in the spelling performance of retarded spellers and by studying the possible psycholinguistic significance of such errors.

Nelson and Warrington (1974) found that a substantial Wechsler Intelligence Scale for Children (WISC) Verbal–Performance IQ discrepancy (in the direction of low Verbal IQ) and retardation in spelling and reading were related to a preponderance of phonetically inaccurate spelling errors in children 8 to 14 years of age. The results of studies by Newcombe (1969) and Kinsbourne and Warrington (1964) also reflected a relationship between a generalized impairment in language functioning and phonetically inaccurate spelling errors in adult patients.

THE 1978 STUDY: DESCRIPTION AND RESULTS

A more extensive study (Sweeney & Rourke, 1978) was designed to accomplish the following: (1) elucidate further the adaptive significance of phonetically inaccurate errors; (2) launch investigations into the psycholinguistic implications of the production of a preponderance of phonetically accurate spelling errors; and (3) investigate possible differences in the nature and extent of the psycholinguistic deficiencies associated with phonetically accurate and phonetically inaccurate spelling retardation at two different age levels.

The subjects in this study had attended school regularly from the age of 6 years. There were three groups of children at each of the age levels commensurate with Grades 4 ("younger") and 8 ("older"). Each of the six groups employed in the study consisted of eight children (five males and three females). The control group (normal spellers, or Ns) at each age level was selected on the basis of a centile score of 50 or above on the Spelling subtest of the Wide Range Achievement Test (WRAT; Jastak & Jastak, 1965). Two experimental groups (phonetically accurate spelling retardates, or PAs, and phonetically inaccurate spelling retardates, or PIs) were selected at each age level. The operational definition of "spelling retardation" was a centile score of 20 or below on the Spelling subtest of the WRAT. PAs rendered at least 60% of their misspelled syllables on the WRAT Spelling subtest in a phonetically accurate fashion, whereas 40% or fewer of the misspelled syllables of PIs on the WRAT were phonetically accurate. The WISC Performance IQ (Wechsler, 1949) was employed as a control for psychometric intelligence in order to avoid the imposition of restrictions with respect to language performance.

The means and standard deviations for age, WISC Performance IQ, WRAT Spelling level, and degree of phonetic accuracy of misspellings are presented in Table 7-1. There were no statistically significant differences at each age level in the following: (1) Performance IQ among PIs, PAs, and Ns; (2) WRAT Spelling level between PIs and PAs; and (3) phonetic accuracy of misspelled syllables between Ns and PAs.

The measures employed to assess the perceptual, psycholinguistic, and cognitive abilities of the aforementioned groups were as follows: Goldman–Fristoe–Woodcock Test of Auditory Discrimination (Goldman, Fristoe, & Woodcock, 1970); WISC Digit Span subtest; Sentence Memory Test (Benton, 1965); Auditory Closure Test (Kass, 1964); Verbal Fluency Test (Strong); WISC Similarities subtest; WISC Arithmetic subtest; Peabody Picture Vocabulary Test (PPVT; Dunn, 1965); WISC Information subtest; WISC Comprehension subtest; WISC Vocabulary subtest; WRAT Reading subtest; Higgins–Wertman Test of Visual Closure (Higgins & Wertman, 1968).

In order to permit meaningful comparison among test performances for the three groups, a graphic illustration of mean standardized T scores on each dependent variable for Ns, PAs, and PIs at each age level is presented in Figure 7-1. The T-score means are arranged such that good performance is represented in one direction (above 50) and poor performance is represented in the opposite direction (below 50). Each dependent variable was analyzed through a two-factor (group $\times$ age) analysis of variance. The Newman–Keuls procedure was employed to make comparisons among means. Analyses for simple effects (as suggested by Winer, 1962) were carried out where necessary.

Performances on the Goldman–Fristoe–Woodcock Test of Auditory Discrimination under both quiet and noise conditions, the WISC Digit Span—forward subtest, and the Test of Visual Closure did not discriminate the groups at either age level. The absence of intergroup differences on measures of auditory discrimination and immediate memory for auditory–verbal information would suggest that the deficit(s) underlying the poor spelling performances of PIs and PAs must be other than a deficit in selective attention, such as that suggested by Dykeman, Ackerman, Clements, and Peters (1971) and Kinsbourne (1973). In addition, the similarity in level of performance for PIs, PAs, and Ns on the Test of

TABLE 7-1. Means and Standard Deviations for Age, WISC Performance IQ, WRAT Spelling, Phonetic Accuracy, and the Dependent Measures for Younger and Older Ns, PAs, and PIs

	Normal		Phonetically accurate		Phonetically inaccurate	
	Younger	Older	Younger	Older	Younger	Older
Independent variables						
Age (in months)						
M	118.50	159.87	120.62	161.25	118.87	161.12
SD	4.75	3.09	5.18	2.86	7.05	5.33
WISC Performance IQ						
M	101.62	105.00	101.00	96.37	100.37	95.87
SD	5.12	7.54	8.17	9.07	8.53	8.14
WRAT Spelling (centile)						
M	65.37	67.62	16.50	12.00	12.37	5.62
SD	10.63	10.95	2.39	6.54	4.86	6.20
Phonetic accuracy (percent)						
M	65.37	76.37	76.62	71.37	28.00	31.87
SD	24.47	12.38	12.14	4.37	5.09	6.55
Dependent measure (number correct unless otherwise indicated)						
Test of Auditory Discrimination—quiet conditions						
M	27.12	27.50	27.75	28.00	27.12	28.12
SD	1.64	1.69	0.88	1.85	1.95	1.35
Test of Auditory Discrimination—noise conditions						
M	18.25	21.87	20.87	21.25	19.37	20.37
SD	3.05	1.55	2.23	3.53	2.72	2.38
WISC Digit Span—forward						
M	6.25	6.75	5.87	6.25	5.75	5.62
SD	0.70	0.70	1.45	1.83	1.28	0.91
Sentence Memory Test[d]						
M	14.37	17.12	14.12	15.50	13.25	13.75
SD	2.66	1.35	2.58	2.39	3.37	2.43
Auditory Closure Test[d]						
M	15.50	20.00	14.62	17.50	11.62	14.37
SD	3.89	3.11	3.62	4.30	4.37	5.44
WISC Digit Span—backward[a]						
M	3.87	4.37	3.62	4.00	3.12	3.00
SD	0.99	0.74	0.74	1.06	0.64	0.75
Verbal Fluency Test[a]						
M	7.56	10.06	6.93	8.87	6.81	6.75
SD	2.00	2.33	1.45	2.51	1.98	2.07

TABLE 7-1. (*Continued*)

	Normal		Phonetically accurate		Phonetically inaccurate	
	Younger	Older	Younger	Older	Younger	Older
Dependent measure (number correct unless indicated)						
WISC Similarities[a]						
M	9.50	15.87	9.37	13.00	8.75	10.00
SD	2.07	3.79	2.55	3.16	2.65	2.82
WISC Arithmetic[e]						
M	9.37	11.37	8.50	10.00	6.75	8.00
SD	0.74	1.18	1.30	1.69	1.48	1.69
Peabody Picture Vocabulary Test[b]						
M	79.12	105.00	79.12	92.87	76.12	81.37
SD	9.12	5.80	7.97	8.85	8.40	7.02
WISC Information[c]						
M	12.87	20.25	10.25	13.00	11.25	11.87
SD	1.35	2.43	1.90	2.13	2.49	2.85
WISC Comprehension[c]						
M	12.62	17.12	11.37	12.50	9.50	12.37
SD	3.11	1.80	3.54	2.67	3.58	4.65
WISC Vocabulary[c]						
M	35.75	47.12	31.12	37.12	30.87	33.50
SD	5.41	4.64	4.35	4.61	6.17	5.63
WRAT Reading (grade level)[f]						
M	6.65	11.63	4.27	5.75	3.02	4.60
SD	1.39	1.23	1.09	1.38	1.00	2.42
Test of Visual Closure						
M	58.75	101.25	60.12	83.00	59.00	65.12
SD	28.47	23.92	27.35	31.89	17.76	12.63

[a] Differences among groups at younger age level not significant; Ns and PAs > PIs at older age level ($p < .05$).

[b] Differences among groups at younger age level not significant; Ns > PAs > PIs at older age level ($p < .05$).

[c] Differences among groups at younger age level not significant; Ns > PAs and PIs at older age level ($p < .05$).

[d] Differences among groups at younger age level not significant; Ns > PIs at older age level ($p < .05$).

[e] Ns and PAs > PIs at both age levels ($p < .05$).

[f] Ns > PAs and PIs at younger age level ($p < .05$); Ns > PAs > PIs at older age level ($p < .05$).

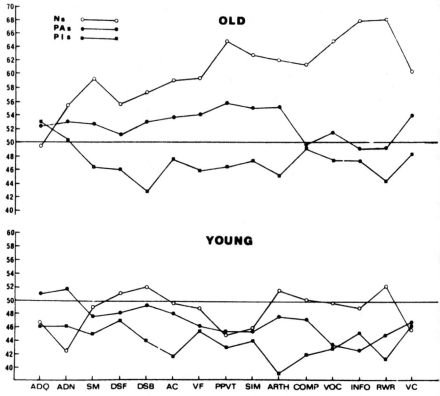

FIG. 7-1. Graphic illustration of mean standardized *T* scores for Ns, PAs, and PIs at each age level. (Abbreviations: ADQ and ADN, Goldman–Fristoe–Woodcock Test of Auditory Discrimination under quiet and noise conditions, respectively; SM, Sentence Memory Test; DSF, WISC Digit Span—forward subtest; DSB, WISC Digit Span—backward subtest; AC, Auditory Closure Test; VF, Verbal Fluency Test; PPVT, Peabody Picture Vocabulary Test; SIM, WISC Similarities subtest; ARTH, WISC Arithmetic subtest; COMP, WISC Comprehension subtest; VOC, WISC Vocabulary subtest; INFO, WISC Information subtest; RWR, WRAT Reading subtest; VC, Higgins–Wertman Test of Visual Closure.) (From J. E. Sweeney & B. P. Rourke, Neuropsychological significance of phonetically accurate and phonetically inaccurate spelling errors in younger and older retarded spellers. *Brain and Language*, 1978, *6*, 212–225. Reprinted by permission.)

Visual Closure (which requires visualizing common objects on the basis of pictorial clues and identifying them verbally) would suggest that a specific deficit in this type of language-related "visualizing" is not responsible for the spelling difficulties encountered by PAs.

Most of the intergroup differences in performance among the Ns,

PAs, and PIs that emerged as statistically significant were evident at the older age level. Older PIs performed at levels significantly inferior to those of older Ns on the following tasks requiring auditory–verbal receptive skills: Sentence Memory Test, WISC Digit Span—backward, and Auditory Closure Test. When the special requirements of each test are examined (i.e., Sentence Memory Test, repetition of meaningful word strings; Auditory Closure Test, blending and synthesis of speech sounds; WISC Digit Span—backward, reversal of numerical sequences), it would seem that only rather basic, straightforward linguistic operations are involved in these tasks. That older PIs are significantly deficient in such relatively elementary skills attests to the profound nature of their psycholinguistic handicap.

Since the performances of PAs were not significantly different from those of Ns at the older age level on the Sentence Memory Test, the WISC Digit Span—backward subtest, and the Auditory Closure Test, and since the performance of older PAs was superior to that of older PIs on the WISC Digit Span—backward measure, it would seem that, at least at the older age level, PAs are as adept as are Ns in these relatively basic psycholinguistic operations.

It would be expected that the apparent deficiency of older PIs in carrying out rudimentary receptive linguistic operations would be extremely debilitating with respect to language development in general. Indeed, this would appear to be reflected by the findings that the performances of the older PIs were significantly inferior to those of older Ns on somewhat more complex measures of psycholinguistic skills: the Verbal Fluency Test, the PPVT, and the WISC Similarities, Arithmetic, Comprehension, Vocabulary, and Information subtests. In addition, the pervasive deficiencies in language functioning exhibited by older PIs are consistent with the reported relationship between a preponderance of phonetically inaccurate spelling errors and a relatively low WISC Verbal IQ in children (Nelson & Warrington, 1974) and dysphasia in adult patients (Newcombe, 1969; Kinsbourne & Warrington, 1964).

The investigation of the possible psycholinguistic deficiencies of PAs in this study was largely exploratory, since very little information was available regarding the adaptive significance of this form of spelling. A review of the pattern of performances of PAs at the older age level revealed some interesting relationships between this pattern and the performances of the Ns and PIs. The performances of the PAs were (1) equivalent to those of Ns and superior to those of PIs on the Verbal

Fluency Test and the WISC Similarities and Arithmetic subtests; (2) inferior to those of Ns and superior to those of PIs on the PPVT; and (3) inferior to those of Ns and equivalent to those of PIs on the WISC Comprehension, Vocabulary, and Information subtests.

PAs performed at levels similar to those of Ns on tests in which the correct responses can be brief, single-word answers. In contrast, the levels of performance of PAs became undistinguishable from those of PIs and inferior to those of Ns on those measures (WISC Comprehension, Vocabulary and Information) in which (1) the formulation of a fairly complex answer to a question is required, and (2) the correct answer cannot be determined by utilizing only information contained in the question itself. It would appear that PAs, at least at the older age level, "join the ranks" of the linguistically deficient PIs when they attempt to encode relatively complex word strings and to extrapolate cognitively beyond the verbal information given. However, such a conclusion would not account satisfactorily for the performance of PAs on the PPVT (which was superior to that of PIs and inferior to that of Ns at the older age level). Since an overt verbal response is not required on the PPVT, the possibility that features of the task other than verbal encoding limit the performance of PAs must be considered. The requirement of this task is to examine visual–spatial pictorial information while using as a basis for such an examination the meaning of a specific word presented through the auditory modality. It may be that PAs, relative to Ns, have particular difficulty in associating the spoken word with visual–spatial information. This requirement may have been enough to begin to mirror the deficiency of this subtype of disabled speller.

To summarize the results of our study (Sweeney & Rourke, 1978) thus far, it would appear that (1) older PIs exhibit a significant deficiency in carrying out very basic, receptive linguistic operations, and (2) older PAs experience significant difficulty in associating the spoken word with an analysis of visual–spatial information, relating the verbal information provided with other information, and encoding relatively complex word strings in response to verbal information provided. It would be expected that PIs would experience considerable difficulty in performing phonemic operations, including phonemic segmentation, in the process of spelling. Luria (1980) describes similar difficulties in adult patients with lesions of the secondary zone of the left temporal lobe, in that they exhibit particular problems in phonemic analysis and synthesis. This linguistic deficiency exhibited by PIs would seem to be so pervasive as to seriously undermine the general development of language skills. The psycholinguistic deficiencies of PAs would appear to be much less debilitating in terms of general language development. The nature of their difficulties is reminiscent of those impairments that Luria (1980) suggests are associated with lesions of the so-called tertiary zone (the parietal–temporal–occipital region) of the left hemisphere. Patients with lesions in this cortical region often have difficulty selecting appropriate graphemes to represent the spoken word, although they can comprehend the word quite well. Furthermore, in the case of PAs, a lack of appreciation for the visual–spatial features of word configurations would seem to result in a rigid adherence to a sound–symbol associational system, with little regard as to whether or not a word "looks right." Such a disturbance would also be expected to interfere significantly with performances on tasks that require (1) the association of the spoken word with visual–spatial pictorial information (e.g., the PPVT), and (2) "visualizing" on the basis of current and previously obtained information (e.g., WISC Arithmetic and Comprehension). At this stage in development, "visualizing" may very well be part of the process of decoding and encoding word strings in order to facilitate the formulation and provision of appropriate, relatively complex verbal responses (as required on the WISC Information, Comprehension, and Vocabulary tests).

The levels of performance of PIs and PAs in the 1978 study were similar to those of Ns at the younger age level on the WRAT Reading subtest. At the older age level, the performances of these three spelling groups on this measure differed in the order PIs < PAs < Ns. These findings are consistent with the results of studies by Nelson and Warrington (1974) and Burgher and Rourke (1976), in which a preponderance of phonetically inaccurate spelling errors was found to be associated with marked reading disability. The latter study was longitudinal in design and compared the number of phonetically inaccurate spelling errors of disabled readers with those of normal readers in Grades 2, 4, 5, and 6. The persistence of a relationship between reading disability and phonetic inaccuracy in spelling over a time span of 4 years in the Burgher and Rourke (1976) study and the poor reading performance of PIs in the 1978 study would suggest that phonetic inaccuracy in spelling is a reliable indicator and predictor of serious reading problems. Furthermore, the impact of phonetic inaccuracy on reading disability seems to have progressively more serious effects over the developmental epochs investigated. In this sense, the dimension that would seem to underlie phonetic inaccuracy in PIs (namely, a deficiency in carrying out receptive linguistic operations, including phonemic synthesis and segmentation) would appear to constitute a "deficit" vis-à-vis reading that does not resolve with age (Rourke, 1976).

Consideration of the apparent deficiency of older PAs in carrying out cognitive processes that involve extrapolating beyond the verbal information provided may be of some assistance in accounting for the oral reading performances of PAs relative to PIs and Ns, at least at the older age level. PAs may encounter difficulty in oral reading when they are required to retrieve a phonemic sequence that is not exactly congruent with the graphic representation of the word, thus rendering them inferior to Ns in reading words with a low phoneme–grapheme correspondence. The superiority of PAs over PIs in reading performance at the older age level may be due to the presumed efficiency with which PAs are able to read words that have a high phoneme–grapheme correspondence. The similarity in degree of deficiency in oral reading for PIs and PAs at the younger age level is not accounted for as readily, given the paucity of differences in levels of psycholinguistic skill development found among the younger PIs, PAs, and Ns in this study. The only measure that discriminated significantly among these groups was the WISC Arithmetic subtest, where the performances of PIs were significantly inferior to those of PAs and Ns. It is of interest that, of all the dependent measures employed, only the Arithmetic subtest would seem to require a well-structured, systematic approach to the analysis of linguistic information that is routinely taught in school. Phonemic segmentation is another well-structured linguistic process that is routinely taught in the academic situation. It may be that younger PIs are relatively deficient in oral reading because they are not able to develop, through instruction, the ability to perform these linguistic operations. The apparent success of PAs in learning such explicit operations and the presumed rigidity that characterizes their application of them may explain the efficient performance of PAs on the WISC Arithmetic subtest (for which, at these fairly elementary levels, cognitive rigidity may be a "positive" attribute) and, at least in part, may explain their inefficient performance on the WRAT Reading subtest (for which rigidity in applying a system of symbol–sound associations may, to some extent, be a handicap).

The marked similarity in levels of psycholinguistic skill development among PIs, PAs, and Ns at the younger age level should also be considered. It may be that a crucial stage of developmental maturity has yet to be reached, and/or that formal instruction in carrying out specific linguistic and psycholinguistic operations is necessary before the differential capacity for the execution of such operations becomes apparent.

RESULTS OF LATER STUDIES

We (Sweeney, McCabe, & Rourke, 1978) carried out a study designed specifically to investigate further the possible difficulty of younger PIs in benefiting from formal instruction in the systematic processing of verbal information. The performances of PIs, PAs, and Ns at the younger age level on a revised version of the Logico-Grammatical Sentence Comprehension Test (Wiig & Semel, 1974) were compared. This test was chosen as the dependent measure for the study because it is composed of subtests that appear to involve the comprehension of linguistic concepts that require logical operations—dimensions that much of the elementary-school program is aimed at enhancing through formal instruction. The test consists of five subtests of 10 questions each, which represent the following grammatical relationships: (1) comparative (e.g., "Are watermelons bigger than apples?"); (2) temporal (e.g., "Does lunch come after breakfast?"); (3) passive (e.g., "John was hit by Eric. Was John hit?"); (4) spatial (e.g., "Pat came after James. Was James first?"); (5) familial (e.g., "Give another name for your mother's father").

The results of this study, as presented in Figure 7-2, were in line with our expectations: The performance of PIs was significantly inferior to the performance of Ns on the subtests of the Logico-Grammatical Sentence Comprehension Test. The performances of PAs did not differ statistically from those of PIs and Ns on this measure, and the relative performances of the groups did not change across subtests (i.e., the PIs < PAs < Ns relationship was maintained). The finding that PIs were deficient, relative to Ns, at the younger age level in comprehending grammatical relationships would lend support to the hypothesis generated on the basis of the results of our earlier study (Sweeney & Rourke, 1978): PIs encounter significant difficulty in carrying out relatively rudimentary operations on language, and this hampers their capacity to benefit from formal academic instruction in the processing of verbal information.

A more direct test of the hypothesis that PIs experience difficulty in carrying out basic linguistic operations was undertaken in another study (Coderre, Sweeney, & Rourke, 1979). Moreover, we attempted in this

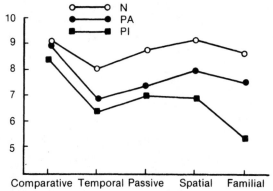

FIG. 7-2. Graphic illustration of mean scores for Ns, PAs, and PIs on subtests of the Logico-Grammatical Sentence Comprehension Test.

study to examine a different hypothesis generated on the basis of the earlier (Sweeney & Rourke, 1978) results: PAs experience a deficiency in transcending or going beyond the verbal information provided when required to do so. The age range of 9–11 years used in this study approximated the "younger" age range (i.e., 9–10.5 years) employed in the 1978 study. The performances of groups ($n = 8$) of PIs, PAs, and Ns on tests of phonemic segmentation and the ability to recognize words with a low grapheme–phoneme correspondence were compared. It was expected that PIs would encounter relative difficulty in segmenting words phonemically, and that PAs would be deficient, relative to Ns, in recognizing the correct graphic representation of words with a low grapheme–phoneme correspondence. Measures of visual memory were also included in this study in order to assess this ability in PAs, since Boder (1973) has suggested that the child who spells in a phonetically accurate manner "has a poor memory for visual 'gestalts.'"

The Phonemic Segmentation Test, constructed for this study, involved presenting to the subject a tape recording of a list of words read by a local elementary-school teacher. Prior to testing, each of these words had been analyzed phonemically, utilizing a symbol system developed for the earlier (Sweeney & Rourke, 1978) study (e.g., "cat" is represented by the phonemic sequence "k/ae/t"). As each word was presented, the subject was required to analyze aloud the phonemic composition of the word. The examiner checked each phoneme produced against the phoneme represented on the scoring form.

The Spelling Recognition Test, also constructed for this study, consisted of items that were made up of four printed words. Three of these words were characterized by a high sound-to-letter correspondence; one of the words was correctly spelled and the other two were incorrectly spelled, but in a phonetically accurate fashion. A fourth word that was unrelated to the other three words was included as a distractor item; this word was included because Boder (1973) suggests that phonetically inaccurate spellers sometimes guess at words on the basis of minimal cues (e.g., word length). A sample item of this test is as follows: "lewse, looss, loose, cake." Each word was presented via the tape-recorded dictation of an elementary-school teacher native to the region where the study was conducted. Each word was dictated, then presented in a sentence, then dictated again. The subject was asked to underline the correct word among the four alternatives presented in random order.

Modifications of the Cloze Procedure (Anderson, 1976) and the Visual Memory Test (Vellutino, Steger, DeSotto, & Phillips, 1975) were employed to assess visual memory or, more specifically, the ability of the subjects to appreciate the "gestalt" of words in reading and to remember the visual–spatial features of graphic configurations. In the modification of the Cloze Procedure for this study, vowels were dropped from words in a sentence (e.g., "The d-g had a b-ne"). The child was required to determine which letters were missing in order to read the sentence aloud. The Visual Memory Test consisted of a sequential presentation of nine cards to the child. On the cards were configurations (which were referred to as "symbols") that the child was instructed to try to remember. Immediately after this presentation, the child was required to attempt to recognize these configurations from a response chart.

The results of this study are presented in Figure 7-3. PIs performed in a statistically inferior manner to PAs on the Phonemic Segmentation Test, suggesting that PIs have significant difficulty, relative to PAs, in analyzing phonemic information in a systematic fashion. It was interesting to note, however, that Ns scored at a level intermediate to that of PIs and PAs on this test, although their performance did not differ significantly from that of PIs or PAs. These results may reflect a propensity of PAs to adhere very strictly to a system of analysis that they have been previously trained to apply. The intermediate performance of Ns may suggest a less stringent application of the system of phonemic segmentation. This flexibility may allow for the utilization of other forms of language-related operations (e.g., "visualizing" the spatial features of the word to be spelled subsequent to phonemic segmentation).

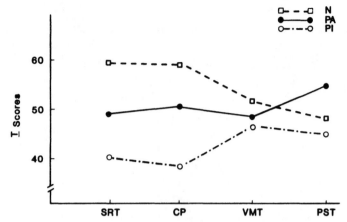

FIG. 7-3. Graphic illustration of mean standardized *T* scores for Ns, PAs, and PIs on measures used in the Coderre, Sweeney, and Rourke (1979) study. (Abbreviations: SRT, Spelling Recognition Test; CP, Cloze Procedure; VMT, Visual Memory Test; PST, Phonemic Segmentation Test.)

In this study, PAs were found to be significantly deficient, relative to Ns, in performance on the Spelling Recognition Test. Hence, it would appear that PAs encounter considerable difficulty in appreciating the correct graphic representations of words. It may be that a "phonetic style" of spelling may reflect an attempt to exploit the usefulness of phonemic information in order to compensate for a deficiency in the ability to assimilate and/or to utilize information regarding the visual features of word configurations.

In addition, it should also be noted that PIs performed in a significantly inferior manner to PAs on the Spelling Recognition Test, which is consistent with the finding that PIs are deficient in the ability to carry out relatively rudimentary operations on language (e.g., phonemic segmentation).

The observations of Boder (1973) that children who spell in a phonetically accurate fashion have deficient memory for the visual–spatial features of word configurations was supported by the deficient performance of PAs relative to Ns on our version of the Cloze Procedure. However, the level of performance of PAs was statistically similar to that of Ns on the Visual Memory Test. This discrepancy in the performance of PAs, relative to Ns, on these two measures may be accounted for by the following: (1) The Cloze Procedure involves an appreciation of the possible meaning of combinations of language (alphabetic) symbols (with which PAs seem to have difficulty, at least in situations that involve words with low correspondences between symbol and sound); and (2) the Visual Memory Test requires that the subject remember visual stimuli that have relatively limited symbolic significance—a task that would seem to have much in common with the requirements of some of the WISC Performance subtests that were used in this study as a control for psychometric intelligence.

The finding that PAs were significantly deficient, relative to Ns, in choosing the correct graphic representation of words with a low grapheme–phoneme correspondence in the Coderre, Sweeney, and Rourke (1979) study is consistent with the observation of Boder (1973) that children who spell in a phonetically accurate manner appear to analyze words in a phonetic fashion when reading. In an attempt to examine this possibility further, we (Sweeney & Rourke, 1982) administered the Diagnostic Screening Procedure for Developmental Dyslexia (Boder, 1973), which was adapted to accommodate Grades 7 and 8, to the groups of PIs, PAs, and Ns used in our earlier study (Sweeney & Rourke, 1978). The modified version of this test consists of 20 words at each of 10 grade levels from the preprimer level to Grade 8. Beginning with the preprimer level, each word on a card was "flashed" in front of the subject for 1 second. If he/she was able to read it, the word was recorded as having been read "by sight." If he/she was unable to read it, the word was presented again for 10 seconds. The word was recorded as having been read by phonetic analysis if the subject was able to read it correctly under the latter condition. Testing was discontinued when the subject failed to read 12 consecutive words under both conditions.

Since PAs may utilize a rigid phonetic style when reading, it was anticipated that PAs would exhibit a significantly higher frequency of correct phonetic reading as compared with Ns on this measure. Correspondingly, it was also expected that PAs would read significantly fewer words correctly "by sight," relative to Ns.

The analyses revealed that, as expected, PAs read significantly more words through phonetic analysis and significantly fewer words "by sight" than did Ns at both age levels. Hence, it would appear that PAs, relative to Ns, rely heavily upon phonetic analysis and de-emphasize a sight-word strategy in reading words.

In this study, it was interesting to note that the relative position of PIs in the frequency of employing a phonetic strategy was different at the two age levels: They did so at a significantly lower level than that of the PAs and Ns at the younger age level, and they did so at a level equivalent to that of PAs and significantly higher than that of Ns at the older age level. In attempting to account for these findings, it should be borne in mind that PIs tend to receive extra intensive instruction in the use of "phonics" in the formal academic situation, and they may develop a "set" to utilize a phonetic strategy in reading by the time they reach the older age level. Older PAs, however, have probably always utilized a rigid phonetic style in reading, and they may not abandon this strategy even when it would be appropriate to do so (as older Ns do).

IMPLICATIONS FOR REMEDIAL EDUCATION AND FURTHER RESEARCH

It would appear that linguistic demands of even an elementary sort (for example, those required for phonemic segmentation or synthesis) are sufficient to render PIs at a disadvantage, relative to PAs and Ns. On the other hand, the deficiencies of PAs do not seem to "emerge" until some extrapolation beyond the verbal information given is required—as, for example, when they are required to appreciate the correct graphic representation of words with a less than one-to-one phoneme–grapheme correspondence–or until they must retrieve factual verbal information and formulate a word string in which to convey the information to a listener. Since language requirements of the latter sort are similar to many of those demanded in the formal academic situation, it would seem quite likely that PIs and PAs would be indistinguishable in terms of a significant proportion of their classroom performances. This being the case, these two groups of disabled spellers would stand a good chance of being provided with similar programs of remedial education, although very different remedial strategies would seem to be warranted on the basis of their distinctive neuropsychological ability profiles.

The limited ability of PIs to carry out very specific operations on linguistic information (e.g., phonemic segmentation) suggests that this subtype of disabled spellers would encounter significant difficulty (1) in learning the rudiments of applying such operations to specific verbal information, including single words, through conventional classroom instruction; and (2) in generalizing from such conventional instruction to new verbal information, including unfamiliar words. Whatever language or language-related operations are being taught in the academic situation, it is unlikely that PIs would be able to execute a specific linguistic operation on any information other than extremely elementary, over-learned, and redundant oral discourse. With this in mind, it may be appropriate to provide PIs with the opportunity to "operate" excessively on each word to be learned (e.g., by synthesizing repeatedly the individual speech sounds of the words presented in sequence, and by segmenting repeatedly the phonemic composition of the word presented orally). Once these operations can be carried out efficiently on a particular word, it would probably also be beneficial to develop the ability to read the word "by sight" in order to promote fluency in reading. However, if concentrated training in the application of these basic operations on unfamiliar words should prove fruitless, it would seem reasonable to consider restricting instruction to intensive involvement in developing a sight-word strategy in reading.

Given that PAs may exploit the usefulness of phonetic and phonemic information (resulting in a slow, "plodding" approach to reading and spelling, with concomitant difficulty in decoding words to be read and assimilating and/or utilizing information regarding the correct graphic forms of words), it may be of assistance to utilize remedial methods involving intensive visual analysis, such as those referred to by Bakker, Moerland, and Goekoop-Hoefkens (1981) as "right hemispheral strate-gies": (1) to focus directly and intensively upon the development of a sight-word strategy in reading; (2) to attempt to increase the salience of the visual–spatial features of word configurations, especially if these are relatively unfamiliar and have a low phoneme–grapheme correspondence; and (3) to encourage the child to "visualize" the graphic features of words to be spelled and to attend deliberately to whether or not a word repro-duced graphically "looks right."

The sight-word vocabulary of PAs may be enhanced through "flash-card" exercises; through activities that require the child to recognize words in tachistoscopic presentations that gradually decrease in exposure time; and through exercises in which the child is required to read aloud simultaneously with the instructor and, as a result of a gradual reduction in reading rate by the instructor, to take the lead in oral reading. Requiring the child (1) to trace repetitiously the spatial features of relatively unfamiliar words made from sandpaper while blindfolded and while repeating the word, and (2) to write out these words correctly and repetitiously while repeating the word may increase the salience of the physical forms of word configurations.

In order to increase the likelihood that PAs will assimilate verbal information and then "go beyond" it, multisensory teaching in conjunction with dramatization should be employed whenever possible. The utilization of previously learned information to extrapolate from limited amounts of verbal information may be enhanced through the multidetermined images that such training may provide.

Investigating the development of linguistic and cognitive abilities in those who exhibit qualitatively distinct spelling disorders would seem to be a fruitful course to follow in delineating underlying deficiencies, with a view to the formulation of a specific plan of remediation. It should be emphasized, however, that the patterns of abilities and deficits emerging from the results of the studies reviewed, and the associated remedial strategies presented herein, are not considered to be exhaustive. Replications of these studies and additional investigations geared to specifying further the nature of the deficits related to different types of spelling disorders would certainly appear to be warranted.

In the case of PIs, questions remain as to whether maximum difficulty is encountered in learning to carry out basic linguistic operations, whether the principal problem is one of generalizing from successful specific applications of linguistic operations, or whether the apparent linguistic handicap of PIs involves major contributions from deficiencies in both of these areas. Furthermore, the possibility should be investigated that some PIs encounter instability rather than a clear deficiency in carrying out rudimentary linguistic operations, and that the achievement of stabilization over time for these PIs encourages a rigid application of such operations similar to that seen for PAs.

In addition, the results of this series of studies of disabled spellers has not, thus far, provided any clear picture as to whether the apparent difficulty exhibited by PAs in "going beyond" the verbal information provided results from a general deficiency in the ability to assimilate useful information, or whether the problem involves difficulty in retrieving and/or utilizing information (primarily of the visual–spatial variety) to which they have previously been exposed. It is possible that both factors may be operative in one subtype of learning-disabled child who exhibits phonetically accurate spelling errors but who spells at a normal level (see Strang & Rourke, Chapters 8 and 14, this volume). Furthermore, it is also possible that PAs themselves are differentiable into two or more sub-types, with each subtype exhibiting a different pattern of neuropsychological abilities and deficits. Finally, it is clear that the suggestions regarding remedial educational strategies for PIs and PAs that have been derived from the results of the research reviewed herein must be subjected to empirical test through well-controlled outcome studies of the sort suggested by Lyon (see Chapter 11, this volume).

REFERENCES

Anderson, J. *Psycholinguistic experiments in foreign language testing.* Queensland, St. Lucia: University of Queensland Press, 1976.

Bakker, D. J., Moerland, R., & Goekoop-Hoefkens, M. Effects of hemisphere-specific stimulation on the reading performance of dyslexic boys: A pilot study. *Journal of Clinical Neuropsychology,* 1981, *3*, 155–159.

Bannatyne, A. D., & Wichiarojote, P. Relationships between written spelling, motor functioning, and sequencing skills. *Journal of Learning Disabilities,* 1969, *2*, 4–16.

Benton, A. L. *Sentence Memory Test.* Iowa City, Iowa: Author, 1965.

Boder, E. Developmental dyslexia: A diagnostic approach based on three atypical reading–spelling patterns. *Developmental Medicine and Child Neurology,* 1973, *15*, 663–687.

Burgher, P. L., & Rourke, B. P. *Comparison of the phonetic accuracy of spelling errors of normal and retarded readers: A four-year follow-up.* Unpublished study, University of Windsor, 1976.

Coderre, D. J., Sweeney, J. E., & Rourke, B. P. *Spelling recognition, word analysis, and visual memory in children with qualitatively distinct types of spelling errors.* Unpublished study, University of Windsor and Windsor Western Hospital Centre, 1979.

Dunn, L. M. *Peabody Picture Vocabulary Test.* Minneapolis: American Guidance Service, 1965.

Dykman, R. A., Ackerman, P. T., Clements, S. D., & Peters, J. E. Specific learning disabilities: An attentional deficit syndrome. In H. R. Myklebust (Ed.), *Progress in learning disabilities* (Vol. 2). New York: Grune & Stratton, 1971.

Goldman, R., Fristoe, M., & Woodcock, R. W. *Goldman–Fristoe–Woodcock Test of Auditory Discrimination.* Circle Pines, Minn.: American Guidance Service, 1970.

Higgins, C., & Wertman, H. *Higgins–Wertman Test of Visual Closure.* Albany, N.Y.: Authors, 1968.

Jastak, J. F., & Jastak, S. R. *The Wide Range Achievement Test.* Wilmington, Del.: Guidance Associates, 1965.

Kass, C. E., Auditory Closure Test. In J. J. Olson & J. L. Olson (Eds.), *Validity studies on the Illinois Test of Psycholinguistic Abilities.* Madison, Wisc.: Photo Press, 1964.

Kinsbourne, M. Mimimal brain dysfunction as a neurodevelopmental lag. *Annals of the New York Academy of Science,* 1973, *205*, 268–273.

Kinsbourne, M., & Warrington, E. K. Disorders of spelling. *Journal of Neurology, Neurosurgery and Psychiatry,* 1964, *27*, 224–228.

Luria, A. R. *Higher cortical functions in man.* New York: Basic Books, 1980.

Nelson, H. E., & Warrington, E. K. Developmental spelling retardation and its relation to other cognitive abilities. *British Journal of Psychology,* 1974, *65*, 265–274.

Newcombe, F. *Missile wounds to the brain.* London: Oxford University Press, 1969.

Newton, B. M. A study of certain factors related to achievement in spelling. *Alberta Journal of Educational Research,* 1961, *7,* 202–208.

Rourke, B. P. Reading retardation in children: Developmental lag or deficit? In R. M. Knights & D. J. Bakker (Eds.), *Neuropsychology of learning disorders: Theoretical approaches.* Baltimore: University Park Press, 1976.

Russell, D. H. A second study of characteristics of good and poor spellers. *Journal of Educational Psychology,* 1955, *46,* 129–141.

Strong, R. T. *Verbal Fluency Test.* Phoenix, Ariz.: Author.

Sweeney, J. E., McCabe, A. E., & Rourke, B. P. *Logical-grammatical abilities of retarded spellers.* Unpublished study, Windsor Western Hospital Centre and University of Windsor, 1978.

Sweeney, J. E., & Rourke, B. P. Neuropsychological significance of phonetically accurate and phonetically inaccurate spelling errors in younger and older retarded spellers. *Brain and Language,* 1978, *6,* 212–225.

Sweeney, J. E., & Rourke, B. P. *Reading strategies of qualitatively distinct disabled spellers.* Unpublished study, District of Parry Sound Child and Family Centre and Windsor Western Hospital Centre, 1982.

Vellutino, F. R., Steger, J. A., DeSotto, L., & Phillips, F. Immediate and delayed recognition of visual stimuli in poor and normal readers. *Journal of Experimental Child Psychology,* 1975, *19,* 223–232.

Wechsler, D. *Wechsler Intelligence Scale for Children.* New York: Psychological Corporation, 1949.

Wiig, E. H., & Semel, E. M. Development of comprehension of logico-grammatical sentences by grade school children. *Perceptual and Motor Skills,* 1974, *38,* 171–176.

Winer, B. J. *Statistical principles in experimental design.* New York: McGraw-Hill, 1962.

8

Arithmetic Disability Subtypes: The Neuropsychological Significance of Specific Arithmetical Impairment in Childhood

JOHN D. STRANG
BYRON P. ROURKE

AN OVERVIEW OF ARITHMETIC DISABILITIES

Mechanical arithmetic is a very complex academic subject. In the case of even rather simple calculations, a mistake made at any point in the operation will most often result in an error. The same does not hold true for reading: It is quite possible to gain an appreciation for the gist of a sentence or passage even when a number of words have been misread or skipped over. In fact, it is often found that the reading comprehension abilities of the young reading-disabled child who tends to perform quite well in mechanical arithmetic will appear to exceed his/her ability to decode individual words. Viewed from another perspective, the latter "type" of learning-impaired child may be able to gain a basic understanding for a sentence or passage even when he/she cannot read all of the words in it.

Performance in mechanical arithmetic is complicated further by two matters: (1) A change in just one digit in a proposed calculation can

John D. Strang. Department of Neuropsychology, Windsor Western Hospital Centre, Windsor, Ontario, Canada.
Byron P. Rourke. Department of Psychology, University of Windsor, and Department of Neuropsychology, Windsor Western Hospital Centre, Windsor, Ontario, Canada.

substantially alter the requirements of the operation; and (2) even seemingly simple mechanical arithmetic calculation involves many steps, rules, and facts about numbers. For instance, there are no less than 33 steps involved in arriving at a correct solution to the problem $62 \times 96 = ?$ (the first step involves "reading the sign," the second step is to "go to the right side of the question," etc.). With this in mind, it would stand to reason that a wide variety of neuropsychological impairments could contribute to a situation in which a child experiences difficulty with the acquisition or application of mechanical arithmetic skills.

Aside from the debilitating effects of central processing deficiencies, children may perform poorly on tests of mechanical arithmetic simply because they have not had enough experience with the subject matter. For example, it is common to find that young learning-disabled children who are referred for special class placement because of reading and/or spelling impairment do not receive the same type, level, or amount of instruction in mechanical arithmetic as do children in the "regular" class setting. In this connection, we have found that children who exhibit rather specific reading and spelling impairments tend (1) to make few errors on the Arithmetic subtest of the Wide Range Achievement Test (WRAT; Jastak & Jastak, 1965) and (2) to leave undone those questions that are obviously beyond their current realm of expertise (Rourke & Strang, 1983). It is most often readily apparent that these (specifically) reading- and spelling-disabled children are quite unfamiliar with those (age-appropriate) mathematical operations that they do not attempt, and that fairly straightforward teaching of the essential aspects of these operations very often eventuates in rapid acquisition of skills.

Children who are poorly motivated, highly anxious, or otherwise emotionally disturbed may also perform particularly poorly on tests of mechanical arithmetic abilities. Slade and Russell (1971) reported that emotionally disturbed children may exhibit very poorly developed mechanical arithmetic abilities (or poor performances on tests of those abilities). We have also witnessed this particular state of affairs frequently in our clinical work.

With all of this in mind, it was not surprising that Badian (1983) found that 6.4% of the children in Grades 1 through 8 in a small ($n = 1476$) U.S. town exhibited poor achievement in mathematics, while only 4.9% were considered to be poor in reading. Along these same lines, we found that three ($n = 20$ in each group) groups of randomly selected (8-, 10-, and

12-year-old) learning-disabled children who were referred to our department for neuropsychological assessment because of academic (primarily reading and spelling) difficulties performed very poorly on the WRAT Arithmetic subtest (Strang & Rourke, 1985). Based on these findings and the other information presented to this point in this chapter, we might expect that many learning-disabled children have less than age-appropriate mechanical arithmetic skills.

The results of a study by Tuoko (1982) offer some insight into the reason for the prevalence of arithmetic underachievers among the population of learning-disabled children at large. She found that children who were hampered by verbal-memory problems (which are commonly exhibited by a number of subtypes of learning-disabled children) were particularly susceptible to having difficulties with the acquisition and utilization of mechanical arithmetic skills. When one considers the number of facts, steps, and procedures that must be remembered in order to complete even a relatively simple mechanical arithmetic calculation, the potential impact of a verbal-memory disorder on performance in arithmetic can be appreciated.

Most children who have verbal-memory problems typically exhibit academic impairments that go beyond mechanical arithmetic difficulties. For example, Rourke and Finlayson (1978) found that a group of children who exhibited evidence of rather outstanding verbal-memory impairment had exceptionally poor reading and spelling skills. Moreover, we have found that virtually any instructional situation that involves the management of relatively large amounts of novel or otherwise complex information can pose particular difficulties for a child who has a memory problem.

If a child's mechanical arithmetic skills are limited as a result of a verbal-memory impairment, it would seem reasonable to propose that the development of these skills would be enhanced simply by providing him/her with a chart containing common arithmetic tables (number facts) and other "key" reminders for the implementation of specific arithmetical operations. It would also be helpful for this type of child to overlearn, by whatever means possible, the steps involved in common mathematical procedures. For the most part, these types of interventions work best when verbal instructions are largely eschewed in favor of demonstrations and other modes of communication that emphasize the delivery of information through the visual (and sometimes tactile) modalities.

SUBTYPES OF ARITHMETIC-IMPAIRED CHILDREN:
A SERIES OF STUDIES

Among the population of children who experience learning difficulties due to central processing deficiencies, we have investigated a group of children who exhibit rather specific difficulties with mechanical arithmetic (Rourke & Finlayson, 1978; Rourke & Strang, 1978; Strang & Rourke, 1983). Remedial recommendations would not appear to be so relatively straightforward for this subgroup of learning-impaired children. The preliminary findings of a follow-up study (Rourke, Young, Strang, & Russell, 1985) of arithmetic-impaired adults ($n = 8$), who exhibited a pattern of neuropsychological strengths and weaknesses that is characteristic of the (specifically arithmetic-impaired) children to be described in this chapter, indicated that not one of these persons scored better than the Grade 7.1 level on the WRAT Arithmetic subtest, even though seven of the eight subjects had received some form of postsecondary education. In fact, four of the arithmetic-impaired adults had earned undergraduate (Bachelor of Arts) university degrees. Certainly, the rather specific and profound arithmetic impairment of this subgroup of persons suggests the need for thorough-going remedial interventions in childhood, which should go well beyond arithmetic tables and "key" reminders.

We have completed three neuropsychological studies that have highlighted the characteristics of the group of children who exhibit specific difficulties with mechanical arithmetic. In the first two studies in this series (Rourke & Finlayson, 1978; Rourke & Strang, 1978), three groups of children selected on the basis of their patterns of performance on the WRAT Reading, Spelling, and Arithmetic subtests were compared. Group 1 was composed of children who were uniformly deficient in reading, spelling, and arithmetic; children in Group 2 were relatively adept (though still impaired, relative to age norms) at arithmetic, as compared with their performance in reading and spelling; Group 3 was composed of children whose reading and spelling performances were average or above, but whose arithmetic performance was quite deficient. The performances of these three groups of children were compared on a number of auditory–perceptual, verbal, and visual–perceptual–organizational variables (Rourke & Finlayson, 1978) and measures of motor, psychomotor, and tactile–perceptual abilities (Rourke & Strang, 1978). There were 15 9- to 14-year-old right-handed children whose Wechsler Intelligence Scale for Children

(WISC) Full Scale IQs fell within the 86–114 range in each group. All subjects had attended school regularly since they were 6 years of age. On the basis of information derived from their social and medical histories and school records, none of the subjects were (1) reported to be in need of psychiatric treatment for an emotional disorder, (2) considered to be "culturally deprived," or (3) hampered by defective vision or hearing.

Group 1 was composed of children whose WRAT Reading, Spelling, and Arithmetic grade-equivalent scores were at least 2.0 years behind their expected grade placement. In no case did the WRAT Reading, Spelling, and Arithmetic centile scores for subjects in Group 1 exceed 18, nor was there more than a 0.9 grade-equivalent discrepancy between any two of the three WRAT subjects for subjects in this group. Group 2 was composed of 15 subjects whose WRAT Reading and Spelling grade-equivalent scores were at least 1.8 years below their WRAT Arithmetic grade-equivalent scores. In no case did the WRAT Reading and Spelling centile scores exceed 14 for subjects in Group 2. Group 3 was composed of 15 subjects whose WRAT Reading and Spelling grade-equivalent scores exceeded their WRAT Arithmetic grade-equivalent scores by at least 2.0 years. These three groups were equated for age and WISC Full Scale IQ. In Group 1, there were 2 girls and 13 boys; all subjects in Group 2 were boys; there were 4 girls and 11 boys in Group 3. The unequal sex distribution in the three groups was not considered to pose any particular difficulty, because the results of a study conducted in our laboratory (Canning, Orr, & Rourke, 1980) would suggest that no sex difference for children with learning disabilities should be expected on measures employed in these two studies or for those employed in the third study (Strang & Rourke, 1983) in this series.

Group 2 and particularly Group 3 children are of most interest to us in this chapter, for the following reasons: (1) They exhibit contrasting patterns of academic abilities; (2) the performances of these two groups of children on our neuropsychological test battery reveal and accentuate the underlying difficulties that can lead to specific and often profound impairment in mechanical arithmetic; and (3) these two groups of children had virtually equally impaired levels of performance on the WRAT Arithmetic subtest, but vastly different levels of performance in word recognition and spelling. With respect to the last-named reason, and based on the combined results of the three studies in this series, it has been suggested strongly that Group 2 and Group 3 children perform poorly (well below age expectation) in mechanical arithmetic for very different ability-based reasons (Strang & Rourke, 1983). Descriptive data for Group 2 and Group 3 children are presented in Table 8-1.

The results of the Rourke and Finlayson (1978) study indicated that children who exhibited relatively poor performances in arithmetic as compared to their levels of achievement in reading and spelling (Group 3) had generally well-developed auditory–perceptual and verbal skills and somewhat deficient visual–perceptual–organizational skills. On the other hand, children who were relatively adept at arithmetic as compared to their level of proficiency in reading and spelling (Group 2) scored well on tests of visual–perceptual–organizational abilities and relatively poorly on measures of verbal and, in particular, auditory–perceptual abilities. With respect to the latter, Group 2 children performed in a markedly impaired manner on tests of word blending (Auditory Closure Test; Kass, 1964), sound–symbol matching (Speech-Sounds Perception Test; Reitan & Davison, 1974), and sentence memory (Sentence Memory Test; Benton, 1965) skills.

We (Rourke & Strang, 1978) found that Group 2 and Group 3 children performed differently on measures of complex psychomotor abilities and on tests designed for the identification of tactile–perceptual impairments. Specifically, Group 2 children (who exhibited better-developed arithmetic than word-recognition and spelling skills) performed in at least an average fashion on measures of psychomotor abilities, although they exhibited relatively poor right-hand performance as compared with their left-hand performance on the Tactual Performance Test (TPT; Reitan & Davison, 1974); children in Group 3 (the group with specific WRAT Arithmetic problems) exhibited bilateral impairment on two measures of psycho-motor abilities (Grooved Pegboard Test and Maze Test; Kløve, 1963). The pattern of performance of Group 3 on the TPT was exactly opposite to that

TABLE 8-1. Means and Standard Deviations for Control Variables and WISC Verbal and Performance IQs

	Age (months)	WISC Full Scale IQ	WISC Verbal IQ	WISC Performance IQ	WRAT Reading	WRAT Spelling	WRAT Arithmetic
Group 2	143.67	99.20	92.27	107.20	2.34	2.51	4.86
	(18.52)	(7.31)	(7.08)	(8.98)	(0.42)	(0.39)	(0.70)
Group 3	140.93	95.00	102.20	87.93	8.47	7.74	4.25
	(18.53)	(5.74)	(6.65)	(7.61)	(1.90)	(1.92)	(1.08)

Note. Standard deviations appear in parentheses.

of Group 2 on this measure: Group 3 children exhibited normal right-hand TPT performance and impaired left-hand TPT performance. When both hands were used conjointly on the TPT, Group 3 children performed at a very poor level. Furthermore, children in Group 3 exhibited evidence of bilateral impairment on a composite measure of tactile–perceptual abilities; this tactile–perceptual impairment was more marked on the left side of the body. Group 2 children performed significantly better than did Group 3 children on this composite measure of tactile–perceptual abilities with the left hand.

In the third study in this series (Strang & Rourke, 1983), performances on the older children's version of the Halstead Category Test (Reitan & Davison, 1974) by Group 2 and Group 3 children were compared. This study was confined to the examination of only two (Group 2 and Group 3) of the three groups employed in the previous studies in this series, because the neuropsychological ability structures of these two groups appeared to be of particular theoretical interest (Rourke, 1982). The results of this investigation revealed that Group 3 children made significantly more errors on this test than did Group 2 children. Furthermore, while the level of performance of Group 2 children on this nonverbal problem-solving measure was quite age-appropriate, the general level of performance of Group 3 children was approximately one standard deviation below the mean, and Group 3 children performed especially poorly on those subtests that require a substantial degree of "higher-order" visual–spatial analysis.

The results of the Rourke and Finlayson (1978), Rourke and Strang (1978), and Strang and Rourke (1983) studies indicated that learning-disabled children who were relatively adept at the WRAT Arithmetic subtest as compared with their performances on the WRAT Reading and Spelling subtests (Group 2) performed poorly on measures of abilities ordinarily thought to be subserved primarily by the left cerebral hemisphere. Group 2 children performed much better (i.e., in an age-appropriate fashion) on measures of abilities ordinarily thought to be subserved primarily by the right cerebral hemisphere. The opposite state of affairs obtained for learning-disabled children who exhibited good performances on the WRAT Reading and Spelling subtests and poor performances on the WRAT Arithmetic subtest. These children (Group 3) performed poorly on measures of abilities ordinarily thought to be subserved primarily by the right cerebral hemisphere, and much better (i.e., in an age-appropriate manner) on measures of abilities ordinarily thought to be subserved primarily by the left cerebral hemisphere.

Figure 8-1 provides an overview of the general level and pattern of performance of Group 2 and Group 3 children on those neuropsychological measures that best differentiate the two groups. For the purposes of comparisons between the two groups and comparisons with normative scores (Knights, 1970; Knights & Norwood, 1980), the summary scores for each measure were converted into *T* scores, based on the normative means and standard deviations. It should be noted that an average score was derived (the mean of normative scores for 11- and 12-year-olds) for each of the dependent measures, because it was thought that this would be an approximate index of age expectation for Group 2 and Group 3 children. The *T* scores are plotted such that good performance is represented in one direction (above 50) and poor performance is represented in the opposite direction.

A qualitative analysis of the WRAT Arithmetic subtest performances of Group 3 children was undertaken to gain further insight into the specific nature of their arithmetic deficiencies. Before reporting the results of this investigation, it should be noted that a child's (or an adult's) errors in arithmetic may vary as a function of such variables as (1) the type of presentation (e.g., written vs. oral), (2) other sources of variability that are inherent in the testing situation itself (e.g., time limits), (3) the type and quality of instruction received in mechanical arithmetic, and (4) the person's age. With this in mind, a detailed qualitative analysis of a child's behavioral productions (e.g., arithmetic errors) can prove to be particularly informative when the productions are interpreted in light of the child's age and his/her particular pattern of neuropsychological strengths and weaknesses (Rourke, Bakker, Fisk, & Strang, 1983).

The results of a qualitative analysis of Group 3 children's arithmetic errors indicated that these children tended to make a large number and wide range of "types" of errors on the WRAT Arithmetic subtest. As would be expected, the type and, in some cases, the quality of errors varied somewhat with age. Nevertheless, it was found that some of the oldest children in Group 3 persisted in making the same types of errors as were found in the WRAT profiles of the younger (9-year-old) children in this group. To provide an overview of the most prevalent types of mechanical arithmetic errors that were found in the WRAT Arithmetic profiles of Group 3 children, these have been classified into seven overlapping categories as follows:

1. Spatial organization. Errors in spatial organization include misaligning numbers in columns (for example, in a two-digit multiplication

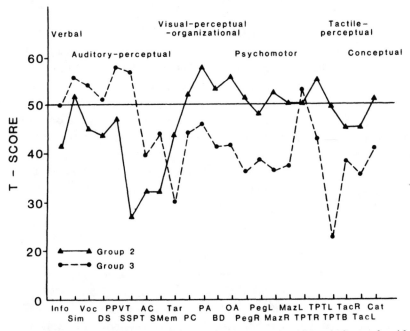

FIG. 8-1. Illustration of the level and pattern of performance for children in Groups 2 and 3 on a selection of neuropsychological measures. (Abbreviations: Info, WISC Information subtest; Sim, WISC Similarities subtest; Voc, WISC Vocabulary subtest; DS, WISC Digit Span subtest; PPVT, Peabody Picture Vocabulary Test; SSPT, Speech-Sounds Perception Test; AC, Auditory Closure Test; SMem, Sentence Memory Test; Tar, Target Test; PC, WISC Picture Completion subtest; PA, WISC Picture Arrangement subtest; BD, WISC Block Design subtest; OA, WISC Object Assembly subtest; PegR, Grooved Pegboard Test, right-hand performance; PegL, Grooved Pegboard Test, left-hand performance; MazR, Maze Test, right-hand performance; MazL, Maze Test, left-hand performance; TPTR, Tactual Performance Test, right-hand performance; TPTL, Tactual Performance Test, left-hand performance; TPTB, Tactual Performance Test, both-hands performance; TacR, Composite Score Tactile–Perceptual Abilities, right-hand performance; TacL, Composite Score Tactile–Perceptual Abilities, left-hand performance; Cat, Halstead Category Test.)

question) and any problem that a child might experience with directionality (e.g., subtracting the minuend from the subtrahend in a subtraction question).

2. Visual detail. Misreading the mathematical sign is an example of an error in visual detail. Failing to include required visual detail in the answer (e.g., a dollar sign or decimal place) may also be classified as a problem related to the appreciation of visual detail.

3. Procedural errors. In some cases, Group 3 children missed a step or added a step to a specific mechanical arithmetic procedure. In other instances, these children applied a learned rule for one mechanical arithmetic procedure to a dissimilar procedure (e.g., applying a rule used for multiplying a two-digit number by a single-digit number to a question involving the addition of a two-digit number to a single-digit number, as in $75 + 8 = 163$).

4. Failure to shift psychological set. When two or more operations of one kind (e.g., addition) were followed by an operation of another kind (e.g., subtraction), Group 3 children sometimes failed to shift set and proceeded to apply the practiced procedure (addition) to the new operation (subtraction). Certainly, some types of procedural errors (see above) can be associated with problems in shifting "psychological set" as well.

5. Graphomotor. It was sometimes observed in the WRAT profiles of Group 3 children that numbers were so poorly formed that they must have been difficult for the child to read. This problem appeared to have contributed directly to errors in some questions. Moreover, since children in this group tend, on the whole, to write with large, rather poorly formed numbers, it was not surprising to find that this led to crowding of a child's work (on the WRAT Arithmetic subtest there is only a fixed amount of space in which to complete each question) and resultant errors.

6. Memory. In some cases, it would appear that a child's error resulted from his/her failure to remember a particular number fact. It should be noted that this type of error was not predominant in the profiles of Group 3 children.

7. Judgment and reasoning. Children in this group typically attempted questions that were clearly beyond their current realm of expertise. In these cases, they produced solutions that were completely unreasonable in view of the task's demands. Unreasonable solutions were also found to be in evidence on questions for which there was some evidence that the child did understand the procedure (i.e., he/she had completed a similar question properly). For example, the answer in a subtraction question was found, in a number of cases, to be in excess of all of the other numbers in the question itself. In other instances, it was quite clear that the child failed to generate a reasonable plan of action when the requirements of a particular mechanical arithmetic question were only slightly different from procedures that the child obviously knew (on the basis of his/her other work). This failure to generalize a particular skill so that it can be adapted to a new, slightly different situation is a predominant feature of the general adaptational characteristics of Group 3 children. With these examples as background, it is evident that some questions can be raised about the (mathematical) judgment and reasoning skills of Group 3 children.

Some of these types of mechanical arithmetic errors can be found in the profiles of other arithmetic-impaired children who exhibit types and degrees of neuropsychological deficiencies that are somewhat different from those of children in Group 3. However, at this point in our investigations of the types of mechanical arithmetic errors exhibited by the various subgroups of children who have problems with arithmetic (e.g., Group 2 children), it would appear that the following characteristics distinguish Group 3 children in general:

1. They tend to make a wider range of types of mechanical arithmetic errors (as described above).

2. On average, they make more errors than do other children who perform poorly on tests of mechanical arithmetic. With respect to the latter, we found that Group 3 children made an average of 7.3 errors on the WRAT Arithmetic subtest. By way of contrast, Group 2 children tended to make few errors on the WRAT Arithmetic subtest, and a number of children were found to have performed without error. The majority of learning-disabled children of this age make no more than 3 or 4 errors on the WRAT Arithmetic subtest.

3. Group 3 children make a preponderance of mechanical arithmetic errors that are directly related to impaired judgment and reasoning. This finding is not particularly surprising when one considers the impaired level of performance obtained by Group 3 children on the Halstead Category Test, a measure that involves complex, nonverbal reasoning and concept-formation abilities (Strang & Rourke, 1983).

On the other hand, the Group 3 Halstead Category Test findings *do not explain* why these children have problems with mathematical concepts. To address this issue, one must consider the information-processing characteristics of Group 3 children (their neuropsychological strengths and weaknesses) from a perspective of developmental neuropsychology, while keeping in mind that it is highly likely that the majority of these children have exhibited the same general type of impairments since birth. To summarize our findings, children in Group 3 exhibited a general configuration of neuropsychological deficiencies that included the following: bilateral tactile–perceptual impairment (more pronounced on the left side of the body); bilateral psychomotor impairment (particularly with the left hand on the TPT); and poorly developed visual–perceptual–organizational abilities. When these impairments are viewed from a perspective of developmental neuropsychology, it would seem that it is precisely those abilities that are impaired in Group 3 children that are most important for the acquisition of adequate sensory–motor experience. Since Piaget (e.g., Piaget, 1928) and others have theorized that the development of nonverbal concept-formation and reasoning abilities are dependent upon the adequacy of a child's sensory–motor experience, it would follow that Group 3 children should exhibit signs of impairment of these abilities. In this view, the conceptual underpinnings and "building blocks" for the development of mathematical reasoning abilities for Group 3 children have failed to develop, at least in part because of inadequate sensory–motor experience.

When the significance of the particular configuration of neuropsychological characteristics exhibited by Group 3 children is considered further in terms of brain–behavior relationships, it is apparent that abilities ordinarily thought to be subserved primarily by the right cerebral hemisphere are impaired. It has been theorized recently (Goldberg & Costa, 1981; Rourke, 1982) that the formation of constructs and concepts is dependent upon right-hemisphere systems for its content. If right-hemisphere systems are dysfunctional from birth, and/or the systems are deprived of necessary experience for their development, then concept and construct development, in general, would be expected to be inadequate. Furthermore, construct- and concept-formation impairments would be expected to persist in the long run. Consequently, we should expect that remedial interventions for Group 3 children would be complex and long-term for academic subjects (such as arithmetic) that appear to require adequately developed right-hemisphere systems for success.

REMEDIATION: WHAT TO DO?

Two underlying principles should be kept in mind when attempting to remediate the arithmetic difficulties of children who exhibit neuropsychological characteristics that mirror those of Group 3 children. The first principle is that mechanical arithmetic should be made as much a verbal task as is possible. In other words, verbal rules and routines should be created for the child, so that he/she can deal effectively with all aspects of each mechanical arithmetic operation that is to be learned. The second principle is that the teaching of such children must be highly systematic and rather concrete. It may be necessary to use concrete (physical) aids to illustrate mathematical concepts, even when the children are older (say, 12 or 13 years of age). In the Rourke *et al.* (1985) follow-up study of eight adult patients who were chosen simply on the basis of the similarities between their neuropsychological characteristics and those of Group 3 children, no subject scored above the grade 7.1 level on the WRAT Arithmetic subtest, even though all of the eight patients had completed high school and had well-developed word-recognition and spelling abilities. All means possible should be used for the remediation of the arithmetic difficulties of Group 3 children when this type of gloomy forecast has been projected.

We have found that the way in which children who exhibit neuro-psychological characteristics similar to those of Group 3 children are taught has a great deal to do with the type and amount of information that they can learn. The following represents a remedial teaching strategy that would seem to suit the specialized instructional needs for the improvement of the arithmetic skills of Group 3 children.

1. Begin by choosing a simple type of mechanical arithmetic calculation that has proven to be problematic for the child.

2. Then, describe the arithmetic calculation to the child in words. Specifically, present an overview of the type and purpose of the operation primarily for orientation purposes, since we have found that Group 3 children may exhibit more difficulties with orientation to new tasks than do other types of learning-impaired children (Rourke, 1982). Describe and emphasize for the child the parts of the operation, and then relate these parts to the whole operation. Note that, at this point in the intervention program, the primary goal would be to have the child come to a point where he/she can describe the mathematical procedure verbally, rather than to attempt to solidify his/her understanding of the underlying mathematical concept.

3. Present the steps involved in the chosen mathematical operation in complete detail. Make certain that each step is described verbally. For example, "Step 1 involves naming the mathematical sign; Step 2 (in the case of a multiplication question) is to move your gaze and hand to the right side of the question," and so on.

4. Once the child seems reasonably well acquainted with the verbal steps involved in arriving at a correct solution for a particular type of mathematical operation, require the child to give a systematic account of the steps involved in the operation.

5. Require the child to write out the rules for that particular operation. After these have been checked for accuracy, allow the child to use this "recipe" as long as it is required. In conjunction with this "cookbook approach," encourage the child to rehearse number facts orally, since children in Group 3 seem to remember best through auditory–verbal feedback.

6. When the verbal steps involved in a particular procedure have been mastered and the child has rehearsed common number facts, it is then time to acquaint him/her with the visual aspects of the operation. That is, work through a sample calculation (of the type learned) by having the child direct the teacher with his/her verbal rules.

7. The teacher might then provide concrete (physical) aids (e.g., number boards, etc.) now and/or later in the remedial process to introduce the underlying mathematical concept. This may prove to be one of the most difficult aspects of remediation for such children.

8. Have the child attempt some trial questions of the type that has been learned. It may be helpful to have him/her work on graph paper to minimize the possibility that graphomotor problems (e.g., crowding of the work) and problems with spatial orientation (e.g., misaligning columns of numbers) will cause errors.

9. If it is needed, color-code the child's graph paper to aid the child with left–right discrimination. For example, there could be a red border on the right side of the page and a green border on the left side of the page.

10. Encourage the child to read each question aloud (at first) before beginning any mathematical operation. This should minimize the chance that the child misses visual detail in the question or in the answer. When it is certain that the child is competent in this skill, have the child read the questions and answers to himself/herself before going on to the next question.

11. Have a hand calculator available for the child for checking the accuracy of his/her answers. If the child finds that the answer is different from that produced by competent use of a hand calculator, he/she should then be required to rework the question by hand, looking for the particular error(s).

12. Record all of the child's mechanical arithmetic errors and task-analyze these errors. Information gained in this exercise will help guide the teacher in making necessary modifications to the remedial arithmetic program to meet the child's current needs in this subject area. In this connection, it is very important to bear in mind that the child's remedial arithmetic needs will change with age.

13. Promote the generalization of mechanical concepts and the proper use of mathematical procedures by using whatever means possible. As mentioned above, it is important to use concrete aids when teaching the child about underlying mathematical concepts. However, if the child is to gain a more functional appreciation for mathematical concepts, it is probably best to relate that operation to some practical aspect of everyday living. For example, addition, subtraction, and multiplication are common mathematical operations that one would use while shopping in a grocery store. Both the child's parents and his/her teachers can be involved with this aspect of the child's remedial arithmetic program.

SUMMARY AND CONCLUSIONS

Mechanical arithmetic is quite complex from an information-processing standpoint, and there are many different reasons why a child might experience difficulties in this subject area. In this chapter, we have highlighted the neuropsychological abilities and deficits of a group of children who exhibit outstanding and rather specific impairment in mechanical arithmetic. We also explained some specific modes of psychoeducational intervention that we have found to be helpful with such children. We should emphasize the following points:

1. The intervention strategy suggested is based rather directly on inferences drawn from the typical pattern of neuropsychological strengths and deficits exhibited by such children, including the type of difficulties that they are likely to encounter in mechanical arithmetic.
2. The efficacy of these intervention modes needs to be tested empirically in a manner similar to that suggested by Lyon (see Chapter 11, this volume).
3. In addition to difficulties in mechanical arithmetic, these children typically exhibit other types of educational handicaps, as well as problems in adaptation of a socioemotional sort (see Strang & Rourke, Chapter 14).
4. These children's pattern of socioemotional abilities and deficits, no less so than in the case of mechanical arithmetic, suggests a

number of specific modes of intervention for their difficulties that are amenable to empirical validation (see Ozols & Rourke, Chapter 13; Strang & Rourke, Chapter 14).

By design, we have given scant attention to these issues as they apply to children within Groups 1 and 2. To do so would have required the subtype differentiation of Group 1 (as suggested by the results of the Fisk & Rourke, 1979, investigation) and the comparisons of these subtypes with Group 2. Such comparisons are the subject of ongoing investigations within our laboratory.

REFERENCES

Badian N. A. Dyscalculia and nonverbal disorders of learning. In H. R. Myklebust (Ed.) *Progress in learning disabilities* (Vol. 5). New York: Grune & Stratton, 1983.

Benton, A. L. *Sentence Memory Test.* Iowa City, Iowa: Author, 1965.

Canning, P. M., Orr, R. R., & Rourke, B. P. Sex differences in the perceptual, visual–motor, linguistic, and concept-formation abilities of retarded readers? *Journal of Learning Disabilities,* 1980, *13,* 563–567.

Fisk, J. L., & Rourke, B. P. Identification of subtypes of learning-disabled children at three age levels: A neuropsychological, multivariate approach. *Journal of Clinical Neuropsychology,* 1979, *1,* 289–310.

Goldberg, E., & Costa, L. D. Hemisphere differences in the acquisition and use of descriptive systems. *Brain and Language,* 1981, *14,* 144–173.

Jastak, K. F., & Jastak, S. R. *Wide Range Achievement Test.* Wilmington, Del.: Guidance Associates, 1965.

Kass, C. E., Auditory Closure Test. In J. J. Olson & J. L. Olson (Eds.), *Validity studies on the Illinois Test of Psycholinguistic Abilities.* Madison, Wisc.: Photo Press, 1964.

Kløve, H. Clinical neuropsychology. In F. M. Forster (Ed.), *The medical clinics of North America.* New York: Saunders, 1963.

Knights, R. M. *Smoothed normative data on tests for evaluating brain damage in children.* Ottawa: Author, 1970.

Knights, R. M., & Norwood, J. A. *Revised smoothed normative data on the neuropsychological test battery for children.* Ottawa: Carleton University, 1980.

Piaget, J. *Judgment and reasoning in the child.* London: Routledge & Kegan Paul, 1928.

Reitan, R. M., & Davison, L. A. (Eds.). *Clinical neuropsychology: Current status and applications.* Washington, D.C.: V. H. Winston & Sons, 1974.

Rourke, B. P. Central processing deficiencies in children: Toward a developmental neuropsychological model. *Journal of Clinical Neuropsychology,* 1982, *4,* 1–18.

Rourke, B. P., Bakker, D. J., Fisk, J. L., & Strang, J. D. *Child neuropsychology: An introduction to theory, research, and clinical practice.* New York: Guilford Press, 1983.

Rourke, B. P., & Finlayson, M. A. J. Neuropsychological significance of variations in patterns of academic performance: Verbal and visual-spatial abilities. *Journal of Abnormal Child Psychology,* 1978, *6,* 121–133.

Rourke, B. P., & Strang, J. D. Neuropsychological significance of variations in patterns of academic performance: Motor, psychomotor, and tactile perception abilities. *Journal of Pediatric Psychology*, 1978, *3*, 212-225.

Rourke, B. P., & Strang, J. D. Subtypes of reading and arithmetical disabilities: A neuropsychological analysis. In M. Rutter (Ed.), *Developmental neuropsychiatry*. New York: Guilford Press, 1983.

Rourke, B. P., Young, G. C., Strang, J. D., & Russell, D. L. Adult outcomes of central processing deficiencies in childhood. In I. Grant & K. M. Adams (Eds.), *Neuropsychological assessment in neuropsychiatric disorders: Clinical methods and empirical findings*. New York: Oxford University Press, 1985.

Slade, P. D., & Russell, G. F. M. Developmental dyscalculia: A brief report on four cases. *Psychological Medicine*, 1971, *1*, 292-298.

Strang, J. D., & Rourke, B. P. Concept-formation/nonverbal reasoning abilities of children who exhibit specific academic problems with arithmetic. *Journal of Clinical Child Psychology*, 1983, *12*, 33-39.

Strang, J. D., & Rourke, B. P. *Personality dimensions of learning-disabled children: Age differences*. Manuscript in preparation, 1985.

Tuoko, H. *Cognitive correlates of arithmetic performance in clinic referred children*. Unpublished doctoral dissertation, University of Victoria, 1982.

IV

Validity Studies of
Learning Disability Subtypes

9

External Validation of
Learning Disability Typologies

JACK M. FLETCHER

The need to develop procedures for classifying children with learning disabilities into homogeneous subgroups is a well-recognized problem (Applebee, 1971; Benton, 1978; Rourke, 1978a; Satz & Fletcher, 1980; Taylor & Fletcher, 1983). A variety of statistical and clinical methods have been used for this research. Regardless of the methods employed, this classification research has uniformly shown that subtypes can be derived from groups of disabled learners. The derivation of subtypes is quite important, because the emergent typologies can form the starting point for more general theories of learning disabilities by identifying descriptively homogeneous subgroups. Unfortunately, the derivation of subtypes is easily misconstrued as the endpoint of the research—as if the mere presence of homogeneous subgroups explains why children have learning problems. The fact that different subtypes emerge through clinical inspection of neuropsychological protocols or the application of a statistical algorithm to the protocols does not establish the validity of the subtypes. Typologies are simply hypotheses concerning the classification of a larger group of individuals into homogeneous subsets. The explanatory value of classification research stems from systematic evaluations of the validity of the typology. In short, a valid typology is reliable (i.e., is not sample- or method-dependent). Furthermore, the typology permits the testing of refutable hypotheses concerning subtype similarities and differences. This hypothesis-testing process may have considerable value for explaining the nature and etiology of learning disabilities.

Jack M. Fletcher. Developmental Neuropsychology Research Section, Texas Research Institute of Mental Sciences, Houston, Texas, USA.

These initial considerations form the basis for a particular view of the role and value of classification research in learning disabilities. According to this view, the goal underlying the derivation of subtypes is simply to define reliable, homogeneous subgroups of disabled learners. The typology resulting from this phase of the research should be descriptively simple and should permit easy categorization of other disabled learners. Theories concerning the etiology and nature of learning disabilities are important for this initial phase of research, particularly in terms of selecting classification attributes and methods. However, theory is merely heuristic at this phase and becomes of primary importance in a later validation phase. In this later phase, hypotheses concerning subtype differences are systematically evaluated against external criteria not involved in deriving the subtypes. This external validity phase represents a potential alternative to the traditional contrasting-groups methodology so characteristic of learning disabilities research (Doehring, 1978; Satz & Fletcher, 1980). The problems with this methodology derive in part from the comparison of heterogeneous groups of disabled learners. A reliable typology that permits identification of new children as members of subgroups would place contrasting-groups methodology into a more meaningful framework.

This view of classification research may differ from subtyping approaches that employ large numbers of variables for deriving subtypes (Doehring, Trites, Patel, & Fiedorowicz, 1981; Fisk & Rourke, 1979; Mattis, French, & Rapin, 1975; Petrauskas & Rourke, 1979). The purpose of this chapter is not to compare the relative merits of any of these approaches; rather, it is to explore the general issue of validating typologies in an effort to show how this point of view has evolved. A general framework for classification research is provided that illustrates the different types of validity that a taxonomy should exhibit (Skinner, 1981). Specific attention is devoted to the validation of taxonomic hypotheses against *external* criteria through a review of studies that can be construed as external validation studies of learning disabilities.

A GENERAL FRAMEWORK
FOR CLASSIFICATION RESEARCH

In a seminal paper, Skinner (1981) provided a framework for conceptualizing and evaluating attempts to classify psychiatric disorders. This framework outlined different components underlying an integrated paradigm for classification research that can be applied to children with learning disabilities. Three components are contained in the framework. First, Skinner (1981) described a "theory formulation component," which involves decisions concerning the kinds of variables that will be used for classification and the theoretical model used to depict subtypes. Second, the "internal validation component" represents studies of the reliability, coverage, and replicability of the subtypes. Third, the "external validity component" concerns the evaluation of a reliable classification system against external criteria. This component addresses whether the subtypes differ from one another in response to treatment, biological markers, and other indices used to study these groups. Although rarely made explicit, each of these components is inherent in classification research in neuropsychology. When each component in turn is considered, examples of how this framework elucidates the nature and purpose of classification research in learning disabilities can be provided.

THEORY FORMULATION COMPONENT

Skinner (1981) described several theoretical and empirical decisions in the theory formulation component. First, a decision concerning the content domain must be made. The content domain concerns the variables to be employed for classification. Most neuropsychological research uses psychometric tests and behavioral observations to classify children. Alternatives could include classification on the basis of history, treatment response, and other characteristics of disabled learners. A second consideration involves the theoretical model used to specify the types and their interrelationships. For example, if Q-type factor analysis and cluster analysis are used, a frequent implicit assumption is that constructs of "ideal types" are desirable. Ideal types are hypothetical individuals displaying a characteristic set of attributes exemplifying a subset of the population. In contrast, hierarchical approaches could be used that would classify children initially according to academic problems and then would attempt to form homogeneous subsets within each academic type. The third concern inherent in the theory formulation component is the *a priori* specification of hypothesized relationships of the subtypes with external variables. Here it should be possible to predict the direction of group differences on remediation outcomes, measures of cognitive skills, or other variables not used to develop the typology. As I indicate later, the attempt to disconfirm these hypotheses systematically in the external validity component is central for evaluating the adequacy of a subtyping solution.

INTERNAL VALIDITY COMPONENT

Internal validity concerns the reliability and replicability of the typology (Skinner, 1981). External validity studies are not meaningful if the typology has low reliability and is difficult to replicate. An ideal typology yields reliable, homogeneous subtypes that can be replicated with different samples and across different techniques (Everitt, 1980). In addition, the typology permits classification of a majority of the subjects in the population (i.e., coverage) and yields a practical way of identifying new members of the subtypes. While there are no widely accepted criteria for evaluating the adequacy of a subtyping solution (Blashfield, 1980; Skinner, 1981), a variety of considerations underlie successful demonstration of internal validity. These considerations include (1) the number of subjects successfully typed (i.e., coverage); (2) the homogeneity of the subtypes; (3) the reliability of the classification attributes; (4) replicability across techniques; and (5) replication with other samples. Morris, Blashfield, and Satz (1981) and Satz and I (see Chapter 3, this volume) provide descriptions of internal validity studies in an attempt to derive learning disability subtypes.

EXTERNAL VALIDITY COMPONENT

This component addresses the degree to which the subtypes can be delineated according to external criteria. Relatively few learning disability studies can be construed as representative of the external validity component. Furthermore, these studies do not always represent explicit attempts to evaluate classification hypotheses. External validity could be represented by the ability of the classification hypotheses to *predict* and confirm the differential effectiveness of various remediation techniques as a function of the type of learning disability (see Lyon, Chapter 11, this volume). The demonstration of a subtype × remediation or subtype × task interaction is a powerful demonstration of external validity. Similarly, *descriptive validity* represents attempts to demonstrate convergent and discriminant validity for the subtypes, usually by using parallel measures (Skinner, 1981). A third source of validity is the extent to which the subtypes are clinically meaningful. A classification system that yields profiles unrecognized by clinicians would receive little acceptance by these practitioners (Skinner, 1981).

A number of validity concerns should be illuminated before the evaluation of specific learning disability typologies against external criteria is discussed. First, hypotheses must be generated on an *a priori* basis and then subjected to experimental tests in which the hypotheses can be refuted. If external validity studies are not conducted from a falsifiable framework permitting refutation, the value of a particular classification hypothesis will not be determined by the results of research, but by the passage of time and loss of interest on the part of researchers (Meehl, 1978; Skinner, 1981).

Second, adequate demonstration of external validity must predict falsifiable differences on variables outside the measurement domain used to establish the subtypes. The demonstration that learning disability subtypes derived from language and visual–spatial measures differ predictably on other language and visual–spatial measures is essentially a self-fulfilling prophecy based on the covariance of tasks within the same measurement domain. To be refutable, differences must be predicted on variables outside the measurement domain, such as a psychophysiological index or measures of cognitive skills involving modalities and processes that differ from the tasks used to derive the subtypes.

Third, external validity can be demonstrated only with criteria besides those used to establish the typology. Showing that groups are different with a discriminant-function analysis using the classification variables is not meaningful for external validity studies. Unless there is poor reliability, the discriminant function will always separate subtypes, since classification methods create homogeneous subsets of individuals.

Fourth, external validity studies are more easily completed when the classification scheme permits easy identification of new members outside of the original sample. If a large number of psychometric tests ($n = 20$) are used to classify the subjects, then external validity studies may be more difficult if the typology is applied to new children. Similarly, the typology should yield procedures for identifying new members. It would be impractical to redo subtype analyses each time new subjects become available. Here it is apparent that external validity studies may be facilitated by the use of a fairly small number of variables. Variable reduction makes for good research by using the most reliable and least redundant variables, as well as for easy identification of new subjects (Fleiss & Zubin, 1969). The use of large numbers of variables, which is apparent in many learning disability subtyping studies, could make systematic external validity studies more difficult to complete. This potential problem reflects the need for careful conceptualization of classification research within this general framework. Deriving subtypes is only the first step in the research: Validity studies should be planned prior to determination of the typology.

EXTERNAL VALIDATION OF LEARNING DISABILITY TYPOLOGIES

In reviewing the burgeoning research on the classification of disabled learners (Lyon, 1982; Satz & Morris, 1981), two distinctions emerge as general characteristics of the research. The first distinction concerns whether the research is based on clinical interpretation of psychometric protocols or on the application of multivariate statistical methods to psychometric data. Clinical approaches to delineating subtypes (e.g., Boder, 1973; Mattis *et al.*, 1975) contrast with statistical approaches based on multivariate statistical procedures (Doehring & Hoshko, 1977; Fisk & Rourke, 1979; Petrauskas & Rourke, 1979; Satz & Morris, 1981; Lyon, 1982). The second distinction concerns whether children are classified according to (1) academic performance (Boder, 1973; Doehring & Hoshko, 1977), (2) processing deficiencies based on a battery of cognitive–neuropsychological tests (Fisk & Rourke, 1979; Lyon, 1982; Mattis *et al.*, 1975), or (3) both dimensions (Doehring *et al.*, 1981; Satz & Morris, 1981). Although these studies have yielded differing results, some initial observations are pertinent.

The classification of children according to patterns of academic deficiency has not always been conceptualized as classification research. However, many studies support the external validity of separating disabled learners according to differences in reading, spelling, and arithmetic performance. Regardless of whether children are classified according to academic performance or processing deficiencies, virtually every study has identified at least one verbal subtype, one spatial subtype, and a mixed verbal–spatial subtype (Lyon, 1982; Satz & Morris, 1981). In contrast to research on academic subtypes, relatively little validation research has been completed for subtypes classified according to processing deficiencies.

Much of this validation research employs measures identical to or highly correlated with tasks used to create the typology (Lyon, 1982). A study that uses a set of measures for subtyping and then employs the same measures for describing the group is an external validation study only from the point of view of clinical relevance. While the fact that subtype profiles have clinical interpretability is important, it can be quite misleading. Good clinicians, like good statistical algorithms, can find patterns in random data, highlighting the need for a systematic evaluation of internal and external validity. In the next section, external validity studies on subtypes of disabled learners are reviewed. Those studies based on academic subtypes are reviewed first, followed by a review of studies based on processing-deficiency subtypes.

EXTERNAL VALIDITY STUDIES

ACADEMIC SUBTYPES

Several approaches have been used to classify disabled learners according to patterns of academic ability. Some studies have employed measures of reading, spelling, and arithmetic (Rourke, 1978b). Other approaches have examined only reading and spelling skills (Boder, 1973), spelling (Sweeney & Rourke, 1978; Sweeney & Rourke, Chapter 7, this volume), and reading (Doehring, Chapter 6, this volume; Doehring *et al.*, 1981). Evaluations of these typologies against external criteria have yielded some interesting findings.

Wide Range Achievement Test Typologies

A series of studies by Rourke (1975, 1978b, 1982) has shown differences in disabled learners according to patterns on the Reading, Spelling, and Arithmetic subtests of the Wide Range Achievement Test (WRAT; Jastak & Jastak, 1978). In these studies, three groups of disabled learners aged 9–14 with IQ scores between 86 and 114 were formed. Group 1 (reading-, spelling-, and arithmetic-disabled) was composed of children with WRAT scores below the 19th centile on all three subtests. Group 2 (reading- and spelling-disabled) contained children with WRAT Arithmetic scores at least 1.8 years higher than their Reading and Spelling scores, which were below the 15th centile. Group 3 (arithmetic-disabled) had WRAT Reading and Spelling scores at least 2 years above their Arithmetic scores. It is important to recognize that Group 1 and Group 2 were equated on Reading and Spelling scores, while Group 2 and Group 3 were equated on (deficient) Arithmetic scores.

These groups were compared on a variety of neuropsychological tests measuring language, visual–spatial, motor, and tactile–perceptual skills (Rourke, 1975). In accordance with *a priori* hypotheses, Rourke and Finlayson (1978) and Rourke and Strang (1978) showed that the Group 3 children had well-developed verbal skills, but poorer visual–spatial, psycho-motor, and tactile–perceptual skills (with the psychomotor and tactile–perceptual skills being particularly poor with the left hand). Group 2 children had problems with a variety of auditory–linguistic skills, but better visual–spatial skills. Children impaired in all three areas (Group 1) had predominant problems in processing verbal material (Rourke, 1982).

These findings have been replicated using different types of measures in at least two studies outside Rourke's laboratory. I (Fletcher, 1983) defined four groups of children aged 9–12 years, using Wechsler Intelligence Scale for Children—Revised (WISC-R) and WRAT criteria slightly more liberal than those employed in the Rourke studies. The four groups included controls ($n = 18$) and disabled learners in Group 1 (arithmetic-, reading-, and spelling-disabled; $n = 24$), Group 2 (reading- and spelling-disabled; $n = 10$), and Group 3 (arithmetic-disabled; $n = 14$). Figure 9-1 presents the WRAT profiles for these groups.

Each child received two memory tasks representing verbal and spatial analogues of Buschke's (1974) selective-reminding procedure. This procedure is based on free-list learning tasks that repeat only those items not remembered on previous trials. The verbal task consists of 12 animal names that are read to the child, who is asked to repeat as many words as possible. On subsequent trials, only words that are not remembered are read to the child, who must then attempt recall of all words on the list. The spatial task consists of eight randomly arranged displays of five dots. The child must remember the location of one dot on each display, with administration and scoring identical to the verbal task. This format permits separate scores for acquisition and retrieval components of memory. Although several scores can be computed for these tasks, only the results for long-term storage (LTS) and consistent long-term retrieval (CLTR) are reported here. The LTS score represents the number of items (words or dots) remembered on two consecutive trials (i.e., without reminding) and is counted cumulatively across trials. In contrast, the CLTR score represents

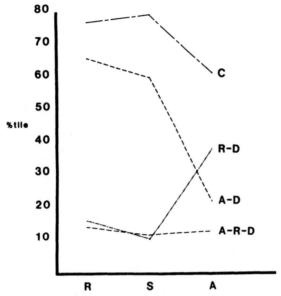

FIG. 9-1. Centiles for WRAT Reading (R), Spelling (S), and Arithmetic (A) subtests by achievement subgroups (C, control; R-D, reading- and spelling-disabled, or Group 2; A-D, arithmetic-disabled, or Group 3; and A-R-D, arithmetic-, reading-, and spelling-disabled, or Group 1).

the number of items remembered on two consecutive trials and across all subsequent trials. According to Buschke (1974), LTS indicates encoding of the item into long-term memory storage, while CLTR indicates the degree to which items stored into long-term memory can be retrieved.

Figure 9-2 plots LTS and CLTR scores for verbal and spatial tasks across the four groups of children. To permit comparisons of verbal and spatial scores, LTS and CLTR scores were standardized with a mean of 10 and a standard deviation of 3 on the basis of the control group's scores. Figure 9-2 shows that the direction of group differences was in the direction predicted by Rourke (1978b, 1982). While no group differences emerged on the verbal LTS index, Group 1 was impaired, relative to controls and Group 3, on verbal CLTR scores and on scores for both spatial tasks. In contrast, Group 2 children performed significantly better than Group 1 and Group 3 children on the spatial task, but more poorly than the controls on the verbal CLTR index. Finally, Group 3 scores were

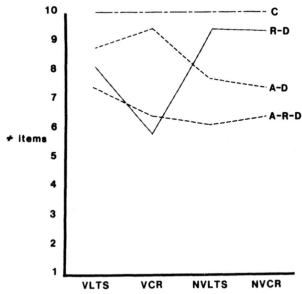

FIG. 9-2. Standardized memory performance (items remembered) on verbal (V) and nonverbal (NV) selective-reminding indices (LTS and CR) for achievement subgroups (see Figure 9-1 for subgroup abbreviations).

comparable to Control scores on the verbal task, but much poorer on spatial LTS and CLTR tasks.

Siegel and Linder (1984) also found differences in the organization of memory among WRAT-defined subgroups of reading-, spelling-, and arithmetic-disabled (i.e., Rourke's Group 1), arithmetic-disabled (i.e., Rourke's Group 3), and control children at several ages. In this study, different measures of phonemic coding in short-term memory (i.e., recall of rhyming and nonrhyming letters) were presented in visual and auditory modalities. Results revealed that the youngest Group 1 children were equally impaired for recall of rhyming and nonrhyming letters, while older Group 1 children had poorer recall of rhyming versus nonrhyming letters. Control children showed the same dissociation as did the older Group 1 children, but performed at much higher levels. The Group 3 children had difficulty with recall in the visual modality, but not in the auditory modality. Again, the visual–auditory dissociation is consistent with Rourke's results (1978b). However, recall of phonetically coded material (i.e., language) was difficult for the Group 3 children in the visual modality. Considering the results of the Fletcher (1983) and Siegel and Linder (1984) studies together, visually presented material may be difficult for arithmetic-disabled children even when the stimuli are linguistic, particularly if the material is novel (Rourke, 1982).

Additional research is needed to explore these hypotheses. The studies summarized in this section support the WRAT subtypes developed by Rourke (1978b). More important in the present context, these studies represent consistent examples of discriminative validity on the basis of *a priori* hypotheses, using external measures that are different from the classification attributes. Finally, as Satz and I (see Chapter 3, this volume) have noted, similar subtypes have emerged in three independent cluster-analytic studies of the WRAT in large samples of disabled and nondisabled learners. The emergence of these subgroups in the absence of *a priori* assumptions concerning the nature of learning disabilities further highlights the importance of these academic patterns. The WRAT can be criticized for its relatively limited assessment of academic skills and the absence of reading comprehension measures. However, WRAT scores correlate highly with more specific academic measures (Jastak & Jastak, 1978; Taylor, Fletcher, & Satz, 1982), and the addition of reading comprehension measures in the three cluster-analytic studies mentioned above did not alter the resultant WRAT subgroups (see Chapter 3, this volume).

Reading and Spelling Patterns

One of the early clinical approaches to subtyping (Boder, 1973) has led to a number of external validity studies. Boder (1973) defined three "dyslexic" subtypes according to patterns of reading and spelling errors. These subtypes include (1) dysphonetic dyslexics, representing children with a deficit in sound–symbol integration; (2) dyseidetic dyslexics, representing children with a deficit in the perception of visual "gestalts"; and (3) mixed dysphonetic–dyseidetic dyslexics, representing children with both problems. In essence, the distinction between dysphonetic and dyseidetic subtypes concerns the degree to which reading and spelling errors are phonetically constrained.

Few studies have used cognitive or neuropsychological measures to try to dissociate these subgroups. One example is a study by Obrzut (1979), who administered an auditory dichotic-listening task and a bisensory (auditory and visual) digit task to normal children and to disabled learners falling into the three Boder subtypes. In general, results demonstrated that the dyseidetic group performed similarly to the controls, while the dysphonetic and mixed subtypes performed more poorly on both tasks. It should be noted that the dyseidetic group did not have difficulty on visually presented tasks. Furthermore, the only group that showed a right-ear advantage on the dichotic test was the dysphonetic group, which was contrary to what was predicted. Finally, the dysphonetic groups had difficulty in both the visual and auditory modalities. This study has additional limitations because of sampling and interpretative problems pointed out by Lyon (1982) and Doehring *et al.* (1981), so that the results provide only limited support for the Boder typology.

Other studies have employed typologies that should yield subtypes similar to those defined by Boder (1973). Sweeney and Rourke (1978) compared poor spellers whose errors could be classified as phonetically accurate and phonetically inaccurate. Since the classification scheme should separate children into subgroups similar to those of Boder (1973), the neuropsychological results are pertinent. Briefly, Sweeney and Rourke (1978) showed that phonetically inaccurate misspellers performed more poorly on language measures than did phonetically accurate misspellers. However, there were few differences on nonlinguistic tasks. Hence, this study provides some indirect support for the Boder typology. Sweeney and Rourke (see Chapter 7, this volume) provide additional evidence supporting the value of classifying children according to types of spelling errors.

At least three electrophysiological studies have compared disabled learners classified according to the Boder typology. Rosenthal, Boder, and Callaway (1982) classified 33 *adult* disabled learners into dysphonetic ($n = 12$), dyseidetic ($n = 11$), and mixed ($n = 10$) subtypes. Event-related potentials (ERPs) were recorded while these adults performed tasks requiring the counting of visual and auditory stimuli under different attentional states. Although results were difficult to interpret, the distributions of the endogenous components of the ERPs were apparently different between the dyseidetic and the dysphonetic subgroups. Rosenthal *et al.* (1982) concluded that the results supported the Boder typology. However, more specific presentation of results would be needed to determine the extent to which the study produced the subgroup $\times$ task interactions necessary to validate the typology.

Fried, Tanguay, Boder, Doubleday, and Greensite (1981) collected ERPs in a study of hemispheric asymmetries in 13 "dyslexic" boys and age-matched controls. Within the "dyslexic" group, the boys were also classified using Boder's (1973) distinction between dyseidetic (visual–spatial) and dysphonetic (auditory–verbal) subtypes. Results revealed the expected hemispheric asymmetries in the controls and the dyseidetic children. No asymmetries were apparent in the dysphonetic subtype, leading Fried *et al.* (1981) to hypothesize an absence of left-hemisphere specialization for language in these children. This conclusion was limited by the sample size of the dysphonetic group ($n = 5$), which may have produced insufficient statistical power for group comparisons.

In a third study, Leisman and Ashkenazi (1980) compared electro-encephalogram (EEG) spectral coherence in Boder-defined "dyslexic" subtypes and normal controls. Although subtype differences did not emerge, the "dyslexic" group showed less coherence between hemispheres and more coherence within hemispheres on parietal and occipital recording sites. However, questions concerning these analyses arise when reported coherence values are examined, because the scores ranged beyond those appropriate for normalized score distributions as defined in the coherence function (Saltzberg, Burton, Fletcher, Michael, & Burch, 1981).

At best, the electrophysiological studies provide mixed support for the Boder typology. These studies are particularly interesting because of the attempt to validate the typology with measures completely different from the classification attributes. In this respect, the studies could be heuristic for future external validity studies. Unfortunately, while Boder's typology was a pioneering effort in the area, it has been widely criticized because of internal validity considerations (Lyon, 1982; Satz & Morris, 1981). Evaluation against external criteria should not proceed without established reliability, which may contribute to the mixed results of those external validity studies employing the Boder subtypes.

Doehring's Academic Subtypes

Doehring *et al.* (1981) summarized a series of studies addressing patterns of neuropsychological and language abilities in three academic subtypes. These subtypes were defined with Q-type factor analysis of a variety of reading-related measures presented by Doehring (1976). The three subgroups consisted of (1) children with oral reading disability, characterized by deficiencies primarily in oral language; (2) children with associative reading disability, characterized by difficulty in associating printed and spoken letters and words; and (3) children with sequential reading disability, characterized by good letter and number reading, but poorer word and syllable reading. The application of a battery of psycholinguistic and neuropsychological tasks to these subtypes revealed some distinctions on the neuropsychological tasks. Few interpretable linguistic differences emerged when the three subtypes were compared. On the neuropsychological battery, the oral reading subgroup was characterized by difficulties on naming tasks and on tasks involving short-term memory, all of which involved sequential oral responses. In contrast, the associative subtype did not display short-term memory difficulties. However, this subtype had the poorest intellectual and achievement test results of the three subtypes. In addition, the associative subgroup had deficiencies with sensory–perceptual and psychomotor tasks employing the nondominant hand. Finally, the sequential subtype had difficulty with the dominant hand for sensory–perceptual and psychomotor tasks. While short-term memory skills were not impaired, general difficulties emerged on measures of spatial-processing skills.

Doehring *et al.* (1981) emphasized that these subtypes were heterogeneous, and that multiple explanations of their reading problems could be entertained. In fact, as the authors acknowledged, the separation among subtypes was not always striking, and differences were not always in predicted directions. The language measures were particularly disappointing in this regard. However, the value of these studies lies in their attempt to demonstrate interactions among reading, language, and neuropsychological skills.

Processing-Deficiency Subtypes

Studies that attempt classification based on cognitive or neuropsychological skills have been infrequently evaluated against external criteria. The reason for this is unclear, but the infrequency could reflect several factors. There is a tendency simply to accept the subtypes resulting from this approach as *prima facie* evidence for their validity (e.g., Mattis *et al.*, 1975). The general framework described for classification research mitigates against this acceptance, if only because such evidence is circular and nonfalsifiable (Skinner, 1981). These studies have not always been conducted from a framework that would illuminate the different components inherent in classification research. Despite these problems, there are some studies that address the external validity of processing-deficiency subtypes. In essence, these studies compare language and visual–spatial subtypes on other measures of these skills.

Verbal–Performance IQ Discrepancies

Differences in WISC Verbal IQ and Performance IQ scores have been frequently compared in groups of disabled and nondisabled learners (Sattler, 1974). While these studies show some fairly reliable characteristics for groups of disabled learners, other studies have subtyped disabled learners according to these discrepancies and have searched for differences on other cognitive measures. Rourke (1975) summarized several of these studies. Results revealed that older disabled learners with higher Verbal IQ scores had better Reading and Spelling than Arithmetic scores. This group also had poorer psychomotor skills and visual–spatial skills than did the high Performance–low Verbal subtype. The latter group tended to display uniformly poor Reading, Spelling, and Arithmetic scores. In general, language skills were lower than those exhibited by the high Verbal–low Performance group.

Findings of this type are particularly interesting in view of a study by Hier, LeMay, Rosenberger, and Perlo (1978). In this study, cerebral axial tomography was conducted on 24 disabled learners. Inspection of cerebral asymmetries revealed that 10 children had larger right than left parieto-occipital regions, a pattern presumably opposite to that observed in normal adults. Eight children demonstrated expected asymmetries (left greater than right), while six demonstrated no asymmetry. A comparison of Verbal and Performance IQ scores revealed significantly lower Verbal scores in the reversed-asymmetry subgroups, but no differences on the Performance scores. While this study does not show that Verbal–Performance discrepancies predict cerebral asymmetries, the findings represent an interesting correlation. Further support for this relationship stems from Conners (1971), who compared high Verbal–low Performance and low Verbal–high Performance disabled learners on ERP measures. Differences emerged in the amplitude and latency of the ERPs over left and right occipital and parietal electrode placements. While this study has been challenged (Sobotka & May, 1977; Weber & Omenn, 1977), the results do show that these subtypes can be dissociated on electrophysiological indices. Perhaps a major problem is that the nature of the processing deficiencies contained in these IQ subgroups is not sufficiently specific, thereby obscuring possible relationships with academic skills.

Another processing-deficiency approach was reported by Pirozzolo (1979) and Pirozzolo and Rayner (1979). In this study, two groups of "dyslexic" learners were formed. The first group was composed of disabled learners with lower Verbal than Performance IQs, language deficits, and poor phonological reading (i.e., an auditory–linguistic sub-type). The second group had lower Performance than Verbal IQs, spatial-processing problems, and visual-discrimination errors in reading (i.e., a visual–spatial subtype). Comparisons of these two subtypes on tasks involving eye movements (Rayner, 1981) revealed differences in saccadic latencies only in the visual–spatial subtypes. Pirozzolo (1979) emphasized that the deficiencies in eye movement were peripheral in nature, since ocular–motor treatment did not improve reading skills. Rather, these deficiencies were another symptom of the basic problem. Additional evaluation of the auditory–verbal subtype (Pirozzolo & Rayner, 1979) revealed an increased number of fixations per line, longer fixation durations, and other findings that were interpreted in terms of the linguistic demands of reading. Comparison of recognition speed for verbal (words) and nonverbal (faces) material presented to the visual half fields revealed the expected left-field asymmetry for faces, but no asymmetry for words.

Lyon's Study

The studies by Pirozzolo and Rayner do show some interesting differences among "language" and "spatial" subgroups. However, as with the IQ discrepancy studies, more specific measures of verbal and spatial skills could be used to generate these typologies. It is unfortunate that so few studies have truly evaluated this kind of processing-deficiency typology. One exception is the recent study by Lyon, Stewart, and Freedman (1982) which, unfortunately, was marred by a methodological difficulty. In this study, cluster analysis was applied to a set of neuropsychological and cognitive measures obtained from 75 disabled learners and 42 normal controls. Five subtypes of disabled learners emerged from this study, including a spatial group, an auditory–verbal group, an unexpected group, a mixed verbal–spatial group, and a sequencing group. A multi-variate analysis of variance (MANOVA) was applied to the classification attributes, with subsequent interpretation of the resultant discriminant functions to determine the basis for group differences. Not surprisingly, the subtypes could be separated along dimensions that were predictable from the interpretation of the discriminant functions. While interesting, the subtype distinctions are based on a confound, because the classification attributes and the external criteria are identical. Differences of this type would fail to emerge only if the subtypes were poorly defined, which is unlikely, given the reliability of the measures and the internal validity studies completed by Lyon *et al.* (1982).

Bakker's Studies

One final processing-deficiency approach to be reviewed was developed by Bakker and associates (Bakker, 1979; Bakker, Licht, Kok, & Bouma, 1980; Bakker, Moerland, & Goekoop-Hoefkens, 1981; Bakker, Teunissen, & Bosch, 1976). Bakker (1979) described a "balance model" of reading disability, which hypothesizes that children learning to read are required to shift from a perceptual strategy to a language strategy as they become older and more proficient readers. Children using an inappropriate strategy at any point in their development will display impaired reading. Hence, disabled readers can be classified into two subtypes: "P-type," which includes children having problems with right-hemisphere perceptual strategies; and "L-type," which includes children with impairment in left-hemisphere linguistic strategies. Although several criteria are used to form the subtypes, the primary basis for classifying disabled learners is left–right ear asymmetries on dichotic-listening tasks, which Bakker *et al.* (1976) have related to patterns of reading errors. Those disabled learners showing left-ear advantages are classified as P-type, while children with right-ear advantages are classified as L-type. It is important to recognize that these two groups are equally impaired in reading, differing only in strategy.

At least two external validity studies of this typology have been completed. Bakker *et al.* (1980) completed a pilot study in which they collected ERPs for left and right temporal (T_3, T_4) and parietal (P_3, P_4) recording sites during reading from P-type and L-type disabled learners, along with normal controls who were also classified according to ear advantage. Positive and negative ERP amplitudes and latencies were analyzed according to a group (disabled vs. nondisabled) $\times$ ear advantage (left vs. right) $\times$ side (electrode placement over left vs. right hemisphere) analysis of variance (ANOVA). Results revealed a clear trend for a group $\times$ ear advantage $\times$ side interaction that was not statistically significant. The absence of significance is not surprising, given the small cell sizes for third-order interactions, which reduced power for this analysis. Collapsing across groups revealed ear advantage $\times$ side interactions for parietal and temporal recording sites for the nondisabled controls. The disabled readers did not show these interactions for temporal or parietal leads. In addition, interesting differences between groups (not subtypes) emerged for first-order main effects. For example, the reading-disabled group had longer parietal P310 and N440 latencies than the controls. Hence, while disabled readers and controls differed, there were no significant differences between the subgroups of disabled learners.

One reason for reviewing the ANOVA in such detail is to illustrate the importance of these interactions for external validation. The fact that only 13 disabled learners were included in this pilot study reduced the power for interaction tests, particularly since only 4 of the 13 children could be classified as P-type dyslexics. Since Bakker *et al.* (1980) did not obtain significant interactions, the results are essentially null as far as the validation of the typology is concerned. However, the emergence of these interactions in the nondisabled children, as well as the clear trend toward significant interactions for ear advantage and side apparent in visual representation of the results for the group of disabled learners, highlights the importance of power considerations for the Bakker *et al.* (1980) study. The other investigation (Bakker *et al.*, 1981) also supported the validity of the typology. This study showed that activation of right or left hemispheres through lateral visual half-field presentation of words altered ERP waveforms and improved reading scores on pre–post comparisons in directions predicted by the nature of the subtypes.

The Bakker studies illustrate an appropriate way to conceptualize external validity studies through the formation and evaluation of *a priori* hypotheses (i.e., theory formulation) that are tested against external criteria. While results are best considered preliminary because of statistical power considerations, the Bakker studies represent a potential model for typology development. In this instance, hypothetical variables representing differences in neural mechanisms (which presumably underlie different learning disability subtypes) received an independent evaluation by variables (EEG indices) not used in the development of the typology.

DIRECTIONS FOR FUTURE RESEARCH

There are certainly other studies that show variations in the performance of subgroups of disabled learners (Rourke, 1975, 1978b). In addition, a small number of studies have evaluated typologies against remediation outcomes (see Lyon, Chapter 11, this volume); these have not been reviewed here and merit consideration along with the studies summarized in this chapter. The most promising external validity studies have been those based on academic subtypes, particularly the WRAT typologies proposed by Rourke (1978b, 1982). The emergence of subtype × task interactions has been based on refutable *a priori* hypotheses; identifying new children as members of academic typologies is a simple matter; and hypotheses have been formulated concerning relationships of the types with a biological substrate (Rourke, 1982). The key for the evaluation of these hypotheses is to apply measures like those used in the electro-physiological studies of the Boder (1973) and Bakker (1979) typologies. Measures of this type clearly depart from the initial classification attributes and form the basis for *a priori* hypotheses concerning subtype differences. As Benton (1978) noted, application of infrabehavioral indices that, presumably, more directly reflect central nervous system (CNS) factors may help establish whether different brain mechanisms underlie the behavioral and cognitive manifestations of learning disabilities.

The development of future typologies must be conceptualized within a framework that permits the design of internal and external validity studies prior to the initiation of the research. While researchers in this area can debate forever the relative merits of clinical versus statistical methods, or *Q*-analyses versus cluster analyses, the only way to resolve these issues is to evaluate emergent typologies against internal and external criteria. Morris *et al.* (1981) have provided a good example of a systematic approach to internal validity, while this chapter has tried to suggest guidelines for external validity. To summarize these guidelines, external validity studies should predict the direction of subtype differences on variables not used to form the typology. These predictions should stem from a typology that leads to the development and evaluation of *a priori* refutable hypotheses concerning similarities and differences among subtypes. In particular, the nature and direction of subtype × task interactions must be predicted and confirmed to demonstrate that a typology has external validity. More generally, conducting external validity studies is one way to replace the outmoded contrasting-groups methodology traditionally employed in learning disabilities research (Doehring, 1978; Satz & Fletcher, 1980). When reliable typologies can be developed that permit simple identification of subtype members, comparisons of subgroups along dimensions used in more traditional approaches may have more meaning.

Recent critical reviews of learning disability research have called for "multiple covariance models" that attempt to account for the heterogeneity of disabled learners (Doehring, 1978; Satz & Fletcher, 1980). The subtyping research provides a genuine opportunity to apply these models in a systematic fashion. If homogeneous subgroups can be reliably defined, external validity studies can explore more directly the meaning of subgroup differences. The value of the Skinner (1981) framework derives in part from the integration of the different phases of classification research into a coherent and general model for research. In some respects, classifying disabled learners is not so much a problem of "discovering" subtypes as it is of developing procedures for identifying children as members of subtypes for which there already exists some consensual agreement among clinicians and researchers. If external validity studies are viewed as part of a confirmatory hypothesis-testing framework, the initial step in the development of typologies could be seen as an attempt to develop simple, reliable identification procedures for placing disabled learners into subtypes. To a certain extent, this view favors relatively simple classification systems that permit the accumulation of large numbers of children into subtypes. Such a system could be adopted by researchers in different settings and could lead to intensive cross-validation studies, with replication of results as a real possibility. This research would continue to compare groups, but comparisons would be made from a hypothesis-testing framework. Presently, virtually any dependent measure yields deficiencies in comparative studies of disabled and non-disabled learners. This factor is one reason why most theories of learning disabilities can be supported by simply reviewing the literature. If this research is carefully approached from a framework of classification theory, it may be possible to alter predominant paradigms and to develop a data base that would permit formation and refutation of different hypotheses. In line with this viewpoint, subtyping studies would not be the province of those individuals who can collect a large data base on many disabled learners; rather, any researcher could conduct external validity studies, provided that appropriate typologies were available.

In developing these typologies, some additional considerations are pertinent. In order to reconcile typologies based on academic patterns and processing deficiencies, a hierarchical approach may be helpful. The selection of children as "learning-disabled" based on *a priori* selection criteria is plausible, but not necessarily consistent with the development of more general typologies of children. Classification could begin at the level of academic patterns and could include nondisabled children in an attempt to classify those children with learning problems (e.g., Satz & Morris, 1981). Since this approach would foster the identification of children who fall into specific academic subtypes, this typology could form the initial level of classification. Subsequent application of measures of cognitive and neuropsychological skills could form the second hierarchically related level of classification and could help specify types according to processing deficiencies. In the absence of careful assessments of academic skills, processing-deficiency typologies combine children with different academic problems into similar subtypes. For example, some children with arithmetic disabilities have spatial-processing problems that also characterize some children with reading problems, but the two groups are very different. Similarly, subgroups of children with arithmetic disabilities that differ in reading levels are clearly distinct subtypes, despite equal levels of arithmetic achievement (Rourke, 1978b). Perhaps one finding that may emerge is that processing-deficiency typologies are more meaningful for children who do not display *specific* academic problems, since specific academic subtypes may already represent relatively homogeneous subsets of the population.

If typologies of learning disabilities were established, there is no guarantee that the children in these subtypes would differ from children with other behavioral disabilities. When groups of children with specific developmental disorders have been compared with children who, for example, have emotional disorders, null results frequently emerge on many of the indices, presumably demonstrating that the developmental disorders are brain-related (Rapoport & Ferguson, 1981; Taylor & Fletcher, 1983). Consequently, not only is it important to develop a typology for learning disabilities, but it is also important to determine how this typology fits into the broader classification of childhood disorders, including psychopathology. This highlights the importance of beginning classification at a level that attempts to determine the types of academic failure. If children with learning disabilities are truly unique, subgroups of disabled learners should emerge as distinct from children with academic problems that presumably reflect low intelligence, emotional problems, and other difficulties.

At this level of classification, the goals are primarily descriptive. The classification and subsequent identification of disabled learners into subtypes are primarily attempts to deal with intrasubject variability. The application of cognitive and neuropsychological measures will permit more detailed descriptions of the subtypes. In addition, studies of the interaction of academic patterns and processing skills will be facilitated. Even here, however, such studies address only the covariance among the measures employed, and there are few implications for directionality (i.e., causality) in this type of correlational research. Furthermore, the substantial covariance among measures of academic skills and cognitive–neuropsychological skills will not provide conclusive evidence that the subtypes are truly different. This evidence will accrue from the demonstration of subtype × remediation technique interactions, or of subtype differences on measures clearly different from those used to develop the typology. While this demonstration is an exciting possibility, perhaps the most pressing need is for reliable typologies. With these typologies, children could be identified as members of subtypes, so that virtually all research could represent an external validity study. In this respect, classification research with learning-disabled children is more than a simple search for subtypes. If appropriately conceptualized, this research could potentially alter predominant research paradigms along the lines suggested by critical reviews of the literature (Applebee, 1971; Benton, 1978; Doehring, 1978; Rourke, 1983; Satz & Fletcher, 1980). While there is no assurance that classification research will lead to this shift, there is certainly little point in continuing to pursue traditional contrasting-groups methodologies that assume a similar deficiency for every disabled learner.

REFERENCES

Applebee, A. N. Research in reading retardation: Two critical problems. *Journal of Child Psychology and Psychiatry and Allied Disciplines*, 1971, *12*, 91–113.

Bakker, D. J. Hemispheric differences and reading strategies: Two dyslexias? *Bulletin of the Orton Society*, 1979, *29*, 84–100.

Bakker, D. J., Licht, R., Kok, A., & Bouma, A. Cortical responses to word reading in right- and left-eared normal and reading-disturbed children. *Journal of Clinical Neuropsychology*, 1980, *2*, 1-12.

Bakker, D. J. Moerland, R., & Goekoop-Hoefkens. Effects of hemisphere-specific stimulation on the reading performance of dyslexic boys: A pilot study. *Journal of Clinical Neuropsychology*, 1981, *3*, 155-160.

Bakker, D. J., Teunissen, J., & Bosch, J. Development of laterality—reading patterns. In R. M. Knights & D. J. Bakker (Eds.), *The neuropsychology of learning disorders*. Baltimore: University Park Press, 1976.

Benton, A. L. Some conclusions about dyslexia. In A. L. Benton & D. Pearl (Eds.), *Dyslexia: An appraisal of current knowledge*. New York: Oxford University Press, 1978.

Blashfield, R. K. Propositions regarding the use of cluster analysis in clinical research. *Journal of Consulting and Clinical Psychology*, 1980, *3*, 456-459.

Boder, E. Developmental dyslexia: A diagnostic approach based on three atypical reading-spelling patterns. *Developmental Medicine and Child Neurology*, 1973, *15*, 663-687.

Buschke, H. Components of verbal learning in children: Analysis by selective reminding. *Journal of Experimental Child Psychology*, 1974, *18*, 488-496.

Conners, C. K. Cortical visual evoked response in children with learning disorders. *Psychophysiology*, 1971, *7*, 418-428.

Doehring, D. G. Acquisition of rapid reading responses. *Monographs of the Society for Research in Child Development*, 1976, *41*, 1-54.

Doehring, D. G. The tangled web of behavioral research and developmental dyslexia. In A. L. Benton & D. Pearl (Eds.), *Dyslexia: An appraisal of current knowledge*. New York: Oxford University Press, 1978.

Doehring, D. G., & Hoshko, I. M. Classification of reading problems by the Q-technique of factor analysis. *Cortex*, 1977, *13*, 281-294.

Doehring, D. G., Trites, R. L., Patel, P. G., & Fiedorowicz, C. *Reading disabilities*. New York: Academic Press, 1981.

Everitt, B. *Cluster analysis*. London: Heinemann Educational Books, 1980.

Fisk, J. L., & Rourke, B. P. Identification of subtypes of learning disabilities at three age levels: A neuropsychological, multivariate approach. *Journal of Clinical Neuropsychology*, 1979, *1*, 289-310.

Fleiss, J. L., & Zubin, J. On the methods and theory of clustering. *Multivariate Behavioral Research*, 1969, *4*, 253-260.

Fletcher, J. M. *Verbal and spatial selective reminding in learning disability subtypes*. Paper presented at the Society for Research in Child Development, Detroit, Michigan, April 1983.

Fried, I., Tanguay, P., Boder, E., Doubleday, C., & Greensite, M. Developmental dyslexia: Electrophysiological validation of clinical subgroups. *Brain and Language*, 1981, *12*, 14-22.

Hier, D. B., LeMay, M., Rosenberger, P. B., & Perlo, V. B. Developmental dyslexia: Evidence of a subgroup with reversal of cerebral asymmetry. *Archives of Neurology*, 1978, *35*, 90-92.

Jastak, J., & Jastak, S. *The Wide Range Achievement Test*. Wilmington, Del.: Guidance Associates, 1978.

Leisman, G., & Ashkenazi, M. Aetiological factors in dyslexia: IV. Cerebral hemispheres are functionally equivalent. *Neuroscience*, 1980, *11*, 157-164.

Lyon, R. Subgroups of LD readers: Clinical and empirical identification. In H. R. Myklebust (Ed.), *Progress in learning disabilities* (Vol. 5). New York: Grune & Stratton, 1982.

Lyon, R., Stewart, N., & Freedman, D. Neuropsychological characteristics of empirically derived subtypes, of learning disabled readers. *Journal of Clinical Neuropsychology*, 1982, *4*, 343–466.

Mattis, S., French, J. H., & Rapin, I. Dyslexia in children and adults: Three independent neuropsychological syndromes. *Developmental Medicine and Child Neurology*, 1975, *119*, 121–127.

Meehl, P. E. Theoretical risks and tabular asterisks: Sir Karl, Sir Ronald, and the slow progress of soft psychology. *Journal of Consulting and Clinical Psychology*, 1978, *46*, 806–834.

Morris, R., Blashfield, R., & Satz, P. Neuropsychology and cluster analysis: Problems and pitfalls. *Journal of Clinical Neuropsychology*, 1981, *3*, 179–199.

Obrzut, J. G. Dichotic listening and bisensory memory skills in qualitatively diverse dyslexic readers. *Journal of Learning Disabilities*, 1979, *12*, 304–314.

Petrauskas, R., & Rourke, B. P. Identification of subgroups of retarded readers: A neuropsychological, multivariate approach. *Journal of Clinical Neuropsychology*, 1979, *1*, 17–37.

Pirozzolo, F. J. *The neuropsychology of developmental reading disorders.* New York: Praeger, 1979.

Pirozzolo, F. J., & Rayner, K. Cerebral organization and reading disability. *Neuropsychologia*, 1979, *17*, 485–489.

Rapoport, J. L., & Ferguson, H. B. Biological validation of the hyperkinetic syndrome. *Developmental Medicine and Child Neurology*, 1981, *23*, 667–682.

Rayner, K. Eye movements and the perceptual span in reading. In F. J. Pirozzolo & M. C. Wittrock (Eds.), *Neuropsychological and cognitive processes in reading.* New York: Academic Press, 1981.

Rosenthal, J. H., Boder, E., & Callaway, E. Typology of developmental dyslexia: Evidence for its construct validity. In R. N. Malatesha & P. G. Aaron (Eds.), *Neuropsychological and neurolinguistic aspects of reading disorders.* New York: Academic Press, 1982.

Rourke, B. P. Brain–behavior relationships in children with learning disabilities: A research program. *American Psychologist*, 1975, *30*, 911–920.

Rourke, B. P. Neuropsychological research in reading retardation: A review. In A. L. Benton & D. Pearl (Eds.), *Dyslexia: An appraisal of current knowledge.* New York: Oxford University Press, 1978. (a)

Rourke, B. P. Reading, spelling, arithmetic disabilities: A neuropsychological perspective. In H. R. Myklebust (Ed.), *Progress in learning disabilities* (Vol. 4). New York: Grune & Stratton, 1978. (b)

Rourke, B. P. Central processing deficiencies in children: Toward a developmental neuropsychological model. *Journal of Clinical Neuropsychology*, 1982, *4*, 1–18.

Rourke, B. P. Outstanding issues in learning disabilities research. In M. Rutter (Ed.), *Developmental neuropsychiatry.* New York: Guilford Press, 1983.

Rourke, B. P., & Finlayson, M. A. J. Neuropsychological significance of variations in patterns of academic performances: Verbal and visual-spatial abilities. *Journal of Abnormal Child Psychology*, 1978, *6*, 121–133.

Rourke, B. P., & Strang, J. D. Neuropsychological significance of variations in patterns of academic performance: Motor, psychomotor, and tactile-perceptual abilities. *Journal of Pediatric Psychology*, 1978, *3*, 62–66.

Saltzberg, B., Burton, W. D., Jr., Fletcher, J. M., Michael, R. L., & Burch, N. R. *Measures of regional neural connectivity.* Paper presented at the Thirty-Fourth Annual Conference on Engineering in Medicine and Biology, 1981.

Sattler, J. M. *Assessment of children's intelligence.* Philadelphia: W. B. Saunders, 1974.

Satz, P., & Fletcher, J. M. Minimal brain dysfunctions: An appraisal of research concepts and methods. In H. Rie & E. Rie (Eds.), *Handbook of minimal brain dysfunctions.* New York: Wiley-Interscience, 1980.

Satz, P., & Morris, R. Learning disability subtypes: A review. In F. J. Pirozzolo & M. C. Wittrock (Eds.), *Neuropsychological and cognitive processes in reading.* New York: Academic Press, 1981.

Siegel, L. S., & Linder, A. Short-term memory processes in children with reading and arithmetic disabilities. *Developmental Psychology,* 1984, *20,* 200–207.

Skinner, H. A. Toward the integration of classification theory and methods. *Journal of Abnormal Psychology,* 1981, *90,* 68–87.

Sobotka, K. R., & May, J. G. Visual evoked potentials and reaction time in normal and dyslexic children. *Psychophysiology,* 1977, *14,* 18–24.

Sweeney, J. E., & Rourke, B. P. Neuropsychological significance of phonetically accurate and phonetically inaccurate spelling errors in younger and older retarded spellers. *Brain and Language,* 1978, *6,* 212–225.

Taylor, H. G., & Fletcher, J. M. Biological foundations of specific developmental disorders: Methods, findings, and future directions. *Journal of Clinical Child Psychology,* 1983, *12,* 46–65.

Taylor, H. G., Fletcher, J. M., & Satz, P. Component processes in reading disabilities: A neuropsychological approach. In R. N. Malatesha & P. G. Aaron (Eds.), *Neuropsychological and neurolinguistic aspects of reading disorders.* New York: Academic Press, 1982.

Weber, B. A., & Omenn, G. S. Auditory and visual evoked responses in children with familial reading disabilities. *Journal of Learning Disabilities,* 1977, *10,* 153–158.

10

Subgroups and Subtypes of Learning-Disabled and Normal Children: A Cross-Cultural Replication

HARRY VAN DER VLUGT

PAUL SATZ

The search for subytpes of learning-disabled children is of recent origin. Most of this research, which has been confined to the past decade, has been critiqued in a recent review by Satz and Morris (1981). The present chapter, and the volume as a whole, are testimony to the increasing interest in and recognition of the subtype problem in reading and learning disabilities. In the past decade, investigators have begun to recognize the heterogeneity that exists in these disabilities and have become increasingly skeptical of those who treat the concept of reading or learning disability as a homogeneous diagnostic entity. Traditionally, these views have fostered rather simplistic explanations concerning biological and/or psychological substrates of the disability. Some examples include the synaptic-transmission theory of Smith and Carrigan (1959), Delacato's (1959) central-neurological-organization theory, Bender's (1958) maturational hypothesis, Cruickshank's (1977) perceptual-deficit hypothesis, and Vellutino's (1978) verbal-mediation hypothesis.

Harry van der Vlugt. Department of Developmental Psychology, University of Tilburg, Tilburg, The Netherlands.

Paul Satz. The Neuropsychiatric Institute, University of California at Los Angeles, Los Angeles, California, USA.

THE FLORIDA STUDY

One of the larger subtype studies reported to date was carried out in Florida by Satz and his associates (Morris & Satz, 1983; Satz & Morris, 1981, 1983). Unique features of these studies included (1) the use of an *unselected* sample of learning-disabled children at the Grade 5 level and a smaller *selected* sample of age-matched controls, both of which samples had been followed longitudinally since kindergarten; and (2) the use of a multivariate statistical procedure (i.e., cluster analysis) to determine, at Grade 5, whether these procedures could initially identify different *subgroups* of learning-disabled and normal subjects using Wide Range Achievement Test (WRAT) subtests, and, subsequently, could identify different *subtypes* within the learning-disabled subgroups.

These objectives were accomplished by first analyzing the WRAT scores of a large and generally unselected sample ($n = 236$) of white boys who remained in Alachua County, Florida, at the end of Grade 5 (6 years later).[1] The sample (mean age = 11 years) included children at all levels of achievement. This approach represented the first attempt to use cluster analysis to define the target subgroup and comparison subgroups prior to the search for subtypes. The advantages of the approach are (1) that it avoids the use of exclusionary criteria in the selection of learning-disabled subjects, and (2) that it provides a more objective and statistical classification of index cases. Cluster analysis is a procedure designed to facilitate the creation of classification schemes. It has been defined as a procedure that groups individuals into homogeneous clusters based on each subject's performance on the clustering variables.

The WRAT Reading, Spelling, and Arithmetic subtests were first converted into discrepancy scores by comparing a child's grade level with the grade-equivalent score obtained on each subtest. These scores were then subjected to cluster analysis in order to group individuals most similar to each other on these discrepancy scores.

The WRAT data were subjected to an average-linkage hierarchical agglomerative clustering method, utilizing a squared Euclidean distance measure of similarity. The average-linkage method combined with the Euclidean distance measure was used because of the high correlation

1. The sample comprised *all* of the *remaining* learning-disabled boys from the original standardization population who continued to reside in Alachua County, plus their primary and sometimes secondary age-matched controls. This selection procedure resulted in a larger number of learning-disabled subjects; we discuss this result below.

among the WRAT subtests (Jastak & Jastak, 1976), and because of its sensitivity to elevation in a data set. This method was thought likely to permit clusters that differed in their levels of achievement to emerge.

Nine clusters (subgroups) emerged, which were then subjected to a K-means iterative partitioning method of clustering. This additional method was used because of the fact that an individual, once placed in a given cluster by a hierarchical agglomerative method, cannot be reassigned to a later-forming cluster, even if his/her similarity to the members of the later-forming cluster is greater.[2] This method attempts to reduce within-cluster variance (i.e., to increase homogeneity) while increasing between-cluster variance (i.e., decreasing overlap), thus attempting to clarify the cluster solution.

The nine subgroups, which included 230 of the 236 subjects, revealed a number of interesting patterns of reading, spelling, and arithmetic skill.[3] These results are presented in Figure 10-1, in which the discrepancy scores on each WRAT subtest are expressed on a scale with a population mean of 0 and a standard deviation of 1. This method permits visualization of the subgroups in terms of both pattern and elevation. Subgroups 1 and 2 both obtained superior scores in Reading, and Subgroup 3 achieved uniformly high Reading, Spelling and Arithmetic scores. Subgroup 4 emerged as a group with adequate Reading and Spelling scores, but standard performance in Arithmetic. Subgroup 5 constituted a unique group by virtue of its average Reading, slightly below-average Spelling, and severely depressed Arithmetic scores. Subgroup 6 showed average Reading and Spelling scores, but was superior in Arithmetic. Subgroup 7's performance in all areas was the most nearly average of all the subgroups.

At the lower end of the achievement spectrum, Subgroups 8 and 9 each contained a large number of children. Reading and Spelling scores for these two subgroups could be arranged according to decreasing levels of performance. Arithmetic scores were below average for both subgroups. The overall achievement levels of subgroups 8 and 9 were sufficiently

2. During each iterative partitioning phase, each individual is statistically removed from his/her parent cluster, and his/her similarity to members of all other clusters is computed. If the individual's similarity to members of another cluster is greater, he/she is placed in that cluster.

3. Three small clusters, consisting of only six subjects, resisted incorporation into the larger clusters until a four-cluster solution. Following the recommendation of Everitt (1974), they were considered "outliers" and were dropped from further analysis.

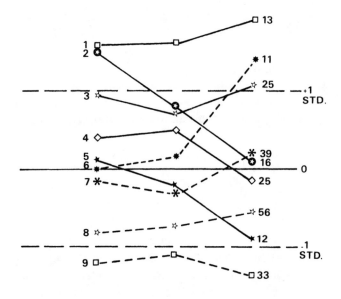

READ   SPELL   ARITHMETIC

FIG. 10-1. WRAT Discrepancy scores for achievement subgroups; mean based on Florida population.

depressed (2-year deficit) to suggest that these children could be labeled "learning-disabled." There were 89 boys in these two subgroups.

The validity of the cluster subgroups was examined by performing a multivariate analysis of variance (MANOVA) to determine whether any group differences existed in terms of IQ (Peabody Picture Vocabulary Test, or PPVT), neuropsychological performance, neurological status, and socioeconomic status (SES). Robust differences were shown for each of these analyses. For example, the PPVT IQ scores ranged from 90 (Subgroup 9) to 116 (Subgroup 1), with an overall sample mean of 103, which closely approximates the standardization mean for this test. Similar subgroup differences were also found for the language and cognitive–perceptual tests of the neuropsychological battery; again, Subgroups 8 and 9 showed lower performances on each of these tests. Chi-square tests of independence were also significant between subgroups in terms of neurological and SES. Subgroups 8 and 9 contained a much larger proportion of children with "soft" neurological signs and lower SES.

These results lend support to the use of cluster-analytic techniques as an objective method of identifying different *subgroups* of learning-disabled *and* normal children, prior to the search for *subtypes* within the learning-disabled subgroups. The learning-disabled subgroups (i.e., 8 and 9) were then subjected to additional cluster analysis, using neuropsychological variables, to search for homogeneous subtypes of learning-disabled children. This second phase of the study is described later in this chapter.

THE DUTCH STUDY

METHOD

Our first purpose in a study conducted in The Netherlands was to determine whether these initial *subgroup* classification methods would yield similar results in a cross-cultural sample of Dutch schoolchildren. The Dutch subjects were 234 white male children who were enrolled in either regular classes or one of two special schools for the learning-disabled, according to IQ level: mild (IQ $\geq$ 90) or severe (IQ $\leq$ 90). The sample distribution was as follows: regular school ($n = 130$), special school—mild ($n = 61$), and special school—severe ($n = 43$). The ages closely matched those in the Florida sample; they ranged from 10 years, 9 months to 11 years, 9 months, with a mean age of 11 years, 3 months. Sample size was also the same between studies (Florida, $n = 236$; The Netherlands, $n = 234$), as were race and sex (white males).

The children were administered a Dutch translation of the WRAT (Jastak & Jastak, 1976).[4] The Reading, Spelling, and Arithmetic subtests were first converted into discrepancy scores by comparing a child's grade level with the grade-equivalent score obtained on each subtest. These scores were then subjected to cluster analysis in order to group individuals most similar to each other on these discrepancy scores. Exactly the same statistical approaches were employed as in the Florida study, in order to achieve a fairly objective cross-cultural replication.

A hierarchical agglomerative method was employed, utilizing an average-linkage method for combining subjects into clusters and a squared

---

4. A reading comprehension test was also administered, but these results were not included in the cluster analysis because of their high correlation (see Table 10-1) with results of each of the WRAT subtests (Reading = .72; Spelling = .72; Arithmetic = .76). The deletion also permitted a more direct replication of the Florida study.

Euclidean distance measure to determine similarity. The latter measure was selected because of the high correlation reported among WRAT subtests (Jastak & Jastak, 1976) and confirmed in previous studies (Satz & Morris, 1981) and the present study (see Table 10-1). The squared Euclidean distance measure was also employed because of its sensitivity to elevation in a data set that included children of varying levels of performance. This approach also permitted the search for subgroups of children whose performance (achievement scores) might vary in terms of pattern as well as level (Morris, Blashfield, & Satz, 1981).

RESULTS

As in the Florida study, nine clusters (subgroups) emerged; these were then subjected to a K-means iterative partitioning cluster analysis to determine whether an optimal solution was obtained. This method, which attempts to reduce within-cluster variance while increasing between-cluster variance, has been strongly recommended by Morris *et al.* (1981) as an important prevalidation check on the cluster solution.

The nine subgroups, which included 231 subjects, revealed patterns and levels of performance quite similar to those in the Florida study. Note also that the coverage was again extremely high (231/234 = 99%), with only three subjects resisting incorporation into the primary clusters. Following the recommendation of Everitt (1974), these "outliers" were dropped from further analyses. The results for each of the nine subgroups are presented in Figure 10-2, where the discrepancy scores on each WRAT subtest are expressed on a scale with a population mean of 0 and a standard deviation of 1. This method permits visualization of the subgroups in terms of both pattern and elevation.

TABLE 10-1. Pearson Product–Moment Correlations among Spelling, Reading, and Arithmetic Subtests of the WRAT, and a Reading Comprehension Test

	Spelling	Reading	Arithmetic
Reading	.86		
Arithmetic	.75	.68	
Reading comprehension	.72	.72	.76

Note. Sample size = 231.

Subgroups 2 and 4 of the Dutch study (Figure 10-2), like Subgroups 1 and 2 of the Florida study (Figure 10-1), obtained superior WRAT Reading scores, but Subgroup 4 (like Subgroup 2 in the Florida study) revealed only average performance in Arithmetic. Subgroup 3 (like Subgroup 3 in the Florida study) achieved high Reading, Spelling, and Arithmetic scores. Subgroup 1 (like Subgroup 7 in the Florida study) emerged as a group with uniformly average performance on each of the WRAT subtests. In fact, the first four subgroups, while varying largely in terms of pattern, could be characterized by their average to superior achievement on the WRAT subtests. These subgroups included 138 of the subjects in the study sample; more is said on this point later.

The remaining subgroups (5-9), while also varying in terms of pat-

FIG. 10-2. WRAT Discrepancy scores for achievement subgroups; mean based on Dutch population.

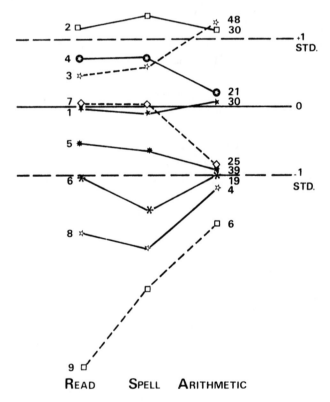

tern, could be characterized by decreasing levels of achievement on the WRAT subtests. These subgroups included 93 of the subjects in the study sample; more is said on this point later. Subgroup 7 (like Subgroup 5 in the Florida study) revealed a pattern of average performance on Reading and Spelling, but very low performance on Arithmetic. This pattern indicated a *specific* arithmetic disability problem. Subgroups 5, 6, 8 and 9 (like Subgroups 8 and 9 in the Florida study), in contrast to the *specific* arithmetic disability subgroup (7), revealed increasingly low performance on each of the WRAT subtests. The patterns in these subgroups would be compatible with a *nonspecific* learning disability, characterized by increasing deficiencies in reading, spelling, and arithmetic. Although performance on the Arithmetic subtest was higher than on the Reading and Spelling subtests in Subgroups 8 and 9, all of these subtest performances were significantly depressed (deficits ≥ 2 years).

VALIDATION

These nine subgroups, based on their respective patterns and elevations, included four that were characterized by average–superior achievement (Subgroups 1–4) and five that were characterized by specific and/or general delays in achievement (Subgroups 5–9). If one compares these subgroup classifications (predictions) with the actual school settings in which the children resided (external criteria), one could determine the accuracy or validity of the clustering solution. Such comparisons can be seen in Table 10-2. The table presents the means and standard scores for each of the three WRAT subtests across the nine subgroup clusters. Inspection of this table reveals that, out of the 138 children classified as belonging to Subgroups 1–4, only 8 of the children in Subgroup 1 and 5 of the children in Subgroup 4 were misclassified as learning-disabled (in fact, as only mildly learning-disabled); this represents a valid negative rate of 91% (125/138) and a false positive rate of 9% (13/138). Conversely, of the 93 children who were classified as belonging to Subgroups 5–9, only 1 child in Subgroup 5, 1 child in Subgroup 6, and 2 children in Subgroup 7 were misclassified as average students. These outcomes represent a valid positive rate of 96% (89/93) and a false negative rate of only 4% (4/93). In terms of overall classification accuracy, the clustering solution, based on the three WRAT subtests, managed to classify correctly 93% of the total study sample (214/231).

TABLE 10-2. Validation of Classification Method Using WRAT Subtests (Nine-Cluster Solution) by Type of School

Cluster	n	Mean WRAT subtest scores			Type of school		
		Reading	Spelling	Arithmetic	Regular	Mild	Severe
1	39	76.92	44.77	38.44	31	8	0
2	30	90.40	53.07	47.70	30	0	0
3	48	82.12	48.31	47.94	48	0	0
4	21	84.95	49.24	39.19	16	5	0
5	39	70.77	40.95	29.02	1	22	16
6	19	65.10	35.74	28.79	1	6	12
7	25	77.72	45.16	29.12	2	18	5
8	4	55.75	32.50	26.75	0	1	3
9	6	32.17	29.00	22.00	0	0	6
Total	231	76.98	45.02	37.66	56%	26%	18%

COMMENTS

The results described above closely approximate the findings reported in the Florida study. Essentially the same number and type of achievement *subgroups* were derived from two cross-cultural samples of 11-year-old white males, based on cluster analysis of their WRAT subtest performances. In each study, a number of different subgroups emerged for the normal and learning-disabled children. Generally, the subgroup patterns were more varied in the normal subjects in both studies. These patterns included some subgroups of children who obtained superior performance levels on each of the WRAT subtests, others of children who obtained average performance on each of the subtests, and still others of children whose achievement patterns varied from average to superior on each subtest. Both the Florida and the Dutch studies also revealed a specific subgroup of children who showed average Reading and Spelling scores, but marked deficits in Arithmetic. This specific arithmetic disability subgroup should come as no surprise to clinicians or investigators familiar with learning-disabled children (see Strang & Rourke, Chapters 8 and 14, this volume). What is important to note, however, is that this specific subgroup of children could be inadvertently screened *out* of intervention programs or screened *into* normal comparison groups in programs or studies in which only reading recognition or comprehension measures were employed.

The remaining learning disability subgroups, by contrast, showed decreasing levels of performance in both studies on each of the WRAT subtests. In fact, there was no subgroup among the remaining subjects whose pattern consisted of average performance on at least one of the WRAT subtests. That is, if Reading and Spelling scores were down, so was the Arithmetic score. In this respect, both studies failed to identify a specific reading disability subgroup. If this finding was valid, it would suggest that the remediation of reading problems may be hampered by the presence of other learning difficulties in a child. These problems might hamper the remediation process if not well understood.

Why should the fact that a specific reading disability subgroup did not emerge in either study cause concern? Most studies have long noted that delays in word recognition and comprehension are intrinsically associated with difficulties in a number of cognitive and linguistic information-processing domains (Doehring, Hoshko, & Bryans, 1979; Mattis, French, & Rapin, 1975; Rourke, 1976, 1978; Rutter, 1978; Satz & Van Nostrand, 1973). These associated deficits, whether correlative or causative, will significantly increase the likelihood of other learning difficulties—namely, arithmetic disability, especially if problems in visual–spatial organization are present (Petrauskas & Rourke, 1979; Rourke & Finlayson, 1978; Satz & Morris, 1983).

SUBTYPE CLASSIFICATION: FLORIDA AND DUTCH FINDINGS

METHOD

In an attempt to replicate the second phase (the *subtype* phase) of the Florida study, we used identical neuropsychological measures as the clustering variables in the investigation of the Dutch learning disability subgroups (5–9). These five subgroups, it will be recalled, were severely impaired on at least one of the WRAT subtests.

The subjects in these five subgroups ($n = 93$) were then subjected to cluster-analytic techniques, based on their performance on four neuropsychological tests. These tests (clustering variables) were selected in the Florida study from a larger group of measures that were based on high factor loadings on a language factor (WISC Similarities subtest; Verbal Fluency Test) and a perceptual factor (Beery Test of Visual–Motor Integration; Recognition–Discrimination). A discussion of the tests and the factor analyses can be found in Fletcher and Satz (1979).

The rationale for this procedure was to restrict the number of tests to a few highly independent factors that would reduce test redundancy and random error variance, and thus would increase subtype interpretability. Reliable variables were, therefore, expected to yield a more reliable classification. The variables also provided the opportunity to employ a number of clustering techniques to insure that the subtypes were replicable across different clustering methods. Replication at this level was felt to be mandatory, in view of the controversy surrounding the potential uses and misuses of cluster analyses (Everitt, 1974).

In the Dutch study, the four-cluster and the seven-cluster solutions appeared to be highly replicable. The subtypes (see Figs. 10-3 and 10-4) are based on performances on the four neuropsychological tests (as in the

FIG. 10-3. Neuropsychological test discrepancy scores for learning disability subtypes; mean based on Florida population. (Abbreviations for tests: SIM, WISC Similarities subtest; VF, Verbal Fluency Test; VMI, Test of Visual–Motor Integration; RD, Recognition–Discrimination. Abbreviations for subtypes: UNX, unexpected; SV, specific verbal deficiency; GV, general verbal deficiency; VPM, visual–perceptual–motor deficiency; GD, general deficiency.)

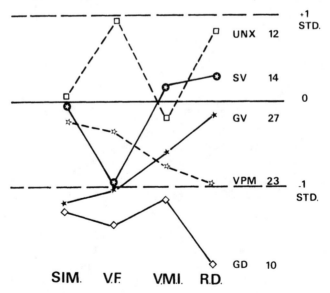

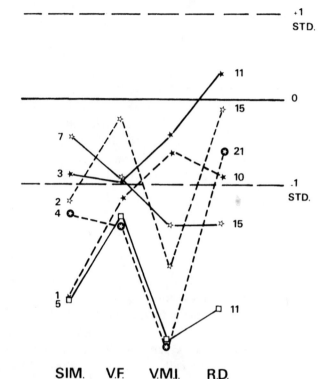

SIM.   V.F.   V.M.I.   R.D.

FIG. 10-4. Neuropsychological test discrepancy scores for learning disability subtypes; mean based on Dutch population. (For key to abbreviations, see Fig. 10-3.)

Florida study), which have been converted to standard scores with a population mean of 0 for the control group ($n = 34$) and a standard deviation of 1.

RESULTS

The six-cluster solution of the Florida study is presented in Figure 10-3, and the seven-cluster solution of the Dutch study is presented in Figure 10-4. Comparing the Dutch seven-cluster solution with the Florida six-cluster solution, it is obvious that the visual–perceptual–motor deficiency subtype of the Florida study is highly similar to Subtype 7 of the Dutch study. Also, the general verbal deficiency Subtype of the Florida study shows a strong resemblance to Subtypes 1 and 3 of the Dutch study. However, Subtype 1 exhibits lower scores for Similarities and Recognition–Discrimination than does Subtype 3. The general deficiency subtype of the Florida study is highly comparable to Subtypes 4 and 5 of the Dutch study. The specific verbal deficiency subtype and the unexpected subtype of the Florida study are not represented in the Dutch study. Instead, a subtype (Subtype 2) with specific deficiencies on the Similarities subtest and the test of Visual–Motor Integration is found; this subtype has no counterpart in the Florida study. Except for this last subtype ($n = 15$), all subjects belonged to subtypes comparable with the Florida study (82%).

COMMENTS

The results reported above closely approximate the findings reported in the Florida study. However, assigning an interpretation to these subtypes should be done with extreme caution. Subtypes 1, 3, 4, 5, and 7 are comparable to those established in other studies, which have typically reported a language-disabled, a perceptually disabled, and/or a mixed subtype of learning-disabled children. In these studies, the language-disordered subtype has more frequently been observed (Doehring & Hoshko, 1977; Mattis, 1978; Mattis et al., 1975; Petrauskas & Rourke, 1979). In the present study, at least 82% (68/83) of the children evidenced some type of language difficulty on the neuropsychological tests (Subtypes 1–5). However, the clustering methods classified these children into different types of language-disordered groups, some with more global language difficulties (Subtypes 1 and 3), some with more selective language and perceptual difficulties (Subtype 2), and some with both global language and global perceptual handicaps (Subtypes 4 and 5). Such profile differences are familiar to clinicians working with learning-disabled children.

    The derivation of Subtype 7 (children with a visual–perceptual–motor disability) should give pause to those who postulate a unitary language deficit for learning-disabled children (Vellutino, 1978). At least 18% of the children in this relatively unselected sample of learning-disabled children showed no impairment in language skills. Most subtype studies have identified a subgroup of learning-disabled children who continue to show selective cognitive deficiencies in processing visual information. To ignore this subtype of learning-disabled children could retard progress in the search for differential causes, as well as subject these children to inappropriate methods of remediation (see Strang & Rourke, Chapter 14, this volume).

CONCLUSIONS

Despite the promise that this cross-cultural replication holds, particularly for establishing an approach for classification, the results should be viewed as preliminary. The following concerns should be noted. First, one must question the use of the WRAT, with its restricted range and highly correlated subtests, as an achievement measure to identify learning-disabled children. However, the classifications obtained with the WRAT were in high concordance with the schools to which the children had been assigned. Second, one could fault the use of such a small number of neuropsychological tests and could ask whether the same subtype clusters would have emerged with a larger number of "different" neuropsychological variables. For example, the study would have been strengthened by the use of more formal psycholinguistic measures. Third, each of the subtypes was derived from a highly homogeneous group of children with respect to age (average 11 years), sex (male), and race (white). Finally, the use of cluster analysis as a multivariate classification method has its own inherent limitations. Cluster analysis includes numerous methods, many of which have been neither critically examined nor clearly defined.

Despite these concerns, the findings described in this chapter provide some assurance that cluster-analytic methods can be applied to a broader segment of school populations, using achievement measures, in order to identify different subgroups of normal and learning-disabled children. When identical neuropsychological measures were used in a Dutch sample as clustering variables in the search for subtypes, 82% of the learning-disabled children were assigned to subtypes that were highly similar to the subtypes obtained in the Florida study.

ACKNOWLEDGMENT

We gratefully acknowledge the conceptual and methodological contributions of Robin Morris in the preparation of this chapter.

226 / *Validity Studies of Learning Disability Subtypes*

REFERENCES

Bender, L. Problems in conceptualization and communication in children with developmental alexia. In P. H. Hock & J. Zubin (Eds.), *Psychopathology of communication.* New York: Grune & Stratton, 1958.

Cruickshank, W. M. Some issues facing the field of learning disabilities. *Journal of Learning Disabilities,* 1977, *10,* 57–64.

Delacato, C. H. *The treatment and prevention of reading problems.* Springfield, Ill.: Charles C Thomas, 1959.

Doehring, D. G., & Hoshko, I. M. Classification of reading problems by the Q-technique of factor analysis, *Cortex,* 1977, *13,* 281–294.

Doehring, D. G., Hoshko, I. M., & Bryans, B. N. Statistical classification of children with reading problems. *Journal of Clinical Neuropsychology,* 1979, *1,* 5–16.

Everitt, E. *Cluster analysis.* London: Heinemann, 1974.

Fletcher, J. M., & Satz, P. Developmental changes in the performance correlates of reading achievement. *Journal of Clinical Neuropsychology,* 1979, *1,* 23–37.

Jastak, J. F., & Jastak, S. R. *The Wide Range Achievement Test Manual of Instruction* (Rev. ed.). Wilmington, Del.: Guidance Associates of Delaware, 1976.

Mattis, S. Dyslexia syndromes: A working hypothesis that works. In A. L. Benton & D. Pearl (Eds.), *Dyslexia: An appraisal of current knowledge.* New York: Oxford University Press, 1978.

Mattis, S., French, J. H., & Rapin, I. Dyslexia in children and adults: Three independent neuropsychological syndromes. *Developmental Medicine and Child Neurology,* 1975, *17,* 150–163.

Morris, R., Blashfield, R., & Satz, P. Neuropsychology and cluster analysis: Potentials and problems. *Journal of Clinical Neuropsychology,* 1981, *3,* 79–99.

Morris, R., & Satz, P. Classification issues in subtype research: An application of some methods and concepts. In H. A. Whitaker & R. N. Malatesha (Eds.), *Dyslexia: A global issue.* New York: Academic Press, 1983.

Petrauskas, R. J., & Rourke, B. P. Identification of subtypes of retarded readers: A neuropsychological multivariate approach. *Journal of Clinical Neuropsychology,* 1979, *1,* 17–37.

Rourke, B. P. Issues in the neuropsychological assessment of children with learning disabilities. *Canadian Psychological Review,* 1976, *17,* 89–102.

Rourke, B. P. Reading, spelling, arithmetic disabilities: A neuropsychological perspective. In H. R. Myklebust (Ed.), *Progress in learning disabilities* (Vol. 4). New York: Grune & Stratton, 1978.

Rourke, B. P., & Finlayson, M. A. J. Neuropsychological significance of variations in patterns of academic performance: Verbal and visual–spatial abilities. *Journal of Abnormal Child Psychology,* 1978, *6,* 121–133.

Rutter, M. Prevalence and types of dyslexia. In A. L. Benton & D. Pearl (Eds.), *Dyslexia: An appraisal of current knowledge.* New York: Oxford University Press, 1978.

Satz, P., & Morris, R. Learning disability subtypes: A review. In F. G. Pirozzolo & M. C. Withock (Eds.), *Neuropsychological and cognitive processes in reading.* New York: Academic Press, 1981.

Satz, P., & Morris, R. The search for subtype classification in learning disabled children. In R. Tarter (Ed.), *The child at risk.* New York: Oxford University Press, 1983.

Satz, P., & Van Nostrand, G. Developmental dyslexia: An evaluation of a theory. In P. Satz & J. Ross (Eds.), *The disabled learner: Early detection and intervention.* Rotterdam: Rotterdam University Press, 1973.

Smith, D. E. P., & Carrigan, P. M. *The nature of reading disability.* New York: Harcourt, Brace & World, 1959.

Vellutino, F. R. Toward an understanding of dyslexia: Psychological factors in specific reading disability. In A. L. Benton & D. Pearl (Eds.), *Dyslexia: An appraisal of current knowledge.* New York: Oxford University Press, 1978.

11

Educational Validation Studies of Learning Disability Subtypes

G. REID LYON

Recent advances in the application of multivariate classification methods (e.g., cluster analysis) to neuropsychological and/or achievement test data obtained from learning-disabled children have shown that the learning-disabled population can be most adequately conceptualized as being comprised of a number of discrete subtypes or subgroups. When using "clustering" techniques, investigators have attempted to partition learning-disabled youngsters into optimally homogeneous subtypes on the basis of the natural multidimensional structure inherent within a set of test data. Thus, subtypes are obtained by maximizing within-subtype homogeneity (the profiles of neuropsychological and/or achievement test scores for children in each subgroup are very similar) and between-subtype heterogeneity (the test-score profiles of children in different subtypes are very different from one another). To date, applications of these "clustering" and other statistical procedures have resulted in the identification of reliable and meaningful subtypes within samples of disabled readers (Doehring & Hoshko, 1977; Fisk & Rourke, 1979; Lyon, Rietta, Watson, Porch, & Rhodes, 1981; Lyon, Stewart, & Freedman, 1982; Lyon & Watson, 1981; Petrauskas & Rourke, 1979; Satz & Morris, 1981), disabled spellers (Sweeney & Rourke, Chapter 7, this volume), and youngsters who manifest arithmetic disabilities (Rourke & Strang, 1978, 1983; Strang & Rourke, Chapter 8, this volume).

G. Reid Lyon. Center for Language and Cerebral Function, and Departments of Neurology and Communication Sciences and Disorders, University of Vermont, Burlington, Vermont, USA.

The theoretical and educational advantages of analyzing the learning-disabled population via multivariate classification methods are numerous. First, exploration of natural subtypes that exist within samples of learning-disabled children may provide insights into possibly useful clinical syndromes (see Lyon, 1983; Rourke, 1982; and Satz & Morris, 1981, for a discussion of this concept). Second, delineation of specific subtype patterns of neuropsychological organization and academic ability structures in learning-disabled children, in combination with assessment of subtype neurophysiological characteristics, can enhance extant knowledge of meaningful continuities of development, especially in reference to brain–behavior relationships (see Duffy, Denckla, Bartels, & Sandini, 1980).

Finally, identification of subtypes of children with putative learning disabilities provides a research framework for the design of studies to investigate two practical questions. First, do different patterns of neurobehavioral deficits influence the acquisition of reading, written language, and arithmetic skills? Second, do relationships exist between a learning-disabled child's neuropsychological pattern of impairment and that youngster's response to a particular teaching approach or intervention? To date, our clinical and research experiences (see Lyon, 1983; Lyon & Wiss, in press; Lyon & Watson, 1981; Lyon *et al.*, 1981, 1982) have suggested that there are some systematic relationships between various learning disability subtype neuropsychological profiles and the types of errors made by subtype members as they engage in reading and written language tasks. In addition, preliminary pilot research conducted in our laboratory (see Lyon, 1983) has indicated that knowledge of the learning characteristics of subtypes can provide an enabling step toward identifying some disabled readers who might benefit more from one type of teaching approach than another.

Research concerned with the relationships among the neuropsychological characteristics of learning disability, the academic learning characteristics of these subtypes, and differential subtype responses to teaching can be considered to be in its early stages. However, these investigations represent a step toward the educational validation of empirically derived subtypes of learning-disabled children. In a practical sense, while identified subtypes can be shown to be "real" or meaningful in a number of ways (e.g., correspondence with known clinical entities, cross-validation, multivariate significance tests), the actual utility of subtype identification procedures lies in our ability to understand and use such classification schemes to optimize learning-disabled children's responses to various forms of teaching. Until specific interactions between patterns of impairment in learning disability subtypes and responses to educational interventions can be identified consistently, the pedagogical value of subtype classification remains open to question.

Within this context, the remainder of this chapter is designed to review the results of studies that have attempted to validate empirically derived learning disability subtypes through investigation of how subtypes either (1) differ with respect to performance on external educational criteria or (2) differ in response to some form or method of teaching. It should be kept in mind that such studies are limited and, at present, generally restricted to investigations of disabled readers. In the main, the studies reviewed in this chapter are those that my associates and I have carried out at Northwestern University. It should also be pointed out that the assessment of the educational validity of empirically derived subgroups can be applied to learning disability subtypes identified by clinical-inferential methods. Since it is beyond the scope of this chapter to review studies associated with clinically derived subtypes and their validation, the reader is referred to Lyon (1983) and Satz and Morris (1981) for a discussion of this information.

ASSESSING THE EDUCATIONAL VALIDITY OF LEARNING DISABILITY SUBTYPES

In general, the *educational* validity of empirically derived learning disability subtypes can be assessed in two major ways. In the first procedure, members of subtypes that have been identified via empirical classification procedures (e.g., cluster analysis or Q-type factor analysis) are administered a series of academic or educational tasks that were not included in the original statistical classification analysis. Then, a series of additional statistical analyses are carried out—analyses of variance (ANOVAs) or multivariate analyses of variance (MANOVAs)—to determine whether significant differences exist among the identified subtypes on these "external" educational tasks. If, for example, significant differences are found among subtypes with respect to how their members perform on a series of oral reading measures, then the subtypes might be considered to be "real," or, more specifically, to have some educational relevance. This form of educational validation can be labeled "determination of subtype differences in educational skills."

In the second procedure, subtype members are assigned to one or more teaching conditions to determine whether interactions exist among subtype characteristics and magnitude of response to type(s) of teaching methods. Obviously, if subtypes respond differentially to various forms of teaching, and if these interactions are systematic and replicable, then the educational validity of the subtypes is well established. This form of validation can be labeled "determination of subtype response to instruction."

As pointed out earlier in this chapter, the number of studies attempting to validate learning disability subtypes educationally by employing either one or both of the procedures described above is limited and generally restricted to investigations of disabled readers. However, although the following review examines only subtypes of disabled readers with respect to differences in their educational skills and their responses to reading instruction, it should be kept in mind that similar procedures could be extended to validation of arithmetic, spelling, and social-personality subtypes.

EDUCATIONAL VALIDATION OF SUBTYPES
OF DISABLED READERS

BACKGROUND

Since 1975, I and several of my colleagues at the University of New Mexico, the University of Alabama at Birmingham, and Northwestern University have carried out a series of studies designed to determine whether samples of school-verified disabled readers could be clustered into independent and homogenous subtypes on the basis of their performance on neuropsychological test batteries. Initially, we were particularly interested in whether the neuropsychological subtypes identified by Mattis, French, and Rapin (1975), who used clinical-inferential subtyping methods, could be replicated using empirical classification techniques (cluster analysis). Later, we became interested in the identification of academic behavioral differences among subtypes and the exploration of differential subtype responses to various forms of teaching. Within this context, our research program to date has done the following: (1) identified six subtypes of disabled readers at the 11- and 12-year-old levels (Lyon, 1978a, 1978b); (2) replicated these subtypes using a new subject sample (Lyon & Watson, 1981); (3) identified some differences among these replicated subtypes on measures of oral reading, reading comprehension, and written language skills (Lyon *et al.*, 1981); (4) identified some differences among these six subtypes in terms of response to a teaching method (Lyon, 1983); and (5) identified five subtypes of disabled readers at the 6- through 9-year-old levels, and found some differences among them in component reading behaviors (Lyon *et al.*, 1982).

For clarity and brevity, the subtype identification and educational validation studies cited above are reviewed and discussed in two different sections. Specifically, the investigations concerned with subtype identification (Lyon & Watson, 1981; Lyon *et al.*, 1982) and educational validation via determination of subtype differences in educational skills (Lyon *et al.*, 1981, 1982) are reported in the next section. This is followed by a discussion of our attempts to validate LD subtypes educationally by assessing differential subtype responses to instruction (Lyon, 1983).

DIFFERENCES IN EDUCATIONAL SKILLS

The Lyon and Watson (1981) Study

The purpose of the Lyon and Watson (1981) investigation was to identify independent subtypes within a school-verified sample of disabled readers. Accordingly, 100 11- and 12-year-old readers, diagnosed according to prevailing U.S. Government guidelines (U.S. Office of Education, 1977), and 50 normal readers were administered a series of auditory receptive, auditory expressive, visual–spatial, visual–motor integration, and visual-memory measures (see Table 11-1). These specific measures were selected for use because of their resemblance to those that have been shown to be deficient in disabled readers in previous studies (Lyon, 1978a, 1978b; Mattis *et al.*, 1975), their common use in the public schools, and their usefulness in assessing those linguistic and perceptual processes hypothesized to subserve the reading process (Luria, 1973; Lyon, 1983). Only 11- and 12-year-old subjects were included in the sample to control for the effects of varying chronological ages and developmental levels. The normal readers were included in the study in order to use their test data in the

TABLE 11-1. Tests and Measures Used in the Identification of Subgroups of Learning-Disabled Readers

Test name and abbreviation	Author(s)
The Naming Test (Naming)	Mattis, French, & Rapin (1975)
The Auditory Discrimination Test (Wepman)	Wepman (1973)
The Token Test, Short Form (Token)	Spellacy & Spreen (1969)
The Auditory Attention Span for Related Syllables subtest of the Detroit Tests of Learning Aptitude (Detroit)	Baker & Leland (1958)
The Sound Blending subtest of the Illinois Test of Psycholinguistic Abilities (ITPA)	Kirk, McCarthy, & Kirk (1968)
The Developmental Test of Visual–Motor Integration (VMI)	Beery & Buktenica (1967)
The Raven's Coloured Progressive Matrices (Raven's)	Raven (1960)
The Memory-for-Designs Test (MFD)	Graham & Kendall (1960)

construction of standard (z) scores. Standard scores were calculated by subtracting each disabled reader's raw score for each of the eight diagnostic measures from the mean score of the normal-reading group and dividing this value by the standard deviation for that measure. The decision to use scores obtained by normal readers rather than the normative data for each diagnostic measure was based on several considerations: (1) the lack of appropriate test statistics for many of the diagnostic measures (e.g., Naming, Detroit, Wepman); (2) the need to compare disabled readers from specific geographic regions and school systems with their normal-reading classmates; and (3) the desirability of using local norms to control for differences in dialect and exposure to different reading curricula.

In order to determine the existence of independent and homogeneous subtypes within the sample of disabled readers, their standard (z) scores were cluster-analyzed using a Euclidean distance average-linkage formula and a minimum variance criterion. Following an initial cluster solution, additional cluster analyses were performed using various subsets of the diagnostic variables to insure that the initial solution was not a function of the disabled readers' performance on one or two diagnostic measures.

The results of all the cluster analyses yielded six subtypes. Figure 11-1 shows the standard score profiles for the six subtypes and indicates the number of children in each. For each profile, the mean line (0) represents the normal-reading group's performance and provides an indication of

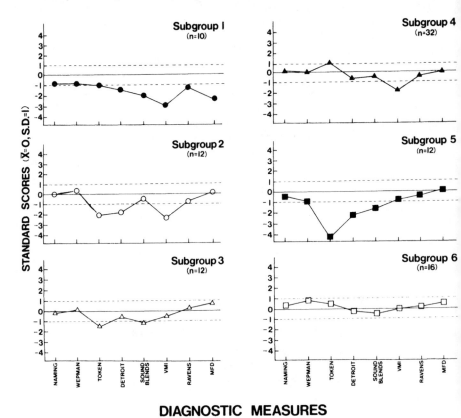

DIAGNOSTIC MEASURES

FIG. 11-1. Standard score profiles for each learning-disabled subtype among 11- to 12-year-old subjects. (From R. Lyon & B. Watson, Empirically derived subgroups of learning disabled readers: Diagnostic characteristics. *Journal of Learning Disabilities*, 1981, *14*, 256–261. Reprinted by permission of The Professional Press.)

how each learning-disabled subtype performed, relative to normal-reading age-mates, on the neuropsychological battery. Neither subtype (cluster) membership nor profile shape differed extensively as a function of the variable subset used. There were also minimal differences between the profile shapes identified in our pilot studies (Lyon, 1978a, 1978b) and the profile shapes in the Lyon and Watson (1981) study (the reader is referred to Lyon, 1983, for a discussion of the similarities and differences in the results of these investigations). The cluster-analytic procedures used in this study accounted for 94% of the disabled readers. Six "outliers" could not be located in any subgroup, and their scores were excluded from further data analyses. Subsequent ANOVAs indicated significant differences among the six subtypes for all diagnostic measures. In addition, a multivariate significance test (Wilks's lambda) showed that the six subtypes were significantly different from one another with respect to their performance on a linear combination of the diagnostic measures, and a post hoc classification analysis (discriminant analysis) indicated a 98% correct hit rate for the classification of subjects into subgroups. An 88% classification hit rate was obtained when these data were "jackknifed."

The results of the cluster analyses, the univariate ANOVAs, and the multivariate analyses indicated that a six-subtype solution was the "best fit" for the data obtained in the Lyon and Watson (1981) study. Prior to describing differences among these subtypes with respect to their educational characteristics, a brief analysis of their linguistic and perceptual behaviors is in order. This analysis should provide a base for an understanding of the differences found among the subtypes in their oral reading and written language skills.

Subtype 1 ($n = 10$) exhibited significant deficits in receptive language comprehension (Token), auditory memory (Detroit), sound blending (ITPA), visual–motor integration (VMI), visual–spatial skills (Raven's), and visual–memory (MFD) skills, with some strengths in naming (Naming) and auditory discrimination (Wepman) skills. This pattern of mixed deficiencies in auditory receptive, auditory expressive, visual–perceptual, and visual-memory skills corresponds to the global language and perceptual deficit subtype identified by Satz and Morris (1981).

Children in Subtype 2 ($n = 12$) also exhibited a pattern of mixed deficits, but in a milder form than observed in Subtype 1. Specifically, significant problems in receptive language comprehension (Token), auditory memory (Detroit), and visual–motor integration (VMI) were observed and may have accounted for the reading problems of these subjects. No deficits were seen in these youngsters' performances on tasks involving naming, auditory discrimination, sound blending, visual–spatial skills, and visual memory.

Members of Subtype 3 ($n = 12$) manifested selective deficits in receptive language comprehension (Token) and sound blending (ITPA) abilities, with corresponding strengths in all other linguistic and visual–perceptual skills measured. Since these children manifested both receptive and expressive oral language deficiencies, it was expected that both oral reading accuracy and comprehension would be limited.

Children in Subtype 4 ($n = 32$) displayed significant deficiencies on the visual–motor integration task (VMI) and average performances on all other measures. This selective deficit in visual–motor behavior was unexpected for two reasons. First, visual–motor behaviors of the type observed in Subtype 4 members have been reported to occur much more frequently in younger children (Mattis *et al.*, 1975; Satz, Rardin, & Ross, 1971). Second, it is not clear why other measures in the diagnostic battery that require the application of visual–perceptual and visual–motor integrative skills did not show similar deficiencies. It could be that the unstructured nature of presentation of the VMI to the children interacted negatively with this subtype's ability to attend to the salient perceptual aspects of the task.

Subtype 5 members ($n = 12$) displayed significant deficits in receptive language comprehension (Token), auditory memory (Detroit), and sound blending (ITPA), with corresponding strengths in all measured visual-perceptual and visual–motor skills. The diagnostic picture observed in Subtype 5 resembles that found among children with global language problems (Mattis *et al.*, 1975; Satz & Morris, 1981; Spellacy & Spreen, 1969) and supports Luria's (1973) hypothesis that necessary behaviors for reading include the adequate retention, synthesis, and expression of sound and word sequences. Given this array of linguistic deficits, it was expected that Subtype 5 would display prominent problems in word-attack and reading comprehension skills.

The pattern of scores obtained by members of Subtype 6 ($n = 16$) indicated a normal diagnostic profile. These results were unexpected, but not inconsistent with present-day notions concerning disabled readers. It is possible, as Larsen (1976) and others (Cohen, 1969; Kirk & Elkins, 1975) have pointed out, that many learning-disabled children read and/or spell poorly because of social, motivational, or educational factors, rather than because of some neurobehavioral deficit. It is of more than passing interest that Satz and Morris (1981) also identified a subtype of disabled readers who performed in a normal fashion on their neuropsychological battery.

The Lyon, Rietta, Watson, Porch, and Rhodes (1981) Study

The specific purpose of the Lyon *et al.* (1981) investigation was to validate educationally the existence and independence of the six subtypes (see Figure 11-1) identified in the Lyon and Watson (1981) study. This educational validation was attempted by comparing the performance of subtype members on measures of oral reading of single words, silent reading comprehension, and written language skills. In this investigation, all subtype members were administered the Reading Recognition and

Reading Comprehension subtests of the Peabody Individual Achievement Test (PIAT; Dunn & Markwardt, 1970) and the Graphic Function, Graphic Names, Graphic Dictation, and Graphic Spelling subtests of the Porch Index of Communicative Ability in Children (PICAC; Porch, 1974).

The results of a univariate ANOVA across subtypes for each PIAT reading measure indicated significant differences among the six subtypes for both Reading Recognition and Reading Comprehension. Post hoc comparisons using the Scheffé method indicated that members of Subtypes 1 and 5 made significantly more errors in oral reading and silent reading comprehension than did children in Subtypes 2, 3, and 4. Members of Subtype 6 scored significantly higher on both reading measures than did the subjects in all other subtypes.

Similarly, the results of a univariate ANOVA across subtypes for each PICAC subtest indicated that each measure successfully differentiated among the six subtypes. Additional post hoc analyses revealed that Subtypes 1, 3, and 5 made significantly more spelling errors than did Subtypes 2, 4, and 6. Subtypes 1 and 3 performed significantly worse than the other subtypes on the Graphic Spelling subtest. Consistent with the reading results was the finding that members of Subtype 1 were the poorest spellers, while the children in Subtype 6 were the most adept.

This educational validation study did indicate a number of subtype differences in educational skills. While all external validation measures did not disciminate significantly between all possible pairs of subtypes, inspection of the statistical data *and* clinical evaluation of subtype differences in reading and written language (spelling) errors reveals interesting relationships between the subtype neuropsychological characteristics described earlier and educational-behavioral development in reading and spelling. These differences and relationships are summarized below.

The reading and spelling errors observed in members of Subtype 1 indicated significant deficits in the development of both a sight-word vocabulary and word-attack skills. For example, when reading single words orally from the PIAT, many Subtype 1 youngsters tended to confuse visually similar letters and words (e.g., "d/b," "n/m," "play/bay," "jump/pond"), to invert letters ("m/w"), and to make reading errors involving internal details ("lodge/ledge," "rain/run"). These oral reading problems appeared to be related to the youngsters' deficiencies in visual–spatial and visual-memory skills. However, the majority of children in Subtype 1 also manifested oral reading deficits that seemed to be associated with their significant deficits in auditory memory and sound blending. For example, frequent vowel errors were noted (e.g., "wagon/wiglin," "colt/callip"), as well as problems in reading words with consonant blends (e.g., "smile/silo") and in pronouncing all syllables in words (e.g., "elegant/elgan").

Subtype 1 children's spelling behaviors also reflected the significant linguistic and visual–perceptual problems observed in the neuropsychological testing. As in their oral reading errors, many of the children confused visually similar words when spelling (e.g., "brush/dush"), inverted letters (e.g., "comb/cowp"), made frequent vowel errors (e.g., "key/kal," "ring/tamy"), and at times produced bizzare nonphonetic spellings (e.g., "pencil/erwich," "spoon/pone," "toothbrush/thothurwlhy"). Subtype 1 members were the most deficient oral readers and spellers in the sample and also produced the lowest scores on the reading comprehension measure. This last finding is not surprising, given the errors described above and their deficiencies in receptive language comprehension.

Subtype 2 members also produced mixed visual and phonic errors when reading, but to a much milder degree than did Subtype 1 children. It appeared that their problems with auditory comprehension and auditory memory impeded a strong phonic attack, as many of the oral reading errors reflected labored auditory analysis and blending (e.g., "run/r-a-l," "fishing/figet"). Surprisingly, many of the children could read phonetically irregular words adequately (e.g., "ruin," "yacht").

The spelling errors produced by Subtype 2 children also appeared more related to their auditory receptive and expressive deficits than to their problems in visual–motor integration. Again, many children could approximate the length of the target words dictated to them, but the letters included in the words often bore no relationship to the sound of the word (e.g., "pencil/pillup," "ring/ralg," "spoon/sasen"). Frequent vowel errors were noted (e.g., "toothbrush/tethbras," crayon/kenon"), as were omissions of final sounds (e.g., "toothbrush/totbu," "crayon/cao"). These youngsters did perform significantly better than Subtype 1 children when comprehending material read silently, indicating some ability to utilize known contexts to predict unknown words.

The oral reading errors made by Subtype 3 youngsters were primarily auditory in nature, as would be expected from their neuropsychological profile. Specifically, their significant deficiencies in receptive language comprehension and sound blending appeared to be related to an inability to read words with consonant combinations (e.g., "smile/soll," "blaze/

bus," "flour/fir," "stylish/sold") and multisyllables ("dangerous/ding," "exercise/exen"). The errors cited here also indicate frequent vowel errors.

The spelling errors produced by the majority of Subtype 3 members were also nonphonetic in nature, ranging from misspellings of simple words (e.g., "run/dab," "play/bek") to misspellings of more complex targets (e.g., "fishing/falup," "igloo/ilit"). The impact of poor auditory comprehension and auditory memory on written language skills could also be observed in Subtype 3 members when they attempted to write grammatically correct sentences using the names of objects displayed before them. Their written productions were frequently concrete (e.g., comb—"I do hinl" [hair]) and were characterized by simple syntax (e.g., pencil—"pclin [pencil] to use") and word omissions (e.g., ring—"when [wear] it no" [on]). As would be expected, comprehension of text read silently was also significantly deficient.

Subtype 4 members displayed an assorted sample of oral reading errors, although most errors were made when attempting to read phonetically irregular words. For example, in the majority of cases, the words "run," "jump," "wagon," and "fishing" were read correctly, although laboriously. Conversely, words such as "brook," "gloves," "ruin," "anchor," and "gaudy" were often mispronounced.

Similar error patterns were also observed in Subtype 4 members' spelling behavior. In general, the misspellings were phonetic in nature, especially when the target words were dictated by the examiner (e.g., "pencil/pensl," "ring/rin," "spoon/spune," "crayon/craon"). Some spelling pattern differences were observed, however, when these youngsters spelled the same words spontaneously in sentences (e.g., "pencil/peole," "ring/rige," "spoon/spon"). This difference in topography of spelling errors could be due to the removal of the auditory cues that are provided by the examiner in dictated spelling. As one might expect, the silent reading comprehension of Subtype 4 children was relatively strong, probably because they could deploy some auditory strengths while reading to help in predicting unknown words from context.

Subtype 5 manifested the most severe deficits in auditory comprehension, auditory memory, and sound blending during neuropsychological testing, and these problems appeared related to the severity of their oral reading and written spelling errors. The major characteristic that distinguished Subtype 5 youngsters from the other children was their consistently poor application of word-attack (phonetic) skills to the reading and spelling process. Quite frequently, even when reading high-frequency one-syllable words, Subtype 5 children could not approximate the correct pronunciation of the word (e.g., "run/wag," "play/ban"). As would be expected, frequent mispronunciations also occurred when they attempted to read more complex words (e.g., "wagon/winter," "brook/ball," "smile/silno").

Analysis of Subtype 5 members' spelling performance revealed similar error patterns. However, in addition to frequent vowel errors (e.g., "brush/blen," "comb/kim"), omission of final sounds (e.g., "pencil/pen," "crayon/caly"), and omission of syllables (e.g., "toothbrush/toth," "penny/pol"), these children also produced poor spacing of letters and words and frequently confused letters (e.g., "brush/dus," "pencil/danit," "spoon/stom").

The significant deficits in auditory comprehension and auditory memory displayed by Subtype 5 also appeared to influence reading comprehension in a negative fashion. These youngsters scored lower on the PIAT comprehension subtest than did any other subtype except Subtype 1.

As would be expected from their neuropsychological test data, children in Subtype 6 were the best readers and spellers in the sample. Both reading and spelling errors were mixed in terms of topography, and no specific error patterns could be discerned. Oral reading errors involved faulty pronunciation of multisyllabic, phonetically irregular words. Although spelling was below age and grade expectation, written formulation and syntax were generally intact with these youngsters.

In summary, the Lyon and Watson (1981) and Lyon *et al.* (1981) studies indicated that subtypes of disabled readers could be identified by empirical means and validated by educational means. The results of these studies indicated a need to determine whether subtypes could be identified within a sample of younger disabled readers, and, if so, whether significant differences would be found among subtypes on measures of component reading skills. The results of the identification and educational validation aspects of this investigation are presented next.

The Lyon, Stewart, and Freedman (1982) Study

The Lyon *et al.* (1982) investigation was initiated in 1980 and was carried out in two phases. The first phase of the study was designed to identify independent subtypes of disabled readers, and the second phase was designed to validate the subtypes educationally against a series of external oral and silent reading criteria. Our subject-sampling procedures in this study differed from those used in the Lyon and Watson (1981) investigation. Specifically, 75 6- through 9-year-old disabled readers, rather than 100 11- and 12-year-olds, were selected for study. However, similar to the Lyon and Watson (1981) study, we also selected a group of normal readers ($n = 42$) from the same classrooms as the disabled readers in order to provide a contrast group for the calculation of standard (z) scores (the rationale for this procedure has been presented earlier in the chapter).

The neuropsychological test battery employed in the first phase of this study (identification of subtypes) also differed from the Lyon and Watson (1981) battery. Specifically, the MFD was replaced by the Benton Visual Retention Test (Benton, 1974), and two additional measures were added—the Grammatic Closure subtest of the ITPA (abbreviated here as ITPA; Kirk *et al.*, 1968) and the Motor Free Visual Perception Test (abbreviated here as Motor Free; Colarusso & Hammill, 1972). All other measures remained in the neuropsychological battery (see Table 11-1). The rationale for inclusion of the new measures can be found in Lyon *et al.* (1982)

The same statistical procedures used in the Lyon and Watson (1981) study were employed in the subtype identification phase of this investigation. Specifically, after a stable cluster solution was obtained with repeated average-linkage cluster analyses of the learning-disabled subjects' standard (z) scores, a number of ANOVAs were performed to determine differences among subtypes (clusters) for each neuropsychological diagnostic measure. This was followed by a MANOVA to determine between-subtype differences on a linear combination of the diagnostic measures. Finally, a discriminant analysis was performed to determine rates of correct classification of subjects into subtypes.

The results of all cluster analyses yielded five subtypes of disabled readers. Figure 11-2 displays the standard score profiles for the five subtypes and indicates the number of children in each. For each profile, the mean line (0) represents the normal-reading group's performance and indicates how each learning-disabled subtype performed, relative to their normal-reading classmates, on the neuropsychological battery. As in the Lyon and Watson (1981) study, neither cluster (subtype) membership nor profile shape differed significantly as a function of the diagnostic variable subset used. However, 11 of the 75 learning-disabled subjects could not be

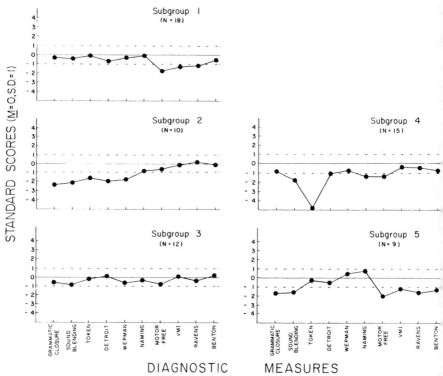

STANDARD SCORES ($\underline{M}$=0,S.D=1)

FIG. 11-2. Standard score profiles for each learning-disabled subtype among 6- to 9-year-old subjects. (From R. Lyon, N. Stewart, & D. Freedman, Neuropsychological characteristics of empirically derived subgroups of learning disabled readers. *Journal of Clinical Neuropsychology*, 1982, *4*, 343–365. Reprinted by permission.)

located consistently in any of the five subtypes. These children were labeled "outliers" and were excluded from further data analyses. The ANOVAS indicated significant differences among the five subtypes for 8 of the 10 neuropsychological measures, and the MANOVA indicated significant differences among the subtypes on the set of these measures as a whole. As in the Lyon and Watson (1981) study, the high classification hit rates that were obtained in the discriminant analysis (92% correct classification) were also observed after "jackknifing" (84% correct classification).

The second phase of this investigation was designed to determine whether, and how, members of the five identified subtypes differed on measures of letter identification, oral reading of single words, word-attack skills, comprehension of word meanings, and comprehension of written passages. Thus, to carry out this educational validation phase, all subjects were administered the five subtests of the Woodcock Reading Mastery Tests (Woodcock, 1973) to assess the reading behaviors cited above. A series of univariate one-way ANOVAs was subsequently computed to determine differences among the subtypes for the five reading measures. Post hoc pairwise comparisons were also computed to determine relationships between subtype membership and Woodcock subtests. The reader is referred to Lyon *et al.* (1982) for a discussion of the rationale for using the Woodcock measures and a description of each subtest.

The results of the univariate one-way ANOVAs across the five subtypes for the Woodcock subtests indicated that significant differences existed for two of the five reading areas measured—word-attack skills and word comprehension. The results of the post hoc comparisons are reported in the context of the following discussion concerning relationships between subgroup neuropsychological characteristics and reading behaviors.

Neuropsychological and Reading Characteristics

Subtype 1 ($n = 18$) manifested significant deficits in visual perception (Motor Free), visual–spatial analysis and reasoning (Raven's), and visual–motor integration (VMI). Visual memory was also below average, but not significantly so. All measured auditory receptive and auditory expressive skills were within the average range. This pattern of impairment corresponds to the characteristics of Johnson and Myklebust's (1967) visual dyslexic subtype, Boder's (1973) dyseidetic subtype, the visual–perceptual–motor subtype described by Satz and Morris (1981), and the visual–motor subtype reported by Lyon and Watson (1981).

The reading errors made by members of Subtype 1 appeared to be related to their profile of neuropsychological deficits. Specifically, their lowest scores were generally obtained when reading phonetically irregular single words aloud. Frequent mispronunciations due to confusion of visually similar words were noted (e.g., "work/word," "what/where," "duck/back"), as were reading errors involving medial vowels and vowel combinations (e.g., "love/live," "watch/witch," "bear/bore"). Several children also made visual errors when attempting to decode phonetically regular nonsense words (e.g., "bim/dim," "beb/ded," "tob/tobe," "laip/

lap," "wips/wids"). On the other hand, a number of Subtype 1 members performed relatively well on this word-attack subtest. Several Subtype 1 members also appeared to deploy their linguistic strengths when reading, as evidenced by relatively high scores on the silent reading comprehension subtests. In fact, Subtype 1 scored second highest of the subtypes on both Woodcock comprehension subtests.

Children in Subtype 2 ($n = 10$) displayed selective deficits in morphosyntactic skills (ITPA), sound blending (ITPA), receptive language comprehension (Token), auditory memory (Detroit), auditory discrimination (Wepman), and naming ability (Naming), with corresponding strengths in all measured visual–perceptual skills. This subtype is similar to the auditory dyslexic subtype reported by Johnson and Myklebust (1967), the dysphonetic subtype described by Boder (1973), the language disorder subtype identified by Mattis *et al.* (1975), the naming disorder subtype described by Satz and Morris (1981), Petrauskas and Rourke's (1979) Subtype 1, and Lyon and Watson's (1981) Subtype 3.

In contrast to Subtype 1, members of Subtype 2 made significantly more errors when attempting to comprehend material read silently than when reading single words orally. In fact, these children obtained the lowest centile ranks on the Woodcock Passage Comprehension subtest and the next to lowest scores on the Word Comprehension measure. Analysis of these children's errors on the Woodcock Word Attack subtest indicated that, in some cases, auditory discrimination, sound blending, and morphological deficits hampered their decoding abilities. For example, frequent substitutions of initial and final consonants were noted (e.g., "maft/naft," "bim/bin," "weet/weed"), as were omissions of word endings indicating tense (e.g., "rayed/nay") and possession (e.g., "wip's/wap").

Members of Subtype 3 ($n = 12$) scored in the normal range on all neuropsychological measures, and thus can be compared to youngsters in the subtypes identified by Lyon and Watson (1981) and Satz and Morris (1981) as scoring significantly below normal on reading tasks without concomitant low performance on neuropsychological test batteries. As suggested earlier in the review of Lyon and Watson's (1981) Subtype 6, it is possible that many children identified as learning-disabled in public school settings may read inefficiently because of social or affective reasons, rather than because of inherent neuropsychological deficiencies.

As was the case with Lyon and Watson's (1981) Subtype 6 (normal neuropsychological profile), members of Subtype 3 scored higher than all other subgroups on all reading measures. These youngsters did have relatively more difficulties in comprehending reading passages than in the other measured reading skills. No systematic patterns of errors could be identified from analysis of their performance on the Word Recognition and Word Attack subtests of the Woodcock.

Children in Subtype 4 ($n = 15$) displayed significant deficiencies in sound blending (ITPA), receptive language comprehension (Token), auditory memory (Detroit), naming ability (Naming), and some aspects of visual perception (Motor Free). This deficit pattern corresponds to the neuropsychological profiles observed in Petrauskas and Rourke's (1979) Subtype 2 (auditory sequencing–visual–spatial memory deficits) and Lyon and Watson's (1981) Subtype 5 (severe auditory comprehension and sequencing deficits).

The difficulties manifested by Subtype 4 members in remembering, analyzing, synthesizing, and correctly sequencing verbal and visual information appeared to have a significant effect on their ability to decode phonetically regular real and nonsense words. For example, on both the Woodcock Word Recognition and Word Attack subtests, a large proportion of Subtype 4 youngsters could not approximate the correct pronunciation of many words (e.g., "my/yip," "water/walk"). Further, most of the children laboriously attempted to "sound out" the individual letters of the nonsense words and then blend them together, making a number of vowel errors (e.g., "weet/wat," "maft/mifl," "lapi/tobe"), sequencing errors (e.g., "plen/pelm," "hets/hest"), and errors of omission (e.g., "telequick/tolchip") in the process.

It appeared that both decoding problems, such as those described above, and deficiencies in auditory comprehension and memory, as observed in neuropsychological testing, significantly impeded Subtype 4 children's comprehension of single words and reading passages. Post hoc analyses indicated the Subtype 4 scored significantly lower on the Woodcock Word Comprehension and Passage Comprehension subtests than did all other subtypes.

Members of Subtype 5 ($n = 9$) manifested significant mixed deficits in morphosyntactic skill (ITPA), sound blending (ITPA), visual perception (Motor Free), visual–motor integration (VMI), visual–spatial analysis (Raven's), and visual memory (Benton). This pattern of neuropsychological impairment is similar to those displayed by Johnson and Myklebust's (1967) mixed dyslexic subtype and Boder's (1973) combined dysphonetic and dyseidetic subtype, but more specifically mimics Satz and Morris's

(1981) Subtype 3 (mixed-deficit type) and Lyon and Watson's (1981) Subtype 1 (mixed-deficit subgroup).

Children in Subtype 5 made primarily "visual" errors when reading single words (both real and nonsense), apparently reflecting their deficiencies in visual analysis and memory. Specifically, a large number of these youngsters confused visually similar words (e.g., "of/on," "work/word," "bed/ded," "nudd/nupp") and some confused letters in the letter identification tasks (e.g., "m/n," "U/W," "J/L"). It also appeared that the combined auditory and visual deficits manifested by Subtype 5 members significantly hampered their comprehension of material read silently.

In summary, results of the Lyon *et al.* (1982) investigation indicated that subtypes of disabled readers could be identified at these tender age levels by empirical methods, and that some "educational relevance" could be attributed to the subtypes as a function of educational validation procedures. However, it is clear from our statistical and clinical analyses of subtypes' oral and silent reading behaviors that a number of children across subtypes made similar errors when decoding words and comprehending written material. That is, not all subtypes differed significantly from one another on all subtests of the Woodcock Reading Mastery Tests. This lack of "total" educational validation of these subtypes points out a need to include more comprehensive reading *and* written language measures in further subtype identification and validation studies. As we observed following the Lyon *et al.* (1981) investigation, comparisons of subtypes against both reading and spelling criteria allows for much greater confidence in inferring the independence of the subtypes than does validating them against either criterion alone. Obviously, the strongest evidence of subtype independence will be provided when studies can both investigate subtype differences in educational skills and determine subtype response to instruction. An initial attempt to explore the latter is reviewed next.

RESPONSE TO INSTRUCTION

Background

The number of studies that have systematically explored differential subtype responses to different forms of teaching is limited. For several reasons, most recent subtype identification studies have not included within their research designs methods for determining interactions between subtype neuropsychological characteristics and types of teaching methods and/or materials. Judging from our own subtype research experience, many practical factors impede the study of subtype response to instruction. For example, many times the youngsters who are included in subtype identification studies are simply not available for instructional follow-up. In other cases, when subtype members are available for study, schools and parents are sometimes reluctant to have their children receive some form of instruction with which they may disagree, or instruction that reduces the time a youngster spends in regular and/or special class settings.

However, it seems that the major reason why there have been so few studies of subtype × teaching method interaction relates to the methodological demands inherent within this type of investigation. Specifically, aptitude (subtype) × treatment (teaching method) research requires either regression analysis (Cronbach, 1967) and/or ANOVA designs (Bracht, 1970). In the case of the regression design, subjects are assigned to their respective treatment (teaching) groups and administered one or more aptitude (e.g., neuropsychological) measures. Following a teaching condition, the aptitude scores are used to predict the achievement scores obtained by the members of each group. The regression lines are then examined for parallelism and plotted to determine whether they interact within the effective range of the aptitude measure.

In the ANOVA design, subjects are administered the aptitude or neuropsychological measures and then assigned, according to their scores, to one of several levels of the aptitude (subtype) factor in a factorial analysis of variance. Bracht (1970) has recommended that, following the teaching intervention(s), an ANOVA be computed to assess possible disordinal interactions among levels of the aptitude (subtype) factor and levels of the intervention (teaching method) factor. A disordinal interaction exists if the analyses of simple effects are significant *and* the mean cell differences have different algebraic signs.

The methodological requirements of these two designs in terms of subject numbers are extensive. Specifically, with both designs, subjects must be equated on preintervention achievement and preintervention regression between achievement and aptitude, *or* must be randomly assigned to the different teaching conditions if the results of the data analysis are to be interpretable (Ysseldyke & Salvia, 1980). Both the matching of subjects on preintervention achievement variables and the random assignment of subjects to teaching conditions require that sample sizes be large. This is especially true if the researcher is interested in randomly assigning subjects from each of several subtypes to several teaching methods or conditions. A review of the subtype literature indicates that such methodological considerations have impeded the interpretation of subtype × teaching interaction studies (see Tarver & Dawson, 1978) or the initiation of new studies. In fact, the reader will note that, in the following review of a subtype × teaching method study, the research design had to be modified because of an inability to meet the methodological criteria discussed above.

The Lyon (1983) Study

Following the Lyon (1978b) and Lyon and Watson (1981) subtype identification studies, we initiated a pilot study to determine whether subtypes identified in these investigations of 11- and 12-year-old disabled readers would respond differently to reading instruction. However, because of the limited number of subjects available to us from the Lyon (1978b) and Lyon and Watson (1981) studies (combined $n = 200$), it was decided to explore the possibility that the six identified subtypes would respond in a significantly different fashion to one teaching condition. Since the subjects in this study had to be matched for preintervention achievement levels and other relevant variables (e.g., age, IQ, sex, race), the initial subject pool of 200 was reduced to 30. Thus, random assignment of youngsters from each of the subtypes to several teaching conditions was impossible.

In light of these logistical difficulties, five subjects were selected from each of the six subtypes identified in the Lyon (1978b) and Lyon and Watson (1981) studies, and were matched on PIAT Reading Recognition grade equivalents, age, IQ, race, and sex. All 30 subjects were white males ranging in age from 12.3 years to 12.7 years and in Full Scale IQ from 103.5 to 105.4. PIAT Reading Recognition preintervention grade equivalents ranged from 3.0 to 3.3. Unfortunately, the subjects could not be equated for amount of previous instruction in phonics, type of curriculum or amount of time spent in their special classrooms, or type of curriculum in their regular classrooms. In addition, the Hawthorne effect was not systematically controlled.

The teaching method selected for the study was s synthetic phonics program developed by Traub and Bloom (1975). This program was chosen because of its well-sequenced format, its coverage of major phonics concepts, and its familiarity to the teachers in training who were providing the instruction. All subjects were provided 1 hour of reading instruction per week (in addition to their special and regular classroom instruction) for 26 weeks.

In the Traub and Bloom (1975) program, children are first required to supply the appropriate sounds for all single letters and letter combinations learned. This is followed in the instructional sequence by naming and writing the letters that correspond to letter sounds given by the teacher. Children are then introduced to consonant–vowel–consonant (CVC) words made up of letters learned to date. All children are taught to write the CVC words from dictation prior to reading them. The instructional sequence then progresses through writing and reading words with different consonant and vowel combinations (CCVC, CCVCC, CVVC) and then writing and reading sentences constructed from known, phonetically regular words and "sight" words. Systematic movement from one level of the reading program was made possible in the present study by requiring that all children meet a 90% accuracy criterion on all lesson components before moving to an instructional objective at a higher level. If a younster did not meet this 90% criterion for moving from one lesson component to the next (e.g., from providing letter sounds to writing CVCs), he was given multisensory exercises and other drills.

Following the 26 weeks of phonics instruction, the 30 subjects were posttested with the PIAT Reading Recognition subtest. Significant differences were found among the six subtypes for gain scores achieved from preintervention testing to posttesting. An analysis of subtype PIAT gain scores indicated that Subtype 6 made the most progress ($M = 11.2$ months), followed by Subtype 4 ($M = 7.8$ months). Subtypes 2 and 3 were similar in achieving moderate gains ($M = 5.1$ and 4.4. months, respectively), while Subtypes 1 and 5 did not appear to improve ($M = 1.0$ and .8 months, respectively).

The results of this pilot educational validation study generally confirmed the predictions made by our experienced clinicians and teachers after they inspected the neuropsychological diagnostic profiles for each subtype (discussed earlier in the chapter) and before intervention was initiated. For example, the significant deficits in auditory comprehension, auditory memory, and sound blending observed in Subtypes 1 and 5 would appear to impede these subtypes' response to synthetic phonics instruction. In fact, two of the five children in Subtype 1 obtained lower PIAT scores on posttesting than on preintervention testing. The strong gains made by Subtypes 6 and 4 were also expected, since these children appeared to possess strengths in the majority of the measured skills necessary for both phonics development and sight-word vocabulary development (e.g., auditory discrimination, auditory and visual memory, sound blending). The moderate responses of Subtypes 2 and 3 to the phonics instruction was not unexpected, given their relative strengths in auditory discrimination, sound blending, and visual memory.

The data obtained in the Lyon (1983) investigation seem to suport the hypothesis that the neuropsychological diagnostic profiles for the six subtypes represent meaningful descriptions of behavior that appear related to the magnitude of response to one teaching method. However, several notes of caution must be stated in reference to the results obtained in this pilot study. First, even though children within and between subtypes were matched on preintervention reading recognition levels, no preintervention regression between achievement and aptitude was computed. Thus, the interpretation of these data remains tenuous. Further, it is difficult to assess the influence that previous phonics instruction and teaching in both special and regular classrooms may have had on posttesting. It is obvious to us that future subtype validation studies involving educational interventions need to be carried out with younger subjects in order to minimize the effects of previous and ongoing instruction on gain scores. In addition, although we observed significantly different responses to a phonics program as a function of subtype membership, we still do not know what other teaching interventions might have been equally or more efficacious for the children in the study. Finally, it is clear to us that the reading measure (PIAT Reading Recognition Subtest) used to assess reading gains was limited and did not adequately reflect the children's application of phonics concepts at either the pre- or postintervention stages. Future studies should include more comprehensive measures of phonics behaviors as well as measures of oral and silent contextual reading and comprehension. The PIAT Reading Recognition subtest does have high test–retest reliability for the grade levels of the children in the study ($r = .89$), and this did allow us to interpret gain scores with some degree of confidence.

SUMMARY

The studies reviewed in this chapter have indicated that subtypes of learning-disabled readers can be identified empirically and validated educationally by observing how subtype members differ in regard to performance on academic tasks (e.g., oral reading, spelling) and response to some form of teaching. However, it seems clear from our investigations that significant improvements need to be made in our research applications of these validation procedures. Specifically, after initial identification, subtypes should be compared on a comprehensive array of academic variables that is sufficient to indicate more specific and illuminating relationships between subtype patterns of impairment and patterns of educational deficits. In addition, special care must be exercised when conducting subtype × teaching interaction studies to control, as much as possible, for extraneous influences (e.g., differences in instructional presentation, amount of previous instruction) that may spuriously inflate or deflate gain scores.

REFERENCES

Baker, H. J., & Leland, B. *Detroit Tests of Learning Aptitude*. Indianapolis: Bobbs-Merrill, 1958.

Beery, D. C., & Buktenica, N. *Developmental Test of Visual–Motor Integration*. Chicago: Follett, 1967.

Benton, A. L. *The Revised Visual Retention Test*. New York: Psychological Corporation, 1974.

Boder, E. Developmental dyslexia: A diagnostic approach based on three atypical reading–spelling patterns. *Developmental Medicine and Child Neurology*, 1973, *15*, 663–687.

Bracht, G. H. Experimental factors related to aptitude–treatment interactions. *Review of Educational Research*, 1970, *40*, 627–645.

Cohen, S. A. Studies in visual perception and reading in disadvantaged children. *Journal of Learning Disabilities*, 1969, *2*, 498–503.

Colarusso, R., & Hammill, D. D. *The Motor Free Test of Visual Perception*. San Rafael, Calif.: Academic Therapy Publications, 1972.

Cronbach, L. J. How can instruction be adapted to individual differences. In R. M. Gagne (Ed.), *Learning and individual differences*. Columbus, Ohio: Charles E. Merrill, 1967.

Doehring, D. G., & Hoshko, I. M. Classification of reading problems by the Q-technique of factor analysis. *Cortex*, 1977, *13*, 281–294.

Duffy, F. H., Denckla, M. B., Bartels, P. H., & Sandini, G. Dyslexia: Regional differences in brain electrical activity by topographic mapping. *Annals of Neurology*, 1980, *7*, 412–420.

Dunn, K. M., & Markwardt, F. D. *Manual, Peabody Individual Achievement Test*. Circle Pines, Minn.: American Guidance Service, 1970.

Fisk, J. L., & Rourke, B. P. Identification of subtypes of learning disabled children at three age levels: A neuropsychological, multivariate approach. *Journal of Clinical Neuropsychology*, 1979, *1*, 289–310.

Graham, F. K., & Kendall, B. S. Memory for Designs Test: Revised general manual. *Perceptual and Motor Skills* (Monograph Suppl. No. 2, VII), 1960, *11*, 147–188.

Johnson, D. J., & Myklebust, H. R. *Learning disabilities: Educational principles and practices*. New York: Grune & Stratton, 1967.

Kirk, S. A., & Elkins, J. Characteristics of children enrolled in child service demonstration centers. *Journal of Learning Disabilities*, 1975, *8*, 630–637.

Kirk, S. A., McCarthy, J., & Kirk, W. *Illinois Test of Psycholinguistic Abilities*. Urbana: University of Illinois Press, 1968.

Larsen, S. C. The learning disabilities specialist. Roles and responsibilities. *Journal of Learning Disabilities*, 1976, *9*, 37–47.

Luria, A. R. *The working brain: An introduction to neuropsychology*. New York: Basic Books, 1973.

Lyon, R. *Extension of learning disabled subgroup research: Contrasts with normal readers and varying racial proportions*. Unpublished manuscript, University of Alabama at Birmingham, 1978. (a)

Lyon, R. *The neuropsychological characteristics of subgroups of learning disabled readers*. Unpublished doctoral dissertation, University of New Mexico, 1978. (b)

Lyon, R. Learning disabled readers: Identification of subgroups. In H. R. Myklebust (Ed.), *Progress in learning disabilities* (Vol. 5) New York: Grune & Stratton, 1983.

Lyon, R., Rietta, S., Watson, B., Porch, B., & Rhodes, J. Selected linguistic and perceptual abilities of empirically derived subgroups of learning disabled readers. *Journal of School Psychology*, 1981, *19*, 152–166.

Lyon, R., Stewart, N., & Freedman, D. Neuropsychological characteristics of empirically derived subgroups of learning disabled readers. *Journal of Clinical Neuropsychology*, 1982, *4*, 343–365.

Lyon, R., & Watson, B. Empirically derived subgroups of learning disabled readers: Diagnostic characteristics. *Journal of Learning Disabilities*, 1981, *14*, 256–261.

Lyon, R., & Wiss, C. Learning styles in children. In A Rotatori & R. Fox (Eds.), *Assessment for regular and special education teachers: A case study approach*. Baltimore: University Park Press, in press.

Mattis, S., French, J. H., & Rapin, I. Dyslexia in children and adults: Three independent neuropsychological syndromes. *Developmental Medicine and Child Neurology*, 1975, *17*, 150–163.

Petrauskas, R. J., & Rourke, B. P. Identification of subgroups of retarded readers: A neuropsychological multivariate approach. *Journal of Clinical Neuropsychology*, 1979, *1*, 17–37.

Porch, B. E. *Porch Index of Communicative Ability for Children*. Palo Alto, Calif.: Consulting Psychologists Press, 1974.

Raven, J. C. *Coloured Progressive Matrices*. New York: Psychological Corporation, 1960.

Rourke, B. P. Central processing deficiencies in children: Toward a developmental neuropsychological model. *Journal of Clinical Neuropsychology*, 1982, *4*, 1–18.

Rourke, B. P., & Strang, J. D. Neuropsychological significance of variations in patterns of academic performance: Motor, psychomotor, and tactile–perceptual abilities. *Journal of Pediatric Psychology*, 1978, *3*, 62–66.

Rourke, B. P., & Strang, J. D. Subtypes of reading and arithmetical disabilities: A neuropsychological analysis. In M. Rutter (Ed.), *Developmental neuropsychiatry*. New York: Guilford Press, 1983.

Satz, P., & Morris, R. Learning disability subtypes: A review. In F. J. Pirozzolo & M. C. Wittrock (Eds.), *Neuropsychological and cognitive processes in reading*. New York: Academic Press, 1981.

Satz, P., Rardin, D., & Ross, J. An evaluation of a theory of specific developmental dyslexia. *Child Development*, 1971, *42*, 2009–2021.

Spellacy, F. J., & Spreen, O. A short form of the Token Test. *Cortex*, 1969, *5*, 390–397.

Tarver, S., & Dawson, M. Modality preference and the teaching of reading: A review. *Journal of Learning Disabilities*, 1978, *11*, 17–29.

Traub, M., & Bloom, F. *Recipe for reading.* Cambridge, Mass.: Educator's Publishing Service, 1975.

U. S. Office of Education. Assistance to states for education of handicapped children: Procedures for evaluating specific learning disabilities. *Federal Register,* 1977, *43,* 65082-65085.

Wepman, J. M. *The Auditory Discrimination Test.* Chicago: Language Research Associates, 1973.

Woodcock, R. W. *Woodcock Reading Mastery Tests.* Circle Pines, Minn.: American Guidance Service, 1973.

Ysseldyke, J. E., & Salvia, J. Methodological considerations in aptitude-treatment interaction research with intact groups. *Diagnostique,* 1980, *6,* 3-9.

V

*Personality and Socioemotional
Dimensions of Learning Disabilities
in Children*

12

Socioemotional Functioning of Learning-Disabled Children: A Subtypal Analysis of Personality Patterns

JAMES E. PORTER
BYRON P. ROURKE

BACKGROUND

Although the early notion that learning disabilities are merely symptoms of underlying emotional conflicts has fallen into disrepute, there remains considerable interest in the emotional, social, and behavioral functioning of learning-disabled children. Most of the research in this area has focused on the learning-disabled child's interpersonal environment. Investigators have examined characteristics of parents of learning-disabled children (e.g., Goldman & Barclay, 1974; Grunebaum, Hurwitz, Prentice, & Sperry, 1962; Wetter, 1972) and the communication patterns within these families (e.g., Campbell, 1972; Miller & Westman, 1964, 1966; Peck & Stackhouse, 1973). A second line of research has been an examination of the way in which learning-disabled children are perceived by their parents (e.g., Seigler & Gynther, 1960; Strag, 1972), by teachers (e.g, Bryan & McGrady, 1972; McCarthy & Paraskevopoulos, 1969), by peers (e.g., Bryan, 1974b, 1976; Siperstein, Bopp, & Bak, 1978), and by independent observers (e.g.,

James E. Porter. Department of Psychology, University of Windsor, Windsor, Ontario, Canada.

Byron P. Rourke. Department of Psychology, University of Windsor, and Department of Neuropsychology, Windsor Western Hospital Centre, Windsor, Ontario, Canada.

Bryan, 1974a; Richey & McKinney, 1978). For a thorough review of this literature, see Porter (1980).

This research into the interpersonal environments of children with learning disabilities is characterized by a great deal of confusion. The results of many studies could best be described as trivial; many fail to be supported in replication attempts; the results of some studies directly contradict each other; and it remains unclear how, or even whether, those factors that have been identified and replicated are related to one another. In general, however, this literature does demonstrate that learning-disabled children must deal with an interpersonal environment that differs markedly from that confronting their normally achieving peers. In contrast to normal achievers, learning-disabled children apparently tend (1) to be perceived as less pleasant and desirable by parents, teachers, and peers; (2) to be the recipients of more negative communications from their parents, teachers, and peers; (3) to be ignored and rejected more often by their teachers; (4) to be treated in a notably more punitive and derogatory manner by their parents; and (5) to live in families that resemble in certain crucial ways those of emotionally disturbed children.

One would certainly expect, therefore, to find that learning-disabled children have a particularly difficult time emotionally and socially. Indeed, it is widely held that learning-disabled children are particularly prone to socioemotional difficulties (Bryant, 1966, Connolly, 1971; Natchez, 1968), and many investigators (e.g., Black, 1974; Halechko, 1977; Zimmerman & Allebrand, 1965) have suggested that a particular pattern of socioemotional problems is generally descriptive of the learning-disabled population. Unfortunately, this hypothesized relationship between learning disabilities and socioemotional problems has been directly assessed in only a few well-controlled studies.

Three studies have been conducted into the general social and emotional functioning of learning-disabled children, as compared to that of their normally achieving peers. McNutt (1978) found learning-disabled adolescents to be more poorly adjusted both emotionally and socially; Zimmerman and Allebrand (1965) found more emotional maladjustment among learning-disabled children, but rough comparability on almost every measure of social adjustment; and Connolly (1969) found no between-group differences regarding either personality organization or degree of emotional disturbance. The notion that learning-disabled children tend to have low self-esteem was examined in four studies. Halechko (1977) and Black (1974) found lower self-esteem among learning-disabled children, whereas Silverman (1978), using the same instrument as did Black, found no between-group differences. Ribner's (1978) study failed to clarify the question. He found that normal achievers demonstrated greater self-esteem than as-yet-undiagnosed learning-disabled children in regular classrooms, but that identified learning-disabled children in segregated classes could not be distinguished from normal achievers on the basis of self-esteem. In summary, the direct evidence regarding the socioemotional functioning of learning-disabled children is, at best, equivocal. A coherent and meaningful pattern of personality characteristics of children with learning disabilities does not emerge from the research literature. There are four methodological and conceptual problems apparent in this research that would appear to contribute to this state of affairs.

METHODOLOGICAL AND CONCEPTUAL ISSUES

DEFINITION OF THE POPULATION

> The sine qua non for systematic investigation would seem to be a good operational definition for the phenomenon under study, one which is unambiguous, in some sense meaningful, and capable of being used by independent investigators. There has been no consistent formulation in studies of reading retardation. (Applebee, 1971, p. 91)

Most investigators would agree that a learning-disabled child is one who demonstrates marked academic underachievement that cannot be traced to intellectual limitations, sensory deficits, motor impairments, socioeconomic disadvantage, inadequate instruction, or emotional disturbance. The actual identification of such children, however, is another matter. In many studies, the criteria used to identify learning-disabled subjects have been vague or undefined. Some investigators (e.g., Peck & Stackhouse, 1973) relied on assessments made by school personnel whose criteria remained unreported, whereas others (e.g, Forness & Esteveldt, 1971) selected subjects solely on the basis of teachers' perceptions without any further assessment whatsoever. Even among those studies in which subject selection criteria are clearly specified, however, there is little consistency in the criteria employed. The effects of differences in selection criteria are dramatically illustrated in a study by McNutt (1978). She applied five commonly employed sets of identification criteria to a large sample of schoolchildren, and found that use of the most inclusive set resulted in the identification as learning-disabled of *over nine times* as many children as did application of the most restrictive set! It would seem likely that some inconsistent or contradictory research results reflect this variation in group composition. Clearly, a universally adopted set of specific identification criteria is needed. Until this is accomplished, it behooves researchers to employ and clearly elucidate specific subject selection criteria in order to convey the nature of the population to which their research results apply.

MEASUREMENT OF MALADJUSTMENT

Constructs such as "emotional disturbance," "socioemotional adjustment," "personality characteristics," and "disturbed patterns of family functioning" have been perhaps even less adequately operationalized than the construct of "learning disability." Connolly (1971) emphasized that maladjustment is a subjective phenomenon that varies in connotation from person to person and situation to situation. He pointed out that the methods traditionally thought to be best for assessing maladjustment are often subjective in nature. The difficulty in replicating research that depends upon subjective judgment is readily apparent. Thus, the failure to replicate some research findings might be due in part to the nature of the instruments used to measure maladjustment or disturbance. Studies that employ reliably quantified psychometric instruments would avoid this problem.

DEVELOPMENTAL CONSIDERATIONS

Several studies offer support for the notion that the nature of the ability deficits exhibited by learning-disabled children varies with age (Leong, 1976; Rourke, Dietrich, & Young, 1973; Rourke & Orr, 1977). If their socioemotional functioning also varies with age (not an unreasonable possibility), differences in research results could reflect differences in the ages of the subjects employed. Therefore, it is necessary for the investigator of learning disabilities to allow for this possibility. This can be done either by restricting the age range of subjects employed, or by designing the study so as to enable an evaluation of developmental parameters.

HETEROGENEITY

The fourth and most important methodological issue to be discussed emerges from a consideration of conceptual or statistical models. Applebee (1971), in his outline of possible statistical models of learning disabilities, emphasized the degree to which the models differ from one another in terms both of underlying assumptions about the nature of learning disabilities, and of implications regarding appropriate research methodologies. Virtually all of the studies that have attempted to identify socioemotional correlates of learning disabilities have employed the same basic research design. Undifferentiated groups of learning-disabled children have been compared to equally undifferentiated groups of normal achievers; learning-disabled children have been treated as a unitary group. In other words, the investigations have been designed to examine the notion that learning-disabled children are unusually prone to developing a *particular pattern* of socioemotional disturbance. Among the most serious drawbacks to such an approach is that it tends to obscure within-group differences. As Applebee (1971) pointed out, employment of this "comparative-populations" approach can only be justified if one can safely assume that learning-disabled children are homogeneous in terms of their socioemotional functioning.

However, recent neuropsychological research indicates that, at least in terms of the patterning of their abilities, learning-disabled children constitute a heterogeneous population (Benton, 1975; Fisk & Rourke, 1979; Rourke, 1978), and meaningful subtypes of learning-disabled children have been identified (Doehring & Hoshko, 1977; Fisk & Rourke, 1979; Mattis, French, & Rapin, 1975; Nelson & Warrington, 1976; Petrauskas & Rourke, 1979; Rourke & Strang, 1978; Sweeney & Rourke, 1978). Could it be that learning-disabled children are also heterogeneous with regard to their socioemotional functioning? Until now, this possibility has not been investigated.

THE PRESENT INVESTIGATION

INTRODUCTION

The investigation to be reported at this juncture was designed to assess the heterogeneity hypothesis. More specifically, the aim was to determine whether distinct subtypes, differing from one another in terms of socio-emotional functioning, could be identified within a sample of learning-disabled children. To this end, *Q*-type factor-analytic techniques were applied to data generated in our study of a sample of such children on whom various measures of emotional, interpersonal, and behavioral functioning had been obtained. Further statistical analyses were conducted to shed light on the psychometric reliability of the subtypal analysis, and to ascertain whether the emerging subtypes differed significantly from one another. Full consideration was given to the other methodological issues discussed above: Rather rigorous criteria for subject selection were em-ployed; psychometric (and therefore easily replicable) measures of socio-emotional functioning were used; and age factors were examined.

SUBJECTS

The 100 subjects employed in this investigation were selected from a population of children referred to a large urban clinic for neuropsycho-logical assessment because of apparent learning or "perceptual" problems. The subjects, 87 males and 13 females, ranged from 6.5 to 15.3 years of age. Each subject had obtained a Wechsler Intelligence Scale for Children (WISC) Full Scale IQ of between 85 and 115 (inclusive) and a centile score of ≤ 25 on at least one subtest (Reading, Spelling, or Arithmetic) of the Wide Range Achievement Test (WRAT; Jastak & Jastak, 1965). Defective hearing or vision had been ruled out for all subjects. A Sweep Hearing Test over a wide range of frequencies was administered as part of the routine neuropsychological assessment; no child who exhibited a hearing loss of ≥ 30 decibels with either ear at any frequency in the speech range was selected as a subject. A child was judged to be free of defective vision if both the psychometrist who administered the neuropsychological test battery and the child's parents reported that the child appeared to have normal vision (either with or without corrective lenses). No children suspected of suffering from sociocultural or economic deprivation were included in the subject sample; suspicion of such deprivation arose when indicated in a report from a Children's Aid Society or from the referring party. Primary emotional disturbance was also ruled out: Children in treatment for emotional disturbance, or diagnosed as needing such treat-ment, were excluded from the study. All subjects spoke English as their primary language and had attended school regularly since at least 6 years of age. Table 12-1 contains subject summary statistics regarding age, WISC IQ (Verbal, Performance, and Full Scale), and WRAT Reading, Spelling, and Arithmetic centile scores.

MEASURES

The Personality Inventory for Children (PIC; Wirt, Lachar, Klinedinst, & Seat, 1977) is completed routinely by the parents of children referred to the clinic for neuropsychological assessment. A staff psychometrist gives the PIC to the parents when they bring the children for testing, and the parents complete the inventory in an unsupervised setting. In the present investigation, the inventories were completed by the subjects' mothers.

The PIC is composed of 600 true–false questions regarding a child's behavior, attitudes, and interpersonal relations. It can be scored for 3 validity or response-style scales (Lie, F, and Defensiveness), 1 general screening scale (Adjustment), 12 clinical scales (Achievement, Intellectual Screening, Development, Somatic Concern, Depression, Family Relations, Delinquency, Withdrawal, Anxiety, Psychosis, Hyperactivity, and Social Skills), and 17 supplemental scales (Adolescent Maladjustment, Aggression, Asocial Behavior, Cerebral Dysfunction, Delinquency Prediction, Ego-Strength, Excitement, Externalization, Infrequency, Internalization, Introversion–Extraversion, K, Learning Disability Prediction, Reality Distortion, Sex Role, Social Desirability, and Somatization).

Both empirical (Darlington & Bishop, 1966) and rational (Klinedinst, 1975) strategies were employed in scale construction. Alpha coefficients of internal consistency, reported in one study for 13 scales, ranged from

TABLE 12-1. Subject Summary Statistics Regarding Age, IQ, and Academic Achievement

	M	*SD*	Range
Age	10.5	2.2	6.5–15.3
WISC			
Verbal IQ	95.0	8.3	76–123
Performance IQ	102.7	10.6	80–131
Full Scale IQ	98.5	8.0	85–115
WRAT			
Reading subtest (centile)	23.4	19.1	3–88
Spelling subtest (centile)	14.8	11.2	1–55
Arithmetic subtest (centile)	19.2	13.2	2–75

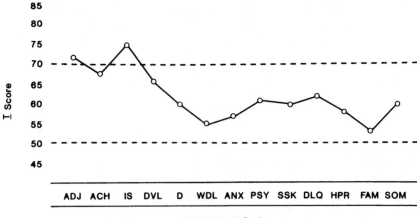

PIC Clinical Scale

FIG. 12-1. Mean PIC clinical profile for total sample. (Abbreviations: ADJ, Adjustment; ACH, Achievement; IS, Intellectual Screening; DVL, Development; D, Depression; WDL, Withdrawal; ANX, Anxiety; PSY, Psychosis; SSK, Social Skills; DLQ, Delinquency; HPR, Hyperactivity; FAM, Family Relations; SOM, Somatic Concern.)

.62 to .84 in a normative sample ($n = 2390$). Test–retest product–moment correlations, reported in another study for all 33 scales, ranged from .68 to .97 ($M = .89$) on a normative sample ($n = 55$). A detailed outline of methods of scale construction and the psychometric properties of each scale is presented in the test manual (Wirt *et al.*, 1977).

SAMPLE MEAN STATISTICS

In order to ascertain whether the data indicated socioemotional disturbance in the sample as a whole, the mean PIC profile for the entire subject sample was plotted (see Figure 12-1). (Scale elevation is associated with disturbed functioning.) Of the specific clinical scales, only the Intellectual Screening scale was markedly elevated (i.e., T score ≥ 70), and only the Achievement scale even approached this level. Scores on those measures designed to evaluate socioemotional functioning were within roughly normal limits. In other words, only those measures associated with intellectual and academic achievement per se were suggestive of disturbance, at least for the sample as a whole. Had a "comparative-populations" research strategy been employed, and had no subtypal analysis been conducted, the present investigation would have provided evidence contrary to the notion that learning-disabled children are particularly prone to socioemotional difficulties.

SUBTYPAL ANALYSIS

In order to test the hypothesis that the population of learning-disabled children is heterogeneous in terms of socioemotional functioning, a subtypal analysis was undertaken. A Q-type factor analysis was conducted on a reduced data set, consisting of the 100 subjects' scores on 15 of the 33 PIC scales. These scales (F, Achievement, Intellectual Screening, Somatic Concern, Family Relations, Withdrawal, Social Skills, Adolescent Maladjustment, Aggression, Asocial Behavior, Internalization, Introversion-Extraversion, K, Learning Disability Prediction, and Reality Distortion) were selected in a manner designed both to minimize the untoward effects of interscale item overlap and to ensure that the set of scales would optimally reflect the major personality dimensions measured by the PIC. Optimal representation was ensured by performing an R-type factor analysis on all of the PIC data and selecting scales that would best reflect each of the emerging factors. (Further details of this and all other statistical procedures are available from us.)

The matrix of the PIC scores was transposed, and product–moment correlational analysis for subjects was performed. The correlational matrix was factored, using an iterated principal-axis solution with initial communality estimates of 1.00 in the diagonal. Orthogonal rotation to a varimax criterion was carried out on emerging factors that yielded eigenvalues greater than the ratio of the number of subjects/number of measures (i.e., 6.67).

Results of this analysis indicated that the subject sample was comprised of four subtypes of learning-disabled children that differed from one another in terms of socioemotional functioning. Four factors accounting for 69.5% of the common variance were identified.

Subjects with at least one factor loading $\geq .50$, and with an interval $\geq .10$ between their highest and next highest loadings, were retained for further analysis. These subjects were divided into groups according to the factor on which they loaded most highly. The groups represent subtypes within the subject sample. Of the 100 subjects, 77 met the criteria for assignment of subtypes. Of the remaining 23 subjects, 13 failed to evidence sufficient separation between their highest and next highest factor loadings, and 10 did not exhibit a factor loading $\geq$ .50. The four factors are clearly unipolar, as all assigned subjects exhibited positive loadings on the factors to which they were assigned. Subject assignment to subtypes was as follows:

- Subtype 1: 34 subjects (44% of those assigned)
- Subtype 2: 20 subjects (26% of those assigned)
- Subtype 3: 10 subjects (13% of those assigned)
- Subtype 4: 13 subjects (17% of those assigned)

The next procedural step was designed to determine whether the differences among subtypes were statistically significant, and to ascertain specifically which variables differed from one subtype to another. A multivariate analysis of variance (MANOVA) was performed, and an overall between-subtype comparison was made. The subtypes were compared with regard to each of the 33 PIC scales, as well as age, sexual composition, WISC Verbal, Performance, and Full Scale IQs, and WRAT Reading, Spelling, and Arithmetic centile scores. Significant differences were found across subtypes overall ($p \leq$ .001), as well as on 28 of the 33 individual PIC scales ($p \leq$ .01). Among the PIC scales, only the Achievement, Intellectual Screening, Development, Cerebral Dysfunction, and Learning Disability Prediction scales did not vary significantly across subtypes. In addition, no significant differences were found regarding age, sexual composition, WISC IQ scores, or WRAT centile scores. In other words, the MANOVA procedure indicates that the four subtypes differed significantly from one another, but only with regard to socioemotional functioning. There was no evidence to suggest any significant differences in ability, school-related functioning, age, or sex among the four subtypes.

The entire subject sample was employed in the final statistical step, which was designed to shed light on the replicability of the subtype analysis. Sixteen PIC scales that had demonstrated high factor loadings in the preliminary R-type factor analysis were employed in this test of psychometric reliability. These scales were divided into two mutually exclusive eight-scale sets in a manner designed to ensure that each set would most closely reflect the factor structure of the PIC. A Q-type factor analysis was performed on subject scores on each of the eight-scale sets (termed "Replication 1" and "Replication 2"); subjects were assigned to factors using the same method as that employed in the subtypal analysis; and a matrix was constructed in which the grouping of subjects in the two analyses was compared.

Sixty-one subjects were assigned to factors in the analysis of both Replication 1 and Replication 2. Table 12-2 presents the matrix in which the grouping of subjects from the two analyses is compared. Considerable agreement is apparent between the two replication analyses. The second replication analysis grouped together 28 of the 35 subjects from Factor I of the first replication analysis, 8 of the 11 subjects from Factor II of the first analysis, 5 of the 6 subjects from Factor III of the first analysis, and 7 of the 9 subjects from Factor IV of the first analysis. In summary, the two analyses demonstrated an agreement or replication rate of 79%. Cramer's index of strength of association, which can range from 0 (complete independence) to 1.0 (complete dependence), provided a statistical measure of the degree of correspondence between the two replication analyses. This index indicated significant and sizable correspondence ($\varphi' = .69$, $p \leq .001$), strongly supporting the psychometric reliability of the subtypal analysis.

In summary, the subtypal analysis offers strong support for the hypothesis that the population of learning-disabled children is heterogeneous in terms of socioemotional functioning. Four subtypes emerged from the multivariate analysis of the personality profiles of 100 learning-disabled children. These subtypes, accounting for 77% of the subjects, differed significantly from one another, and the psychometric reliability of the analysis was confirmed. It would appear that *there is no single learning-disabled personality type.*

TABLE 12-2. Group Comparison Matrix from Replication Analyses

Replication 2 groupings	Replication 1 groupings			
	Factor I	Factor II	Factor III	Factor IV
Factor I	<u>28</u>	1	0	1
Factor II	1	0	<u>5</u>	1
Factor III	1	2	1	<u>7</u>
Factor IV	5	<u>8</u>	0	0

Note. Agreement between the two analyses in subject groupings is indicated by underlined figures.

Replication rate = 79%. $\varphi' = .69$; $p \leq .001$.

SUBTYPE CHARACTERISTICS

The final step was designed to ascertain the most salient socioemotional characteristics of each of the four subtypes. The science (or art) of interpreting PIC profile configurations is still at an early stage of development. There is, however, adequate data on the meaning of individual scale elevations. In the personality descriptions below, each subtype is described according to the characteristics of the criterion validation samples employed in the development of the PIC scales that we found to be elevated for that subtype. The mean scores on the PIC clinical scales were plotted for each subtype (see Figures 12-2 through 12-5), and these subtype personality profiles were compared and contrasted. Table 12-3 provides a brief description of each of the clinical scales.

As one would expect in a sample of learning-disabled children, all four subtypes exhibited at least moderate scale elevations (i.e., T scores ≥ 60) on the Achievement, Intellectual Screening, and Development scales. Thus, in terms of the PIC, all four subtypes demonstrated the following: (1) academic achievement below grade level; (2) behavior similar to that of children with intellectual limitations; and (3) atypical intellectual and/or physical development.

FIG. 12-2. Mean PIC clinical profile for Subtype 1. (Abbreviations: ADJ, Adjustment; ACH, Achievement; IS, Intellectual Screening; DVL, Development; D, Depression; WDL, Withdrawal; ANX, Anxiety; PSY, Psychosis; SSK, Social Skills; DLQ, Delinquency; HPR, Hyperactivity; FAM, Family Relations; SOM, Somatic Concern.)

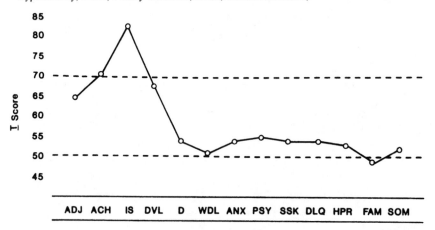

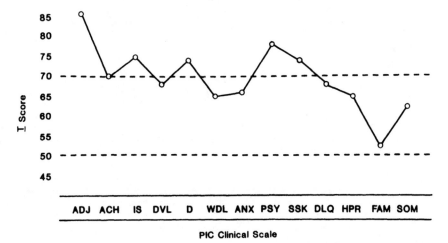

FIG. 12-3. Mean PIC clinical profile for Subtype 2. (Abbreviations: ADJ, Adjustment; ACH, Achievement; IS, Intellectual Screening; DVL, Development; D, Depression; WDL, Withdrawal; ANX, Anxiety; PSY, Psychosis; SSK, Social Skills; DLQ, Delinquency; HPR, Hyperactivity; FAM, Family Relations; SOM, Somatic Concern.)

FIG. 12-4. Mean PIC clinical profile for Subtype 3. (Abbreviations: ADJ, Adjustment; ACH, Achievement; IS, Intellectual Screening; DVL, Development; D, Depression; WDL, Withdrawal; ANX, Anxiety; PSY, Psychosis; SSK, Social Skills; DLQ, Delinquency; HPR, Hyperactivity; FAM, Family Relations; SOM, Somatic Concern.)

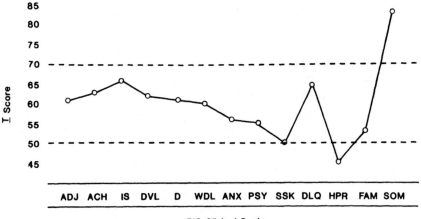

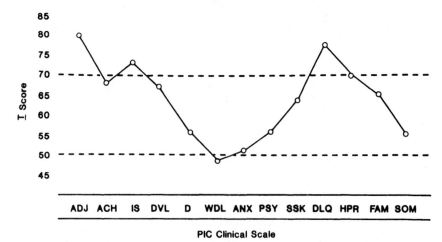

ADJ ACH IS DVL D WDL ANX PSY SSK DLQ HPR FAM SOM

PIC Clinical Scale

FIG. 12-5. Mean PIC clinical profile for Subtype 4. (Abbreviations: ADJ, Adjustment; ACH, Achievement; IS, Intellectual Screening; DVL, Development; D, Depression; WDL, Withdrawal; ANX, Anxiety; PSY, Psychosis; SSK, Social Skills; DLQ, Delinquency; HPR, Hyperactivity; FAM, Family Relations; SOM, Somatic Concern.)

Of greater interest is the total absence of other common areas of disturbed functioning. On none of the personality scales do all four types evidence elevations. Apparently, the four subtypes do not have any specific personality characteristics in common. These results directly contradict the widely held notion that one aspect of the "learning disabilities syndrome" is a particular mode of personality functioning; this offers further support for the heterogeneity hypothesis. The personality characteristics describing each subtype are outlined below.

Subtype 1

The first subtype, comprised of 37 subjects (44% of those assigned to subtypes), represents the most frequently found personality pattern within the learning-disabled sample. The Subtype 1 profile is markedly elevated (i.e., T score ≥ 70) on only two scales (Intellectual Screening and Achievement), and moderately elevated on only one other (Development). On the personality scales, the profile indicates minimal between-scale variation and a total absence of even moderate scale elevations. In other words, the personality profile suggests balanced and well-adjusted socioemotional

TABLE 12-3. Personality Inventory for Children (PIC) Clinical Scales

Scale	Description
Achievement (ACH)	Designed to assist in the identification of children whose academic achievement is significantly below age expectation.
Intellectual Screening (IS)	A screening device to identify children whose difficulties might be due to impaired intellectual functioning. IS is designed to provide an index of need for an in-depth intellectual assessment.
Development (DVL)	Designed to measure poor general intellectual and physical development.
Depression (D)	Composed of items judged to reflect childhood depression (brooding, crying spells, lack of energy, anhedonia, pessimism, poor self-concept, uncommunicativeness, etc.).
Withdrawal (WDL)	Designed to measure withdrawal from social contact.
Anxiety (ANX)	Containing items that measure limited frustration tolerance, exaggeration of problems and concerns, worries that reflect parental concerns, behavioral and physiological correlates of anxiety, irrational fears and worries, and nightmares.
Psychosis (PSY)	Designed to discriminate children with psychotic symptomatology from normal, behaviorally disturbed nonpsychotic, and retarded children. High-scoring children tend to be withdrawn and anxious, have poor social skills, and evidence indications of reality distortion.
Social Skills (SSK)	Composed of items selected to measure various characteristics that reflect effective social relations in childhood (ability to lead and to follow, level of active participation in organized activities, self-confidence and poise in social situations, and social comprehension and tact in interpersonal relations).
Delinquency (DLQ)	A concurrent measure of delinquent tendencies (interpersonal insensitivity, disregard for limits, antisocial tendencies, impulsivity, interpersonal hostility, etc.).
Hyperactivity (HPR)	Designed to identify children who display characteristics frequently associated with the "hyperkinetic syndrome."
Family Relations (FAM)	Designed to assess family effectiveness and cohesion (level of parental role effectiveness, ability to cooperate in making family decisions, family involvement in community affairs, presence of feelings of love and happiness in the home, parental emotional adjustment, appropriateness of discipline, and concern for the rights of the child).
Somatic Concern (SOM)	Composed of items that measure various health-related variables (frequency and seriousness of somatic complaints and illnesses, adjustment to illness, appetite and eating habits, sleep patterns, energy and strength, headaches and stomach aches, and physical basis for symptoms).

Note. The scale descriptions have been adapted and summarized from those presented in the PIC manual (Wirt, Lachar, Klinedinst, & Seat, 1977).

functioning. These children seem to evidence no more personality problems, on the average, than do their normally achieving peers. Apparently, *the school-related difficulties of almost half of the learning-disabled children are not accompanied by socioemotional problems.*

Subtype 2

The personality profile of the second subtype, comprised of 20 subjects (26% of those assigned to subtypes), is the most elevated overall. This profile is markedly elevated on five scales and moderately elevated on six others. Only on the Family Relations scale is the Subtype 2 profile within the normal range. These children appear to constitute the most seriously disturbed subtype within the learning-disabled population. The Subtype 2 profile is markedly elevated on the Achievement and Intellectual Screening scales, as well as on the Psychosis, Depression, and Social Skills scales. In addition, comparative elevations (i.e., T scores ≥ 65 and at least 5 points higher than any other subtype profile) are evident on the Anxiety and Withdrawal scales.

One would expect these children to be moody and brooding, with many of the symptoms of childhood depression (anhedonia, lack of energy, crying spells, concern with death and separation, etc.). Their self-esteem tends to be low, and they are notably more fearful, worried, anxious, and emotionally labile than are their well-adjusted peers. They may evidence a variety of specific symptoms, such as difficulty falling asleep, nightmares, eating disturbances, fear of school, excessive worry, self-blame, or self-criticism. Poor interpersonal functioning is another characteristic of this subtype. Social (even physical) isolation at school and at home, excessive shyness, peer conflict, failure to initiate peer relationships, interpersonal distrust, emotional distance, and a preference for solitary intellectual pursuits are prevalent. It is clear that the school-related difficulties of the children of Subtype 2 are accompanied by a great deal of subjective pain and serious internalized socioemotional disturbance.

Subtype 3

The personality profile of the third subtype, comprised of 10 subjects (13% of those assigned), is the most noteworthy for its marked elevation on only one scale—Somatic Concern. The Achievement, Intellectual

Screening, and Development scales, though moderately elevated, are all notably below those of the other three subtypes.

It would appear that, despite roughly normal functioning in most personality areas, the somatic complaints of Subtype 3 children are sufficiently serious to raise questions about their socioemotional functioning. One would expect to find a disproportionate number of visual problems and a wide variety of somatic complaints among these children. Such symptoms as fainting spells, headaches, dizzy spells, chest pains, sustained fatigue, and gastrointestinal discomfort are particularly prevalent within this subtype. These children clearly focus considerable concern on their physical well-being, and their mothers express a great deal of distress about their children's health. It is not clear whether the somatic complaints of Subtype 3 children reflect a psychogenic component, or whether these are the learning-disabled children with particularly poor physiologically based medical histories.

Subtype 4

The personality profile of the fourth subtype, comprised of 13 subjects (17% of those assigned), is markedly elevated on the Delinquency, Intellectual Screening, and Hyperactivity scales. In addition, it is comparatively elevated on the Family Relations scale.

The academic problems of Subtype 4 children tend to be accompanied by considerable behavioral disturbance. Many of the characteristics commonly ascribed to the "hyperkinetic syndrome" are indicated. These children tend to be overactive, restless, highly distractible, and impulsive. In response to authority, both at home and at school, they are frequently disobedient, disrespectful, unreliable, and argumentative. A limited tolerance for frustration is suggested; this may be associated with temper tantrums, destruction of property, displacement of anger, and typically delinquent behavior during adolescence. Lying and stealing are prevalent as these children readily tend to act out their impulses in an antisocial fashion. They may have histories of problematic peer relations, characterized by physical and verbal aggression and by interpersonal insensitivity. They tend to experience little anxiety or internal discomfort and, in many ways, resemble children diagnosed as having a "conduct disorder." The home lives of these children may reflect separation, divorce, or serious marital strife. Family instability, chronic family conflict, and parental inconsistency in setting limits are suggested.

INTERPRETATION OF NONSIGNIFICANT RESULTS

The principal nonsignificant findings in the present study concern the relationship between the four personality subtypes and nonpersonality variables. No significant between-subtype differences were found with regard to age or sexual composition; WISC Verbal, Performance, or Full Scale IQs; or WRAT Reading, Spelling, or Arithmetic centile scores. Caution is called for in interpreting these findings. It would be inaccurate to assume that these results are simply contraindicative of any relationship between the pattern of personality functioning of learning-disabled children and age, sex, IQ, or patterns of academic achievement. Indeed, studies designed to deal specifically with the relationships between patterns of abilities and deficits and personality and socioemotional functioning (e.g., Ozols, & Rourke, Chapter 13, this volume; Strang & Rourke, Chapter 14, this volume) suggest that such relationships can be quite positive and striking.

The nature of the statistical technique employed to identify subtypes of learning-disabled children has important implications for the interpretation of the apparent lack of relationship between age and personality. The subtypes were generated via an analysis of personality profile *configurations* rather than profile *elevations*. Therefore, the findings with regard to age fail to support the notion of a relationship between age and *personality patterns*. The possible relationship between age and degree of personality disturbance was not examined. (See Strang & Rourke, Chapter 14, this volume, for an explicit test of this relationship.)

The composition of the subject sample did not permit a meaningful investigation of sex differences among personality subtypes. Because only 13% of the subjects were female, between-subtype differences in sexual composition would have had to be extremely large to have reached statistical significance. No females at all (compared to 15% of the males) were assigned to Subtype 3, whereas 58% of the females (compared to 42% of the males) were assigned to Subtype 1. Were this pattern to hold up in a subject sample composed equally of large numbers of males and females, between-subtype differences in sexual composition would be statistically significant. Thus, the results of the present investigation offer neither support nor contrary evidence regarding the hypothesis that there is a relationship between personality subtypes and sexual composition in the learning-disabled population.

The question is somewhat more complex with regard to IQ and academic achievement. The results do not suggest that there is any simple relationship between personality subtype and any of the IQ or achievement scores (taken one at a time). However, the possibility of a relationship between personality subtype and the configuration of IQ or achievement scores was not examined. In fact, post hoc analysis supports the hypothesis that there is a significant relationship between personality subtype and configuration of achievement scores. Whereas no more than 30% of the subjects in Subtypes 1, 2, or 3 demonstrated average or better skills in any academic skill area, 62% of those in Subtype 4 were at least average in one or two skill areas ($\chi^2 = 8.21, p \leq .05$). This suggests a relationship between uneven academic functioning and the personality characteristics of Subtype 4. Too few of the subjects demonstrated any specific pattern of uneven academic skills (e.g., good reading and spelling with poor arithmetic) to permit an examination of the relationship between personality subtypes and patterns of specific learning deficiencies (see Strang & Rourke, Chapter 8, this volume).

Furthermore, data do not suggest a relationship between personality subtype and Verbal–Performance IQ discrepancy. However, only 9% of the total subject sample demonstrated the Verbal IQ > Performance IQ pattern, as compared to 47% who demonstrated the Verbal IQ < Performance IQ pattern. The very small number of subjects exhibiting the former pattern precluded a meaningful investigation of possible relationships between personality subtypes and IQ patterns.

METHODOLOGICAL LIMITATIONS

The principal limitation of the present study is that no test of statistical reliability, in contrast to psychometric reliability, was conducted. Statistical reliability would have been determined by conducting the *Q*-type factor analysis on two different sets of subjects, and then comparing the results of the two analyses. In the present investigation, there were not enough subjects who met the rather rigorous selection criteria to conduct such a procedure.

SUMMARY AND CONCLUSIONS

Educators and mental health professionals have noted frequently that learning-disabled children are particularly prone to socioemotional difficulties. Attempts to validate this notion, however, have failed to yield consistent and conclusive results. An examination of these studies reveals that virtually all of them employed research designs implicitly based on the untested assumption that the population of learning-disabled children is homogeneous in terms of personality functioning. Evidence of hetero-geneity of *ability* patterns in this population raised the question of whether the contradictory findings in pesonality research with learning-disabled children might be a reflection of the inaccuracy of the homogeneity assumption.

The results of the investigation reported in this chapter directly contradict the homogeneity assumption. It would appear that learning disabilities in children are not accompanied by a particular cluster of socioemotional characteristics. On the basis of our findings, it seems reasonable to conclude that the contradictory and inconclusive nature of previous research results in this area is attributable to the design of studies based on the assumption that learning-disabled children constitute a single personality type.

Four distinct personality patterns, accounting for 77% of the sample of learning-disabled children, were identified. The most commonly oc-curring pattern, demonstrated by almost half of these children, indicates quite adequate socioemotional functioning. This clearly refutes the notion that learning-disabled children are also emotionally disturbed. The other three personality patterns appear to be characterized, respectively, by (1) marked psychological disturbance reflected by internalized socio-emotional difficulties (26% of those classified); (2) a disproportionate pervasiveness and/or intensity of somatic concerns, accompanied by otherwise adequate personality functioning (13% of those classified); and (3) behavioral disturbance reflected by overactivity, distractibility, inter-personal insensitivity, and antisocial behavior (17% of those classified).

There is an obvious need to cross-validate the results of this study; such an investigation is currently proceeding in our laboratory. At the same time, the findings of the current study deserve careful attention. Future investigations into the socioemotional functioning of learning-disabled children should take into account the apparent heterogeneity of personality functioning in this population. Furthermore, should these results be confirmed in future studies, it would be incumbent on educators, school psychologists, and others to address the varying social and emo-tional needs of learning-disabled children.

The primary responsibility for the assessment of the personality functioning of learning-disabled children usually falls upon the school psychologist. If the results of our investigation are reliable, it would appear that Subtype 1 children, for example, whose personality functioning is adequate, would be quite amenable to the direct remediation of their learning deficits. It would also be found that children in Subtypes 2, 3, and 4 need special attention for both their learning and socioemotional problems. Although treatment should be offered according to the individual needs of each of these children, several generalizations seem warranted. For the Subtype 2 child, the advisability of family therapy, individual psychotherapy, and/or play therapy in particular should be considered. Special attention for the Subtype 3 child should include a determination of his/her proneness to psychosomatic disorders and physical illness. If psychophysiological reactions to stress are prominent, family therapy, individual play therapy, and parent training groups should be considered. The parent groups could focus on how psychosomatic reactions to stress can be reinforced in the home, and how children can be taught to relieve their stress in adaptive ways. There is, of course, a particular need for close medical monitoring and specific attention to the medical needs of all Subtype 3 children. Low-pressure teaching strategies would seem most important for these children. For the Subtype 4 child, behaviorally oriented approaches (e.g., contingency contracting) in combination with socialization programs in the school would be appropriate. Working with the home through family therapy or a parental counseling program would seem advantageous.

The need for a multidisciplinary approach to ameliorating the complex and varying problems of learning-disabled children is clear. The apparently heterogeneous nature of their socioemotional needs would seem to require the orchestrated application of a number of therapeutic modes and techniques that take into consideration the developmental course of this group of clinical disorders (see Rourke, Bakker, Fisk, & Strang, 1983, for an extended discussion of this topic).

REFERENCES

Applebee, A. N. Research in reading retardation: Two critical problems. *Journal of Child Psychology and Psychiatry*, 1971, *12*, 91–113.
Benton, A. L. Developmental dyslexia: Neurological aspects. In W. J. Friedlander (Ed.), *Advances in neurology* (Vol. 7). New York: Raven Press, 1975.

Black, F. W. Self-concept as related to achievement and age in learning disabled children. *Child Development*, 1974, *45*, 1137–1140.

Bryan, T. H. An observational analysis of classroom behaviors of children with learning disabilities. *Journal of Learning Disabilities*, 1974, *7*, 26–34. (a)

Bryan, T. H. Peer popularity of learning-disabled children. *Journal of Learning Disabilities*, 1974, *7*, 621–625. (b)

Bryan, T. H. Peer popularity and learning-disabled children: A replication. *Journal of Learning Disabilities*, 1976, *9*, 307–311.

Bryan, T. H., & McGrady, H. J. Use of a teacher rating scale. *Journal of Learning Disabilities*, 1972, *5*, 199–206.

Bryant, N. Clinical inadequacies with learning disorders: The missing clinical educator. In J. Helmuth (Ed.), *Learning disorders* (Vol. 2). Seattle: Special Child Publications, 1966.

Campbell, D. M. Interaction patterns in families with learning problem children. *Dissertation Abstracts International*, 1972, *33*, 1783B. (University Microfilms No. 72-25, 252)

Connolly, C. The psychosocial adjustment of children with dyslexia. *Exceptional Children*, 1969, *46*, 126–127.

Connolly, C. Social and emotional factors in learning disabilities. In H. R. Myklebust (Ed.), *Progress in learning disabilities* (Vol. 2). New York: Grune & Stratton, 1971.

Darlington, R. B., & Bishop, C. H. Increasing test validity by considering interitem correlation. *Journal of Applied Psychology*, 1966, *50*, 322–330.

Doehring, D. G., & Hoshko, I. M. Classification of reading problems by the Q-technique of factor analysis. *Cortex*, 1977, *13*, 281–294.

Fisk, J. L., & Rourke, B. P. Identification of subtypes of learning disabled children: A neuropsychological, multivariate approach. *Journal of Clinical Neuropsychology*, 1979, *1*, 289–310.

Forness, S. R., & Esteveldt, K. C. *Classroom observation of learning and behavior problem children*. Los Angeles: Graduate School of Education, UCLA, 1971.

Goldman, M., & Barclay, A. Influence of maternal attitudes on children with reading disabilities. *Perceptual and Motor Skills*, 1974, *38*, 303–307.

Grunebaum, M. G., Hurwitz, I., Prentice, M. M., & Sperry, B. M. Fathers of sons with primary neurotic learning inhibitions. *American Journal of Orthopsychiatry*, 1962, *32*, 462–472.

Halechko, A. D. Self-esteem and perception of parental behavior in children with learning disabilities. *Dissertation Abstracts International*, 1977, *38*, 359B. (University Microfilms No. 77-15, 246)

Jastak, J. F., & Jastak, S. R. *The Wide Range Achievement Test*. Wilmington, Del.: Guidance Associates, 1965.

Klinedinst, J. K. Multiphasic measurements of child personality: Construction of content scales using the Personality Inventory for Children. *Journal of Consulting and Clinical Psychology*, 1975, *43*, 700–715.

Leong, C. K. Lateralization in severely disabled readers in relation to functional cerebral development and synthesis of information. In R. M. Knights & D. J. Bakker (Eds.), *The neuropsychology of learning disorders: Theoretical approaches*. Baltimore: University Park Press, 1976.

Mattis, S., French, J. H., & Rapin, I. Dyslexia in children and young adults: Three independent neuropsychological syndromes. *Developmental Medicine and Child Neurology*, 1975, *17*, 150–163.

McCarthy, J. M., & Paraskevopoulos, J. Behavior patterns of learning disabled, emotionally disturbed, and average children. *Exceptional Children*, 1969, *36*, 69–74.

McNutt, G. L. The identification of learning disabled adolescents. *Dissertation Abstracts International,* 1978, *38,* 4097A. (University Microfilms No. 77-29, 067)

Miller, D. R., & Westman, J. C. Reading disability as a condition of family stability. *Family Process,* 1964, *3,* 66–76.

Miller, D. R., & Westman, J. C. Family team work and psychotherapy. *Family Process,* 1966, *5,* 49–59.

Natchez, G. (Ed.). *Children with reading problems.* New York: Basic Books, 1968.

Nelson, H. E., & Warrington, E. K. Developmental spelling retardation. In R. M. Knights & D. J. Bakker (Eds.), *The neuropsychology of learning disorders: Theoretical approaches.* Baltimore: University Park Press, 1976.

Peck, B. B., & Stackhouse, T. Reading problems and family dynamics. *Journal of Learning Disabilities,* 1973, *6,* 506–511.

Petrauskas, R. J., & Rourke, B. P. Identification of subtypes of retarded readers: A neuropsychological, multivariate approach. *Journal of Clinical Neuropsychology,* 1979, *1,* 17–37.

Porter, J. F. Identification of subtypes of learning disabled children: A multivariate analysis of patterns of personality functioning. *Dissertation Abstracts International,* 1980, *41,* 1125B.

Ribner, S. The effects of special class placement on the self-concept of exceptional children. *Journal of Learning Disabilities,* 1978, *11,* 319–323.

Richey, D. D., & McKinney J. D. Classroom behavioral subtypes of learning disabled boys. *Journal of Learning Disabilities,* 1978, *11,* 297–302.

Rourke, B. P. Neuropsychological research in reading retardation: A review. In A. L. Benton & D. Pearl (Eds.), *Dyslexia: An appraisal of current knowledge.* London: Oxford University Press, 1978.

Rourke, B. P., Bakker, D. J., Fisk, J. L., & Strang, J. D. *Child neuropsychology: An introduction to theory, research, and clinical practice.* New York: Guilford Press, 1983.

Rourke, B. P., Dietrich, D. M., & Young, G. C. Significance of WISC Verbal–Performance discrepancies for younger children with learning disabilities. *Perceptual and Motor Skills,* 1973, *36,* 275–282.

Rourke, B. P., & Orr, R. R. Prediction of the reading and spelling performance of normal and retarded readers: A four-year follow-up. *Journal of Abnormal Child Psychology,* 1977, *5,* 9–20.

Rourke, B. P., & Strang, J. D. Neuropsychological significance of variations in patterns of academic performance: Motor, psychomotor, and tactile–perceptual abilities. *Journal of Pediatric Psychology,* 1978, *3,* 62–66.

Seigler, H. G., & Gynther, M. D. Reading ability of children and family harmony. *Journal of Developmental Reading,* 1960, *4,* 17–24.

Silverman, R. G. An investigation of self concept in urban, suburban and rural students with learning disabilities. *Dissertation Abstracts International,* 1978, *38,* 5398A. (University Microfilms No. 78-01, 877)

Siperstein, G. N., Bopp, M. A., & Bak, J. J. Social status of learning disabled children. *Journal of Learning Disabilities,* 1978, *11,* 98–102.

Strag, G. A. Comparative behavioral ratings of parents with severely mentally retarded, specific learning disability and normal children. *Journal of Learning Disabilities,* 1972, *5,* 631–635.

Sweeney, J. E., & Rourke, B. P. Neuropsychological significance of phonetically accurate and phonetically inaccurate spelling errors in younger and older retarded spellers. *Brain and Language,* 1978, *6,* 212–225.

Wetter, J. Parental attitudes toward learning disability. *Exceptional Children*, 1972, *38*, 490–491.

Wirt, R. D., Lachar, D., Klinedinst, J. K., & Seat, P. D. *Multidimensional description of child personality: A manual for the Personality Inventory for Children.* Los Angeles: Western Psychological Services, 1977.

Zimmerman, I. L., & Allebrand, G. N. Personality characteristics and attitudes toward achievement of good and poor readers. *Journal of Educational Research*, 1965, *57*, 28–30.

13

Dimensions of Social Sensitivity in Two Types of Learning-Disabled Children

EDITE J. OZOLS

BYRON P. ROURKE

The contention that socioemotional problems often occur in conjunction with childhood learning disorders can be noted throughout the history of research on learning disabilities. In this chapter, we review current research exploring social problems of learning-disabled children, and comment on the limitations of this body of research. This is followed by the presentation of a framework that we would suggest for the investigation of these important and complex questions. This framework combines a neuropsychological subtyping approach to learning disabilities with a component analysis of social competence. The focus of this chapter is the presentation of a study derived from this framework, in which two groups of learning-disabled children, classified according to their patterns of neuropsychological abilities, were found to differ in their performance on four exploratory tasks of social sensitivity. In the final portion of this chapter, treatment considerations for dealing with the social problems of these two groups of children are presented.

Edite J. Ozols. Department of Psychology, University of Windsor, Windsor, Ontario, Canada, and Department of Neuropsychology, St. Michael's Hospital, Toronto, Ontario, Canada.

Byron P. Rourke. Department of Psychology, University of Windsor, and Department of Neuropsychology, Windsor Western Hospital Centre, Windsor, Ontario, Canada.

EXPLORING THE SOCIAL COMPETENCE OF
LEARNING-DISABLED CHILDREN

Social competence can be defined as a child's ability to satisfy inter-personal needs in ways that are both effective and acceptable to society (Schneider, 1982). The importance of developing effective social skills has long been supported by evidence that adult mental health is correlated with childhood social competence (Cowen, Pederson, Babigian, Izzo, & Trost, 1973).

Social competence is a very complex concept that is difficult to define operationally. Researchers interested in determining characteristics of socially competent children (e.g., Nakamura & Finck, 1980) acknowledge the variability of effective social behavior, and recognize the importance of situational determinants of behavior. However, others have attempted to clarify this concept by delineating the components of effective social functioning (e.g., Anderson & Messick, 1974). The many skills and abilities outlined by a component analysis of social competence can be classified into three groups: (1) perceptual skills, such as those required in the perception of facial expressions; (2) cognitive abilities, such as the ability to abstract reasons regarding the motivation for an individual's social behavior; and (3) motor and language skills, by which the child manifests his/her social behavior. Although this basic classification of abilities may be useful for theoretical purposes, it is important to recognize that appropriate social behavior results from a complex coordination of these and other variables.

One important social skill that is largely dependent on perceptual analysis is the ability to monitor and evaluate accurately the affective states of others. The ability to perceive nonverbal cues is especially important, as studies have shown that most people rely on nonverbal information as the source of meaning in social situations (Mehrabian, 1972). Aspects of nonverbal communication include facial expression, gaze direction, eye contact, clothing and how it is worn, body movement, posture, interpersonal distance, touch, and vocal variations in speech (Mayo & LaFrance, 1979). An understanding of nonverbal cues is crucial even in infancy, when patterns of mutuality based on gaze direction, touch, "cooing," and so forth, are established between an infant and its caregiver.

Studies with a cognitive focus stress the child's active role in constructing social knowledge, and probe his/her understanding of relations between persons. One example of this approach is a study by Flapan (1968), who examined the development of children's reasoning regarding the feelings of characters in film episodes. The results of this investigation suggested that children progress from providing explanations of these episodes in situational terms (i.e., descriptions of overt actions) to explanations in psychological terms to explanations in terms of interpersonal perceptions.

However, in addition to perceptual, cognitive, and behavioral skills, it is obvious that an individual must also possess certain attitudinal characteristics. In any given social situation, an individual must have the self-confidence and emotional resolve to act in the appropriate manner that he/she has determined by perceptual and cognitive analysis. This motivational set allows an individual to respond effectively, without interference from negative emotions, such as anxiety. Aspects of social competence that figure prominently in this dimension include a differentiated self-concept and consolidation of identity, a concept of oneself as an initiating and controlling agent, and a realistic appraisal of oneself, accompanied by feelings of personal worth (Anderson & Messick, 1974).

Examination of the learning disabilities literature reveals that it is frequently claimed that learning-disabled children experience problems in their social world, and that their socioemotional difficulties persist into adolescence and adulthood (Bryan, Donahue, & Pearl, 1981; Kronick, 1980; Siegel, 1974). Researchers have attempted to elucidate the social characteristics of this group using a variety of measures, such as parent observations (Owen, Adams, Forrest, Stolz, & Fisher, 1971), teacher ratings (Bryan & McGrady, 1972; Keogh, Tchir, & Windeguth-Behn, 1974), peer ratings (T. H. Bryan, 1974), and classroom observations of the interactions of learning-disabled children (T. S. Bryan, 1974; Bryan & Wheeler, 1972). These studies have consistently demonstrated the social failure experienced by this group of children as a whole: In comparison to their peers and siblings, the learning-disabled children tend to be judged in more negative and rejecting terms by parents, teachers, and classmates. Moreover, it has been shown that some of these children are less accurate in perceiving their own social status (Bruininks, 1978).

Investigators interested in determining the etiology of this social rejection have usually focused on one perceptual, cognitive, or behavioral skill that they assert is lacking in learning-disabled children as a whole. For example, Kronick (1980) has proposed that the social problems of learning-disabled children may result from a deficit in schematic judgment, or an inability to realize the organization of an interactional situation. A different perspective is provided by Bryan (1982), who claims that the social problems of learning-disabled children are due to a linguistic deficit. She sees these children as deficient in the pragmatics necessary for interpersonal communication, and believes that they lack an understanding of rules that govern socially appropriate speech (e.g., paying compliments, expressing verbal affection, inviting others' participation).

Other studies have investigated the learning-disabled child's ability to perceive and interpret accurately the affective states of others. For example, Wiig and Harris (1974) found that learning-disabled adolescents were significantly less efficient than normal adolescents at labeling the emotions expressed by a young female's videotaped nonverbal expressions of anger, embarrassment, and other emotions. In another study, Bachara (1976) presented stories to learning-disabled children aged 7 to 12 and had them select appropriate facial expressions from a set of pictures of faces; the learning-disabled children made significantly more errors than did normal children. Bryan (1977) presented a film of an adult female expressing various emotions, and found a significant difference between the performance of the learning-disabled subjects and the normals, with the learning-disabled group being less able to describe the scenario in an accurate fashion. However, this finding was not replicated (LaGreca, 1981).

The research approach of these studies, which typically compared a group of learning-disabled children to a nondisabled group, was perhaps a necessary initial phase in the investigation of social problems of learning-disabled children. However, the contradictory results that have recently been recognized may relate directly to two major limitations of this body of research.

The first major limitation of this research is the lack of a conceptual model to elucidate the skills involved in social competence that are deficient in learning-disabled children. It is impossible to obtain an accurate picture of the incidence of social problems in this group without considering the complexity of this concept, as well as the need for operational definitions of the components. There is no point in continuing a search for the "one" deficit area that interferes with the growth of social competence in learning-disabled children. Just as there are many reasons for academic failure, so there are many reasons for social failure. A component analysis of social competence will help us recognize that, while some children experience social problems because they lack certain perceptual, cognitive, or behavioral skills, others may manifest social difficulties more directly as a result of attitudinal–motivational variables.

Furthermore, it is difficult to draw conclusions from the existing research because different research teams have used different definitions of learning disabilities in selecting subjects to study. It is of particular concern that so many researchers neglect even to report their criteria for subject selection. In addition, the accepted practice of studying learning-disabled children as a uniform population has masked the significant differences within this heterogeneous group. It is crucial that research in this area begin to consider the types of learning disabilities, as different types of social problems may be associated with different types of learning disabilities, and some types of learning-disabled children may have no social problems at all (as suggested by Porter & Rourke, Chapter 12, this volume). The failure to consider criteria for subject selection is probably the principal cause for the many contradictory results in the literature dealing with this and other issues in the field of children's learning disabilities.

A PROPOSED FRAMEWORK FOR STUDYING SOCIAL PROBLEMS OF LEARNING-DISABLED CHILDREN

Although it is likely that the majority of schoolchildren fluctuate in their school performance due to "emotional" factors, such as low motivation, these children are excluded from most definitions of learning disabilities. A learning disability is considered to be a retardation or delayed development in one or more of the processes of speech, language, reading, writing, arithmetic, or other school subjects, which results from factors other than emotional disturbance, mental retardation, sensory deprivation, or cultural or instructional factors (McCarthy & McCarthy, 1969). However, in everyday functioning, "emotional" and "cognitive" factors are in constant interaction. For example, although a learning disability may initially be the "primary" factor in a child's academic failure, it is clear that a "secondary" factor, the resulting loss of motivation, may become a critical factor in the child's continued failure to learn. The assumptions that psychologists and educators make regarding the issue of "primacy" will have important implications for the child's treatment planning.

The approach that we propose focuses on the role that central processing deficiencies play in the social functioning of learning-disabled children. It is unfortunate that the utilization of a neuropsychological framework has so often been interpreted as reflecting an emphasis on static, organismic dysfunction. For this reason, we must emphasize that our approach is an attempt to integrate dimensions of socioemotional development and central processing features in order to fashion a useful model by which to study the crucial aspects of individual human development, including learning disabilities. A neuropsychological model of brain–behavior relationships provides us with a useful method by which to differentiate among types of learning-disabled children. We expect that different patterns of central processing deficits and abilities differentially predispose a child to different patterns of social behavior, as well as to different types of academic disabilities.

Recent neuropsychological studies have isolated the two subtypes of learning-disabled children that we focus on in this chapter. Children in the first group have poor psycholinguistic skills in conjunction with very well-developed abilities in visual–spatial analysis, organization, and synthesis. On academic measures, their outstanding deficiencies appear in reading and spelling. However, they tend to perform very well on tests of nonverbal problem solving and concept formation, and they exhibit no problems with psychomotor coordination or tactile perception. Their speech and language are rather immature and impoverished, and their reading is slow and labored. This pattern of performance on neuro-psychological measures reflects an impairment in abilities ordinarily thought to be subserved primarily by the left cerebral hemisphere, within a context of relatively well-developed abilities that are thought to be dependent upon intact right-hemisphere systems for their satisfactory elaboration and development (Rourke, 1982; Rourke & Finlayson, 1978; Rourke & Strang, 1978).

Children in the second group experience their major academic failure in mechanical arithmetic, while exhibiting advanced levels of word recognition and spelling. These children exhibit outstanding problems in visual–spatial organization and synthesis, in conjunction with bilateral psychomotor deficiencies and bilateral tactile–perceptual difficulties. They have great difficulty in generating and dealing with nonverbal and otherwise novel and/or complex concepts (Strang & Rourke, 1983), and thus they also tend to have problems with school subjects that involve such skills (e.g., many aspects of natural science). They exhibit clear strengths in rote verbal learning, regular phoneme–grapheme matching skills, amount of verbal output, and verbal classification. They exhibit fairly normal simple stereotyped motor movements and simple tactile–perceptual abilities. Behaviorally, it has been noted that they attempt mathematical calculations for which they have little understanding, and that they often neglect to check the adequacy of their solutions. They tend to process print in a rigid, programmatic fashion, and their reading comprehension scores are often much lower than their word-recognition scores. This pattern of test performance typifies children with "nonverbal learning disabilities" (Myklebust, 1975), and it reflects impairment of abilities ordinarily thought to be subserved primarily by the right cerebral hemisphere (Rourke, 1982; Rourke & Strang, 1983; Strang & Rourke, 1983).

Our knowledge of the neuropsychological characteristics of children in these two subtypes allows us to make predictions regarding their social skills and social behavior. Children in the subtype characterized by poor auditory–linguistic processing in conjunction with adequate visual processing skills have many cognitive strengths that will serve them well in social adaptation, when we consider that processing of social information requires good visual–perceptual skills, conceptual abilities, intermodal integration, and processing of novel stimuli. However, we can expect that these children will be at a disadvantage in social situations that involve a heavy reliance on verbal expression for social cue generation. Though children in this group possess many of the cognitive skills crucial for effective social functioning, some of them may also exhibit social problems (usually manifested as "behavior problems"), primarily as a result of attitudinal and motivational variables. Emotionally, some of these children appear to develop a "negative set" toward reading and spelling, and they internalize and generalize this sense of failure in the form of low self-esteem. Unfortunately, the lack of standardized measures of social competence that would allow us to obtain a valid estimate of the incidence of this "socioemotional side effect" of learning disabilities poses obstacles to the testing of this hypothesis.

However, children with nonverbal learning disabilities may be at an even greater risk for the development of social problems, because they lack many of the perceptual and cognitive skills that are crucial in social functioning. Their difficulty in attending to and interpreting visual–perceptual information will render their interpretation of nonverbal social cues (such as facial expressions, hand movements, body postures, and other physical gestures) problematic. Their deficiencies in processing novel stimuli and dealing with informational complexity will also interfere with their performance in social situations. They appear almost to cease exploring their environment motorically, visually, and tactually as a general consequence of their inability to profit from nonverbal experiences.

These issues have received scant attention in the literature. However, Johnson and Myklebust (1967) have provided us with an excellent description of children with "nonverbal disorders of learning," chronicling their social problems as well as their academic difficulties. A recent study by Wiener (1980) provides further support for the assertion that this group of children experiences more severe social problems. Wiener classified learning-disabled children, aged 8–12, as having either a "conceptual disability" (lowest scores on Wechsler Intelligence Scale for Children— Revised [WISC-R] Similarities, Comprehension, and Vocabulary subtests), a "spatial disability" (lowest scores on Picture Completion, Block Design, and Object Assembly subtests), or a "sequencing disability" (lowest scores on Digit Span and Coding). A measure of each child's social competence was then obtained, using counselors' ratings of children's peer relationships, as well as peer ratings. Significant differences among the groups were found, with children in the "spatial disability" group exhibiting the lowest scores on peer acceptance measures.

In summary, the proposed framework for studying social problems of learning-disabled children begins with a thorough analysis of the neuropsychological abilities and deficits of children classified into subtypes. From our knowledge regarding the children's performance on measures of academic and cognitive functioning, we can generate hypotheses regarding their performance on measures of social competence. In forming these hypotheses, it is important to consider the complex interactional nature and the many components of social competence. In the next section, we present a recent study that utilized this framework for comparing subtypes of learning-disabled children with respect to their ability to perceive certain social dimensions.

AN EXPERIMENT INVESTIGATING DIMENSIONS OF SOCIAL SENSITIVITY IN TWO TYPES OF LEARNING-DISABLED CHILDREN

The purpose of this study was to investigate whether two groups of learning-disabled children, classified according to their patterns of neuropsychological abilities, would differ in their performance on four exploratory tasks of social sensitivity. The study was an initial attempt to test the theoretical position that different patterns of central processing abilities and deficits affect learning-disabled children's performance differentially on tasks involving social perception.

SUBJECTS

The learning-disabled subjects had been referred for neuropsychological assessment because of a "learning" and/or a "perceptual" problem to which it was thought that cerebral dysfunction might be a contributing factor. The children had received extensive neuropsychological assessments within 2 years of the time of the study. A description of the comprehensive assessment procedures employed can be found elsewhere (Rourke, 1975, 1976, 1981). A child was excluded from the study if the neuropsychological formulation indicated that the child's pattern of functioning was contraindicative of dysfunction at the level of the cerebral hemispheres, and if emotional problems were thought to be a primary factor interfering with the child's performance. The complete Wide Range Achievement Test (WRAT; Jastak & Jastak, 1965) and five Wechsler Intelligence Scale for Children (WISC; Wechsler, 1949) subtests (Arithmetic, Vocabulary, Comprehension, Picture Arrangement, and Object Assembly) were readministered in this study to ascertain that the child's pattern of performance on these measures remained essentially the same as on the previous neuropsychological assessment.

A combination of criteria from previous studies was used to specify two groups of learning-disabled children: (1) a group with relatively poor auditory–perceptual and language-related abilities, in conjunction with relatively well-developed visual–spatial abilities (these children are referred to here as the "language disorder" group); and (2) a group of children who exhibited poor visual–spatial abilities, in conjunction with relatively well-developed auditory–perceptual and language-related abilities (these are referred to as the "spatial disorder" group) (Rourke & Finlayson, 1978; Rourke & Strang, 1978; Rourke & Telegdy, 1971; Rourke, Young, & Flewelling, 1971). The children ranged in age from 8 to 11 years, and their performances on the dependent variables were compared to a group of average-achieving children of the same age (referred to as the control group). Children in the control group were attending a regular school and had no past history of learning and/or emotional problems. Subject selection criteria for the three groups are presented in Table 13-1, and the means and standard deviations for the selection variables are contained in Table 13-2.

MEASURES

The visual stimuli used in the present study were selected and modified from materials in the "Toward Affective Development" kit (Dupont, Gardner, & Brody, 1974), an educational tool designed to further children's social and affective growth. Four tasks, which varied in their stimulus and response modalities, were developed for the present study.

The first task, Task A, was designed to investigate children's ability to select an appropriate nonverbal gesture on the basis of information provided in a verbal story delivered orally by the examiner. Each child was presented with a matrix of six pictures of a young child who was

TABLE 13-1. Criteria for Group Selection

		Group	
Variable	Control	Language disorder	Spatial disorder
All of the following:			
WRAT Reading (centile)	≥ 45	≤ 20	[b]
WRAT Spelling (centile)	≥ 35	≤ 20	[b]
WRAT Arithmetic (centile)	≥ 30	[b]	≤ 25
WISC Verbal IQ[a]	≥ 90	≤ 90	VIQ–PIQ ≥ 10
WISC Performance IQ[a]	≥ 90	PIQ–VIQ ≥ 10	≤ 90
WISC Full Scale IQ[a]	≥ 85	≥ 85	≥ 85
WISC Vocabulary scaled score	≥ 8	≤ 8	≥ 9
WISC Object Assembly scaled score	≥ 8	≥ 10	≤ 8
Teacher ratings in reading, spelling, and arithmetic	At least average	[b]	[b]
Two of the following:			
Tactual Performance Test—Both Hands (minutes)	[b]	Average	At least 1 *SD* below average
Tactual Performance Test—Left Hand (minutes)	[b]	Average	At least 1 *SD* below average
Tactual Performance Test—Location (*n* correct)	[b]	Average	At least 1 *SD* below average
Target Test (*n* correct)	[b]	Average	At least 1 *SD* below average

[a] IQ scores prorated for control subjects.

[b] Variable not used as criterion for this group.

TABLE 13-2. Means and Standard Deviations for Selection Variables

| Variable | Group (*n* = 7 for each) | | |
	Control	Language disorder	Spatial disorder
Sex			
Male	3	5	3
Female	4	2	4
Age (months)			
M	122.86	119.71	113.57
SD	12.57	13.91	9.25
WRAT Reading (centile)			
M	65.57	9.00	41.57
SD	15.05	3.05	36.70
WRAT Spelling (centile)			
M	58.14	9.85	28.28
SD	11.87	6.47	32.68
WRAT Arithmetic (centile)			
M	41.00	21.57	18.00
SD	16.21	11.44	4.83
WISC Verbal IQ			
M	109.14	83.28	99.00
SD	9.82	4.95	5.16
WISC Performance IQ			
M	105.14	106.14	81.14
SD	9.42	10.71	4.14
WISC Full Scale IQ			
M	107.71	93.57	89.71
SD	8.18	7.39	4.46
WISC Vocabulary (scaled score)			
M	11.57	8.14	10.85
SD	2.23	1.06	1.86
WISC Object Assembly (scaled score)			
M	11.43	12.00	6.57
SD	1.90	1.29	1.27
Tactual Performance Test—Both Hands (minutes)			
M		1.44	4.12
SD		.55	3.17
Tactual Performance Test—Left Hand (minutes)			
M		2.75	6.98
SD		1.24	3.14
Tactual Performance Test—Location (*n* correct)			
M		2.71	1.71
SD		1.25	1.38
Target Test (*n* correct)			
M		13.43	7.86
SD		4.58	4.02

exhibiting the following nonverbal gestures: In the top row, the child was rubbing his stomach, waving his hand, and clenching his fist; in the bottom row, the child was tapping his fingers on a desk, shaking a forefinger, and stretching out his hand. The children were then read six stories, with two stories each relevant to three gestures: waving a hand, clenching a fist, and shaking a forefinger. The story required the subject to infer the next action in the story by pointing to the nonverbal gesture appropriate to the story character's specified experience. The responses were scored as appropriate (1) or inappropriate (0).

Task B was designed as a measure of the child's ability to select an appropriate facial expression on the basis of information provided in a verbal story, in combination with visual information. Each child was presented with four large colored pictures of children involved in social interactions. Each picture was presented separately, and beside the picture were placed six small pictures of a child's face; four of these expressed the emotions of anger, fear, happiness, and sadness, and there were also two "neutral" faces. The faces of the children in the large pictures were covered. Each subject was presented with a story concerning each large picture. The subject's task was to choose the appropriate facial expression for the main character, and to place this face on the large picture. The responses were scored as appropriate (1) or inappropriate (0).

The third task, Task C, was designed as a measure of the children's ability to describe feelings as portrayed in visual representations of social situations. Each child was presented with two large colored pictures of children involved in social interactions. The subjects were asked to state the feelings of three characters in each picture. Responses were scored as follows: 2 for any dominant emotion, 1 for any other appropriate emotion, or 0.

The purpose of Task D was to study the children's ability to make inferences regarding the reasons for feelings that occur in social situations. The visual stimuli were identical to those used in Task C, and subjects were asked to provide an explanation of each character's feelings. Responses were scored as follows: 2 for an explanation of feeling in psychological or interpersonal terms (e.g., "He's worried because the baby might be hurt"), 1 for an explanation of feeling in situational terms (e.g., "He's worried because the house is on fire"), or 0.

The order of task presentation was varied randomly across subjects. The order of story presentation in Tasks A and B was varied randomly, as was the order of picture presentation and questions in Tasks C and D.

The WRAT Spelling, Reading and Arithmetic subtests were administered first, followed by administration of the five WISC subtests. The four dependent variables (Tasks A, B, C, and D) were administered last. Each subject was tested individually; the testing session lasted approximately 1½ hours.

RESULTS

Significant differences among groups were found for the combination of dependent variables: A one-way multivariate analysis of variance (MANOVA) across the four dependent variables yielded a significant main effect for group, $F = 2.96$, $p < .01$. One-way analyses of variance (ANOVAs) yielded significant group effects for the two tasks requiring verbal responses: $F = 5.75$, $p < .01$, for Task C; $F = 3.89$, $p < .04$, for Task D. Testing for simple effects across groups using the Tukey A procedure revealed that the language disorder group differed significantly from the control group on Task C ($p < .01$) and Task D ($p < .05$). The results of the MANOVA, ANOVAs, and analyses of covariance (ANCOVAs) are presented in Table 13-3. Covariate analyses for group effects with age and sex as covariates yielded essentially the same results as those for the analyses where the covariates were not employed.

The pattern of group performance was in the expected direction on all four tasks, favoring the control group on tasks requiring nonverbal responses (Tasks A and B), as well as on tasks requiring verbal responses (Tasks C and D). Furthermore, children in the language disorder group tended to do better than those in the spatial disorder group on Tasks A and B, while children in the spatial disorder group tended to perform at levels superior to those of the language disorder group on Tasks C and D. In addition to the nonsignificant trends, statistically significant differences between groups were found on Tasks C and D: Children with auditory-perceptual and linguistic handicaps performed significantly more poorly than normals on measures of social perception that involved verbal labeling and explanations. Thus, the results of the present study provide preliminary support for the theoretical position outlined earlier: Learning-disabled children can be expected to vary in their performance on at least some tests of social perception as a function of the interaction between their disability characteristics and the task demands.

Some qualitative differences were also noted in the test behavior and social behavior of the children. For example, upon entering the testing

TABLE 13-3. Summary of MANOVA, ANOVA, and ANCOVA Results for Group Effect on Dependent Variables

Variable	F ratio	p	Discriminant vector
Task A	1.66	.22	.092
Covariate sex	1.75	.20	
Covariate age	1.09	.36	
Task B	1.68	.21	.120
Covariate sex	1.58	.23	
Covariate age	2.24	.14	
Task C	5.75	.01	.072
Covariate sex	5.12	.02	
Covariate age	5.30	.02	
Task D	3.89	.04	.056
Covariate sex	3.15	.07	
Covariate age	3.63	.05	
MANOVA	2.96	.01	Root 1.69

Note. The Hotelling–Lawley trace was used for the MANOVA F test.

room, children in the language disorder group appeared alert and interested in their social and visual environment. During the testing itself, they often looked at the examiner for cues and reassurance. In contrast, children in the spatial disorder group generally did not explore their environment upon entering the testing room, and did not attend visually to other objects in the room. They tended to wait for the examiner to provide complete instructions on most tasks, and they made few spontaneous movements. There were also noticeable differences in the physical appearance of the children: Those in the spatial disorder group were often overweight, and their faces had a tired and depressed quality, whereas those in the language disorder group appeared physically healthy and alert.

In general, children in the language disorder group were more responsive to the examiner. They expressed variability in their emotional reactions, and often smiled and laughed as they successfully performed visual–motor tasks. For example, one child in this group smiled as he completed a puzzle and then exclaimed, "I did it! I like them. Can I do some others?" This delight was in contrast to his comments as he completed the WRAT: "I can't spell. I don't know arithmetic. I got them all wrong." However, children in the spatial disorder group often stared at the examiner, and rarely expressed emotion appropriately through their facial expressions. Their voices also had a monotonic or expressionless quality (this was primarily true of the females of the group). However, this general expressionless state was occasionally interrupted by over-dramatized expression. For example, one girl spoke of a planned trip to the zoo in an unusual, animated fashion: She had a high-pitched voice, and raised her eyebrows in excitement during this explanation, in marked contrast to almost all of her other behavior within the testing situation.

Children in the language disorder group rarely initiated conversation with the examiner, and provided very brief and often "concrete" verbal replies to questions. On difficult items they often tended simply to shrug their shoulders and say, "I don't know." In contrast, many of the children with spatial disorders were very talkative, and often expressed resistance to difficult tasks with lengthy verbal statements. For example, some of the "resistance" statements from this group were as follows: "My head hurts when I have to think so much," "I'll have to think about that one. I'm not that sure. It's a little hard," "Let's skip that one. It's a little too hard for me," "I don't know sign language," and "If it's hard, do we still try?" Some of the children in the spatial disorder group frequently interjected comments that were irrelevant to the test situation (e.g., "My hamster died," "Did you notice my glasses?," "Are these all small rooms?," "Oh, I'm so itchy these days!"). However, it is interesting to note that there were within-group differences in the degree of talkativeness of these children: It appeared that those who were talkative were extremely talkative, while those who were withdrawn were extremely withdrawn.

There were also many differences between groups in their test approaches. Children in the spatial disorder group tended to write very slowly, and had large, unskillful handwriting. Most of them did not use a strategy to arrange the puzzles on the WISC Object Assembly subtest: They did not use common lines to match pieces; often pieces and entire puzzles were inverted; and often completely incongruous pieces were joined. For example, on the FACE puzzle, one child joined the eyebrow part to the mouth; on the HORSE puzzle, another child just formed a long string of puzzle pieces. Children in this group took a long time to respond on many tasks, but especially on those of a nonverbal nature. When they were presented with the materials for the social tasks, they did not appear particularly interested and did not scan the materials. In contrast, children in the language disorder group exhibited quick, agile hand movements on motor tasks, and took care to align task materials in a correct fashion. They appeared intent on understanding the visual information in the pictures, and scanned the pictures closely. While these children ranged from an average to a fast reaction time on most measures, they were noticeably slow on tasks requiring verbal responses.

The flexibility of the children's thoughts regarding emotions was probed by asking each child whether the character in a story could feel another way than the one that he/she had initially selected. For example, the examiner would say to a subject, "You said that Johnny would feel this way [examiner would point to child's response] if he fell down and hurt himself. Could he feel this way [examiner would point to happy face] in this situation? Why [not]?" It is interesting to note that four of the seven children in the language disorder group demonstrated flexibility on at least one such question, while none of the children in the spatial disorder group did. As a matter of fact, one girl in the spatial disorder group asked, "What do you mean?" after each flexibility question was presented. This observation supports the notion that children with non-verbal learning disabilities have a tendency to exhibit stereotyped and restricted emotional responses.

LIMITATIONS OF THE STUDY AND DIRECTIONS FOR FUTURE RESEARCH

The primary purpose of this exploratory study was to investigate whether two groups of learning-disabled children, classified according to their pattern of neuropsychological abilities, would differ from each other and from normals in their performance on tasks designed for the measurement of some dimensions of social sensitivity. Statistically significant differences among groups were found for the combination of dependent variables, as well as for the tasks requiring verbal responses (Tasks C and D). The pattern of group performance was in the expected direction on all tasks. Both groups of learning-disabled children tended to perform somewhat less well than the normally achieving group. However, these results suggest that the *particular* difficulties that these children experience in social situations are more a function of their *pattern* of central processing abilities and deficits than of their status as learning-disabled children.

The small number of subjects in each group necessarily limits the generalizability of our results. This restriction in subject size was due to the difficulty in finding children who met the criteria for the spatial disorder group, as children with nonverbal learning disabilities were referred less often for neuropsychological assessment than were their language-disordered peers. In addition, the tender age of subjects in this study may have influenced the variability within the groups. A third possible limitation relates to the particular subject selection criteria for group or subtype composition employed in this study. However, the exact criteria adopted would certainly allow for replication of the study findings.

Limitations in the construction of the four exploratory tasks were also due to a lack of appropriate standardized procedures. Tasks A and B may have been limited by a ceiling effect; an examination of the average scores on these tests suggests that they may have been too easy for the control group. Furthermore, we may have obtained more statistically significant results had these tasks been "purer" measures of verbal and nonverbal skills. Future studies could systematically vary the presentation of social information to the child (either verbal, nonverbal, or both), and vary the modality involved in the child's response (verbal, nonverbal, or both).

The development of reliable and meaningful measures of social competence is the most pressing need in this area of investigation. In addition, the criteria for subject selection and subtype selection need to be further refined. It is also important to determine the incidence of different types of social problems among different subtypes of learning-disabled children, as it is clear that not all children in this group experience social difficulties. Studies utilizing the framework outlined in this chapter will eventually allow us to predict the specific patterns of neuropsychological, emotional, familial, and environmental characteristics that put learning-disabled children "at risk" for the development of socioemotional difficulties.

TREATMENT AND TRAINING CONSIDERATIONS

The development of appropriate remedial techniques to deal with the social problems of learning-disabled children is a largely unexplored area. In this section, we present general principles regarding intervention with the learning-disabled child, and then discuss how these principles may apply in planning treatment for the two subtypes emphasized in this chapter.

First of all, it is vital to pursue an individualized approach in planning remediation. The heterogeneous nature of children with learning disabilities precludes the possibility of ever finding the "one best method" of intervention, whether this method is meant to address academic, social, or any other problems faced by such children.

To this end, a thorough assessment of each child's neuropsychological strengths and weaknesses, as well as his/her social skills, is necessary. While standardized neuropsychological assessment procedures have been available to clinicians for quite some time, there is still a lack of normed and standardized tools for measuring social competence. However, clinicians may obtain basic information regarding a child's interpersonal relations by using teacher and parent ratings of social behavior, as well as direct individualized assessment of the various "skills" and "attitudes" involved in social competence. It is also important to bear in mind that some children may not be experiencing social problems at the time they are assessed, but may be "at risk" for future socioemotional difficulties, due to the predicted interaction of their ability structure and what is for them an inappropriate environment (Rourke, Bakker, Fisk, & Strang, 1983).

Some children in the language disorder group may encounter problems dealing with the linguistic aspects of social communication. Suggestions regarding the training of conversational skills in learning-disabled children have been provided by Bryan (1982) and LaGreca (1981), and such training may be appropriate for this subtype. Other children in this group may manifest inappropriate social behavior more directly, as a result of prolonged experiences of frustration and consequent negative emotional experiences. These children will probably respond well to psychotherapeutic intervention that is nonverbal in orientation, because active participation is always more meaningful to these children than is any discussion of appropriate and inappropriate behavior. For example, in a play therapy situation, this type of child can attempt to resolve conflicts by nonverbal means. Role playing may also be a powerful means of social learning for this group, as it engages their well-developed skills of visual imitation. However, we would predict that many of the children in this subtype will not require any extensive psychotherapeutic intervention, as they already possess most of the skills and attitudes required for effective social functioning.

In contrast, it is likely that many children in the spatial disorder group will require intervention designed to improve their social skills. Their well-developed verbal skills can be used as a means by which to analyze and understand their nonverbal experiences in the social realm. For example, they may benefit from training in problem-solving skills utilizing a verbal approach (Spivack & Shure, 1974). Children in this subtype may also benefit from training in the visual–spatial and visual–perceptual skills essential to social interaction. For example, pictures of facial expressions and social scenes can be presented to these children, who can then be encouraged to describe these visual stimuli, with immediate feedback provided. Remedial suggestions for social skills training for children in this subtype have been provided by several authors (Johnson & Myklebust, 1967; Minskoff, 1980a, 1980b), and can also be extrapolated from social skills training programs that have been established for nonclinical populations (e.g., Fagen, Long, & Stevens, 1975).

CONCLUSION

Given the tentative nature of the findings presented in this chapter, it is evident that we are only at the beginning stages of exploring these complex phenomena. The social problems of learning-disabled children will certainly continue to be an active focus of research for some time to come. We hope that the neuropsychological model described in this chapter, with its emphasis on subtypes of learning disabilities and a component analysis of social competence, will serve to generate new hypotheses and relevant research questions.

The reader is reminded that our emphasis on a cognitive (central) processing model does not preclude the importance of considering all aspects of a child's functioning—the child's behavior is, of course, a result of the interaction among disability characteristics, temperament characteristics, familial and environmental influences, and important emotional variables, such as motivation. In fact, it should be emphasized that the theoretical position outlined in this chapter and elsewhere (Rourke, 1982) is an attempt to eliminate the artificial dichotomy between children's "cognitive" and "affective" functioning that has been espoused in the literature for so long. It remains for future research to test the limits of this approach.

REFERENCES

Anderson, S., & Messick, S. Social competency in young children. *Developmental Psychology*, 1974, *10*, 282–293.

Bachara, G. Empathy in learning disabled children. *Perceptual and Motor Skills*, 1976, *43*, 541–542.

Bruininks, V. L. Peer status and personality characteristics of learning disabled and non-disabled students. *Journal of Learning Disabilities*, 1978, *11*, 29–34.

Bryan, T., Donahue, M., & Pearl, R. Learning disabled children's communicative competence on referential communication tasks. *Journal of Pediatric Psychology*, 1981, *6*, 383–393.

Bryan, T. H. Peer popularity of learning disabled children. *Journal of Learning Disabilities*, 1974, *7*, 621–625.

Bryan, T. H. Learning disabled children's comprehension of nonverbal communication. *Journal of Learning Disabilities*, 1977, *10*, 501–506.

Bryan, T. H. *Social cognitive understanding and language.* Paper presented at the meeting of the Ontario Association for Children with Learning Disabilities, Toronto, April, 1982.

Bryan, T. S. An observational analysis of classroom behaviors of children with learning disabilities. *Journal of Learning Disabilities*, 1974, *7*, 26–43.

Bryan, T. S., & McGrady, H. J. Use of a teacher rating scale. *Journal of Learning Disabilities*, 1972, *5*, 199–206.

Bryan, T. S., & Wheeler, R. Perception of learning disabled children: The eye of the observer. *Journal of Learning Disabilities*, 1972, *5*, 484–488.

Cowen, E. L., Pederson, A., Babigian, H., Izzo, L. D., & Trost, M. A. Long-term follow-up of early detected vulnerable children. *Journal of Consulting and Clinical Psychology*, 1973, *41*, 438–446.

Dupont, H., Gardner, O. S., & Brody, D. S. *Toward affective development.* Circle Pines, Minn.: American Guidance Service, 1974.

Fagen, S., Long, M., & Stevens, B. *Teaching children self-control: Preventing emotional and learning problems in the elementary school.* Columbus, Ohio: Merrill, 1975.

Flapan, D. *Children's understanding of social interaction.* New York: Teachers College Press, 1968.

Jastak, J. F., & Jastak, S. R. *The Wide Range Achievement Test.* Wilmington, Del.: Guidance Associates, 1965.

Johnson, D., & Myklebust, H. R. *Learning disabilities: Educational principles and practices.* New York: Grune & Stratton, 1967.

Keogh, B. K., Tchir, C., & Windeguth-Behn, A. Teachers' perceptions of educationally high risk children. *Journal of Learning Disabilities*, 1974, *7*, 43–50.

Kronick, D. An overview of research relating to the etiology of interactional deficits in the learning disabled. In R. M. Knights & D. J. Bakker (Eds.) *Treatment of hyperactive and learning disordered children.* Baltimore: University Park Press, 1980.

LaGreca, A. M. Social behavior and social perception in learning disabled children: A review with implications for social skills training. *Journal of Pediatric Psychology*, 1981, *6*, 395–416.

Mayo, C., & LaFrance, M. On the acquisition of nonverbal communication: A review. In S. Chess & A. Thomas (Eds.) *Annual progress in child psychiatry and child development.* New York: Brunner/Mazel, 1979.

McCarthy, J. J., & McCarthy, J. F. *Learning disabilities.* Boston: Allyn & Bacon, 1969.

Mehrabian, A. *Nonverbal communication.* Chicago: Aldine-Atherton, 1972.

Minskoff, E. H. Teaching approach for developing nonverbal communication skills in students with social perception deficits: Part I. The basic approach and body language clues. *Journal of Learning Disabilities*, 1980, *13*, 118–124. (a)

Minskoff, E. H. Teaching approach for developing nonverbal communication skills in students with social perception deficits: Part II. Proxemic, vocalic and artifactual clues. *Journal of Learning Disabilities*, 1980, *13*, 203–208.

Myklebust, H. R. Nonverbal learning disabilities: Assessment and intervention. In H. R.

Myklebust (Ed.) *Progress in learning disabilities* (Vol. 3). New York: Grune & Stratton, 1975.

Nakamura, C. Y., & Finck, D. N. Relative effectiveness of socially oriented and task-oriented children and predictability of their behaviors. *Monographs of the Society for Research in Child Development*, 1980, *45*(No. 185).

Owen, F. W., Adams, P. A., Forrest, T., Stolz, L. M., & Fisher, S. Learning disorders in children: Sibling studies. *Monographs of the Society for Research in Child Development*, 1971, *36*(No. 144).

Rourke, B. P. Brain-behavior relationships in children: A research programme. *American Psychologist*, 1975, *30*, 911–920.

Rourke, B. P. Issues in the neuropsychological assessment of children with learning disabilities. *Canadian Psychological Review*, 1976, *17*, 99–102.

Rourke, B. P. Neuropsychological assessment of children with learning disabilities. In S. B. Filskov & T. J. Boll (Eds.), *Handbook of clinical neuropsychology*. New York: Wiley-Interscience, 1981.

Rourke, B. P. Central processing deficiencies in children: Toward a developmental neuropsychological model. *Journal of Clinical Neuropsychology*, 1982, *4*, 1–18.

Rourke, B. P., Bakker, D. J., Fisk, J. L., & Strang, J. D. *Child neuropsychology: An introduction to theory, research, and clinical practice*. New York: Guilford Press, 1983.

Rourke, B. P., & Finlayson, M. A. J. Neuropsychological significance of variations in patterns of academic performance: Verbal and visual–spatial abilities. *Journal of Abnormal Child Psychology*, 1978, *6*, 121–133.

Rourke, B. P., & Strang, J. D. Neuropsychological significance of variations in patterns of academic performance: Motor, psychomotor and tactile–perceptual abilities. *Journal of Pediatric Psychology*, 1978, *3*, 62–66.

Rourke, B. P., & Strang, J. D. Subtypes of reading and arithmetical disabilities: A neuropsychological analysis. In M. Rutter (Ed.), *Developmental neuropsychiatry*. New York: Guilford Press, 1983.

Rourke, B. P., & Telegdy, G. A. Lateralizing significance of WISC Verbal–Performance discrepancies for older children with learning disabilities. *Perceptual and Motor Skills*, 1971, *33*, 875–883.

Rourke, B. P., Young, G. C., & Flewelling, R. W. The relationships between WISC Verbal–Performance discrepancies and selected verbal, auditory–perceptual, visual–perceptual, and problem-solving abilities in children with learning disabilities. *Journal of Clinical Psychology*, 1971, *27*, 475–479.

Schneider, B. H. *Development of an individualized social competence intervention procedure for children with behavior and learning disorders*. Paper presented at the meeting of the Ontario Association for Children with Learning Disabilities, Toronto, April 1982.

Siegel, E. *The exceptional child grows up*. New York: E. P. Dutton, 1974.

Spivack, G., & Shure, M. B. *Social adjustment of young children: A cognitive approach to solving real-life problems*. San Francisco: Jossey-Bass, 1974.

Strang, J. D., & Rourke, B. P. Concept-formation/non-verbal reasoning abilities of children who exhibit specific academic problems with arithmetic. *Journal of Clinical Child Psychology*, 1983, *12*, 33–39.

Wechsler, D. *Wechsler Intelligence Scale for Children*. New York: Psychological Corporation, 1949.

Wiener, J. R. A theoretical model of the acquisition of peer relationships of learning disabled children. *Journal of Learning Disabilities*, 1980, *13*, 506–511.

Wiig, E., & Harris, S. Perception and interpretation of nonverbally expressed emotions by adolescents with learning disabilities. *Perceptual and Motor Skills*, 1974, *38*, 239–245.

14

Adaptive Behavior of Children Who Exhibit Specific Arithmetic Disabilities and Associated Neuropsychological Abilities and Deficits

JOHN D. STRANG

BYRON P. ROURKE

> Hercule Poirot to Captain Hastings (from Agatha Christie's *ABC Murders*): "Speech, so a wise old Frenchman said to me once, is an invention of man's to prevent him from thinking."

We have found that well-motivated children who exhibit specific and outstanding problems with the Wide Range Achievement Test (WRAT; Jastak & Jastak, 1965) Arithmetic subtest (in the context of at least age-appropriate WRAT Reading and Spelling subtest performances) are remarkably similar in their neuropsychological and, in many cases, their general adaptive behavioral characteristics. This chapter has two primary purposes: (1) to describe the common neuropsychological and behavioral characteristics of such children; and (2) to attempt to explain how such behavioral similarities among a group of children could come about. The chapter begins with a case study that serves to illustrate the classic pattern

John D. Strang. Department of Neuropsychology, Windsor Western Hospital Centre, Windsor, Ontario, Canada.

Byron P. Rourke. Department of Psychology, University of Windsor, and Department of Neuropsychology, Windsor Western Hospital Centre, Windsor, Ontario, Canada.

of neuropsychological impairments and strengths that are characteristic of such children, and some frequently noted (and presumably associated) behavioral characteristics.

LAURIE: A CASE STUDY

Laurie, a girl aged 9 years, 6 months, was referred for a complete neuropsychological assessment by her family physician. The chief referral complaint was academic difficulties. Although Laurie was not referred by academic authorities, her school records indicated that she was experiencing difficulties with mathematics and had poor written work. Furthermore, it was noted by her teachers that she required more verbal direction than did other children of her age and in other ways seemed to be overly dependent on the teacher for guidance, direction, and other forms of assistance. For example, she still required the teacher's help in buttoning her coat. Outside the classroom setting, she was often harassed by other children and was the butt of their jokes.

In the testing situation, she presented as a somewhat overweight young girl who prolonged separating from her mother before formal testing began. Her clothes were clean and relatively well coordinated, but her undershirt hung out. Her hair was disheveled slightly at the beginning of the testing session. By the end of the testing sessions (approximately 6 hours later), she was quite unkempt in appearance. She did not seem to take notice of her physical appearance, and some of her other incidental behavior (e.g., burping and then laughing) was also socially inappropriate.

On a number of occasions during this testing session, Laurie's comments were clearly inappropriate for the situation at hand. For example, after she had completed a relatively complex nonverbal problem-solving test in which she was given ongoing feedback regarding the correctness of her performance (the Halstead Category Test; Reitan & Davison, 1974) and she had fared quite poorly, she said, "I like this test, it was fun."

Throughout the day, she required explicit verbal instructions to perform even the simplest of motor and other tasks that were primarily nonverbal in their requirements. For instance, it was necessary to instruct her in a verbal, step-by-step fashion before beginning the Finger Tapping Test (Reitan & Davison, 1974), as she failed to benefit from the initial verbal instructions and visual demonstration. Because of her apparent need for explicit verbal instructions, she required longer to complete testing than do most children of her age.

She was friendly and cooperative, and she appeared to put forth her best efforts during this day-long testing session, despite her apparent social and cognitive inadequacies.

The results of Laurie's neuropsychological assessment were considered to be a "classic" example of this subtype of neuropsychologically impaired children. Briefly, there was evidence of bilateral (right- and left-hand) impairment on relatively complex tests of tactile–perceptual capabilities and bilateral impairment on several tests of psychomotor abilities (e.g., the Grooved Pegboard Test; Kløve, 1963). On the Tactual Performance Test (TPT; Reitan & Davison, 1974), her right-hand (i.e., dominant-hand) performance was normal, but she performed in a severely impaired manner with her left hand. In fact, she required approximately twice as much time to complete this formboard task with her left hand as she did with her right hand, even though the left-hand trial followed the right-hand trial. On a third trial, in which both hands were used conjointly, her performance was also markedly impaired.

In general, this young girl's visual–perceptual–organizational skills were found to be impaired. Her graphic reproductions of geometric forms (particularly a Greek cross) were distorted. Her handwriting was large and somewhat tentative. Some evidence suggested that she tended to scan less well in her left visual field than in her right visual field, although there were no clear signs of visual-field defects.

On the other hand, Laurie performed exceptionally well on tests of "automatic" (in some respects, superficial), primarily receptive language abilities (e.g., word-blending skills, speech-sounds perception), and her vocabulary was quite well developed for her age. Her level and pattern of performance on the WRAT was also considered to be a reflection of her well-developed "automatic" (overlearned) language-related skills. On the WRAT Reading and Spelling subtests, her grade-equivalent scores were superior: Reading, 9.3 (99th centile); Spelling, 6.5 (86th centile). Her misspellings were phonetically accurate in the extreme—that is, while the phonemes were represented by appropriate graphic equivalents in virtually all of her misspelled words, it would appear that she failed to appreciate the exact visual characteristics of the word to be spelled. On the WRAT Arithmetic subtest, Laurie performed very poorly. Her grade-equivalent score of 3.0 (16th centile) was 3.5 years below her WRAT Spelling subtest score.

When Laurie's neuropsychological test results were discussed with her teacher, her school principal, and a special educational consultant in a remedial educational conference setting, there was some resistance to the notion (the neuropsychologist's opinion) that the majority of this girl's adaptive deficiencies were related directly to her particular pattern of neuropsychological strengths and weaknesses. It appeared that these school authorities (who were not responsible for Laurie's original referral for a neuropsychological assessment) were positively impressed, particularly by her WRAT Reading and Spelling performances in conjunction with their personal observations of this girl. With respect to the latter, they viewed her as being an overly dependent, "overprotected" child. In other words, from a school-related standpoint, Laurie's academic deficiencies were not particularly outstanding (i.e., she could read and spell proficiently). Furthermore, they surmised that her inappropriate social behavior and interactional style were the result of inadequate parenting and a general lack of experience. After some deliberation, school authorities conceded that Laurie might benefit from specialized remediation in some academic and other developmental realms; consequently, on the recommendation of the neuropsychologist, she was enrolled in a special center for children who exhibit outstanding learning and other adaptive deficiencies. It was thought that the milieu offered by this specialized institution and the ability of the staff to tailor a program to meet her special education and other needs would be most beneficial to this girl in the long run.

NEUROPSYCHOLOGICAL STUDIES OF CHILDREN WITH SPECIFIC ARITHMETIC DISABILITIES

The case of Laurie is especially instructive for our purposes in this chapter. As was mentioned earlier, this child's neuropsychological test results were "classic" with respect to our studies of children who exhibit a pattern of at least age-appropriate reading and spelling skills and exceptionally depressed mechanical arithmetic skills (as measured by the WRAT). The essential findings of these studies, particularly as they pertain to the neuropsychological status of children like Laurie, are reviewed only briefly here, as they have been described in some detail in a previous chapter of this volume (see Strang & Rourke, Chapter 8).

There have been three studies completed in our laboratory regarding the neuropsychological significance of children whose WRAT Reading and Spelling performances were average or above but whose WRAT Arithmetic performances were relatively deficient (at least 2 years lower than their WRAT Reading and Spelling scores). In the first study in this series, Rourke and Finlayson (1978) found that this group of children performed in at least an age-appropriate level on a wide variety of measures of auditory–perceptual and verbal abilities. These included a sound–symbol matching test (Speech-Sounds Perception Test; Reitan & Davison, 1974), a word-blending test (Auditory Closure Test; Kass, 1964), a test of memory for sentences of gradually increasing length (Sentence Memory Test; Benton, 1965) and two vocabulary tests (the Vocabulary subtest of the Wechsler Intelligence Scale for Children [WISC; Wechsler, 1949, and the Peabody Picture Vocabulary Test [Dunn, 1965]). On the other hand, these children performed in a somewhat impaired fashion on tests of visual–perceptual–organizational abilities. As a group, their most outstandingly poor performances were obtained on the Block Design and Object Assembly subtests of the WISC.

In the second study in this series, we (Rourke & Strang, 1978) conducted an in-depth investigation of the motor, psychomotor, and tactile–perceptual abilities of the children classified as Group 3 by Rourke and Finlayson (1978). The results of this study indicated that, as a group, these children did not exhibit evidence of impairment in any simple motor abilities (e.g., speed and grip strength). However, there was clear evidence of difficulties with each hand on a complex speeded eye–hand coordination test (Grooved Pegboard Test; Kløve, 1963), and on a test of motor steadiness in the kinetic disposition (Maze Test; Kløve, 1963). On a relatively complex problem-solving test that involves tactile-form recognition, manual dexterity, and the ability to benefit from kinesthetic feedback, (the TPT; Reitan & Davison, 1974), these children exhibited a normal level of performance with the right hand (on a first trial). However, on a second trial, which involved the left hand only, this group failed to improve their performance, and the mean score for this trial fell within the impaired range. On a third trial, in which both hands are used together, these children performed at an exceptionally poor level. On other measures of fairly complex tactile–perceptual disabilities (e.g., finger agnosia, finger dysgraphesthesia, astereognosis for coins), there was evidence of impairment on both sides of the body. This tactile–perceptual impairment was most evident on the left side of the body.

In a third study in this series, we (Strang & Rourke, 1983) compared the Halstead Category Test performances of the two groups of children in the previous studies who differed most markedly in their patterns of WRAT scores. We found that the group of children who exhibited very poor WRAT Reading and Spelling abilities and relatively better WRAT Arithmetic abilities (Group 2) performed in an age-appropriate fashion on this complex nonverbal problem-solving test. In comparison, the Category Test performances of the group of children with whom we are concerned in this chapter (the Group 3 children) were significantly impaired. Furthermore, it was found that these children with specific arithmetic impairments performed most poorly on those Category Test subtests that were least amenable to solution by means of a verbal strategy or that required substantial shifting of psychological set.

In summary, children who presented with outstanding and rather specific deficiencies in WRAT Arithmetic (as compared with their performances in WRAT Reading and Spelling) were found to exhibit evidence of bilateral psychomotor impairment, except on the TPT. On the TPT, Group 3 children exhibited normal right-hand performance, impaired left-hand performance, and markedly impaired performance when both hands were used conjointly on a third trial. They also exhibited evidence of poorly developed complex tactile- and visual-perceptual-organizational skills, and their nonverbal concept-formation abilities were impaired as well. As a group, they excelled at language-related skills of the "automatic" or rote variety.

In other words, these Group 3 children would appear to be most clearly disabled in the perception, analysis, organization, and synthesis of nonverbal information (introduced via the tactile and visual modalities), as well as to exhibit psychomotor output and nonverbal problem-solving difficulties. With this in mind, we refer to this particular pattern of neuropsychological strengths and weaknesses as a "nonverbal perceptual-organizational-output disability" (NPOOD).

The incidental behaviors of Laurie in the testing session and the way in which she was perceived and treated by others are typical of Group 3 children. Although we have found that there is some variability in the degree to which children who exhibit NPOOD have developed appropriate social and general adaptational skills, it is most often apparent that such children are not well adjusted from a socioemotional standpoint, and that they are strikingly similar to one another in their general behavioral characteristics (e.g., they tend to be overly talkative in many social situations). The sources of data that have led us to this conclusion are the following: short- and long-term longitudinal studies of individual children; findings from cross-sectional investigations of children (and adults) who exhibit NPOOD; comparisons of the adaptive behaviors and characteristics of NPOOD children with those of other subtypes of neuropsychologically impaired children; and perusals of historical records of NPOOD children and accounts of them given by their parents and teachers.

There have also been two formal, but preliminary, investigations completed in our laboratory that have examined socioemotional and behavioral characteristics of children who exhibit specific neuropsychological characteristics that are considered to be hallmarks of NPOOD. One of these studies is discussed in some detail in another chapter in this book (Ozols & Rourke, Chapter 13). Ozols and Rourke found that those children who bore some of the neuropsychological characteristics that typify NPOOD did not understand pictures depicting various social situations as well as did children who were language-impaired and otherwise exhibited a pattern of neuropsychological strengths and weaknesses quite opposite to that seen in NPOOD children. Based in part on the findings of the Ozols and Rourke study, we hypothesized that this subtype of learning-disabled children may not attend to and/or understand the nonverbal behavior of others in novel social situations, and that this may contribute to their social interaction difficulties.

In another study (Strang & Rourke, 1985), the suspected behavioral insufficiencies of children who exhibited some classic NPOOD (neuropsychological) characteristics were investigated from another point of view. Specifically, their Personality Inventory for Children (PIC; Wirt, Lachar, Klinedinst, & Seat, 1977) profiles were compared with those of two other subtypes of learning-disabled children, one of which (Group 2, in this study) exhibited some evidence of poorly developed language-related skills and much better developed visual–perceptual and visual–organizational abilities.

Valid PIC profiles provide at least a reflection of the parent's (in our study, the mother's) perceptions of the child's personality functioning. With this in mind, we found that the NPOOD-like group of children (Group 3) exhibited a mean PIC profile that was suggestive of the presence of psychopathology. The PIC Psychosis scale, and, in general, those scales that constitute the Psychopathology–Internalization factor identified by Lachar (cited in Wirt *et al.*, 1977)—namely, Psychosis, Social Skills, Anxiety, Withdrawal, and Depression—best characterized and distinguished the PIC profiles of the group of NPOOD-type children. When the degrees of discrepancy between the language-related and visual-perceptual-organizational skills for Group 2 and Group 3 children were increased through a reselection procedure, the PIC results were even more distinct. Figure 14-1 illustrates the mean PIC profile differences for the three groups of children employed in this study. Some of the neuropsychological and academic characteristics of these three groups are listed in Table 14-1.

FIG. 14-1. Mean PIC profiles for Group 1, Group 2, and Group 3 learning-disabled Children (*n* = 7 in each group). (Abbreviations: L, Lie scale; F, F scale; DEF, Defensiveness scale; ADJ, Adjustment scale; ACH, Achievement scale; SOM, Somatic Concern scale; D, Depression scale; FAM, Family Relations scale; DLQ, Delinquency scale; WDL, Withdrawal scale; ANX, Anxiety scale; PSY, Psychosis scale; HPR, Hyperactivity scale; SSK, Social Skills scale.)

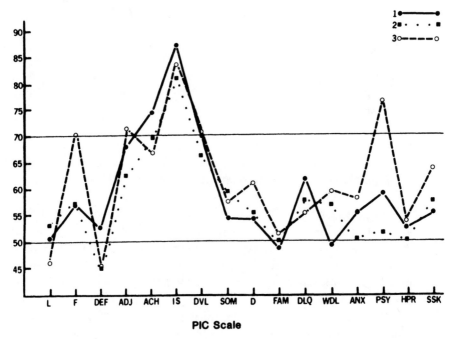

PIC Scale

TABLE 14-1. Means and Standard Deviations for Age, WISC Full Scale IQ, WISC Verbal IQ, WISC Performance IQ, WISC Vocabulary and Similarities Subtests (Combined) Score, WISC Block Design and Object Assembly Subtests (Combined) Score, and WRAT Reading, Spelling, and Arithmetic Centile Scores

Variables	Group 1	Group 2	Group 3
Age (months)	123.85 (14.38)	127.28 (20.85)	121.85 (18.70)
WISC Full Scale IQ	95.71 (5.46)	98.00 (10.64)	95.85 (8.00)
WISC Verbal IQ	93.00 (5.53)	87.00 (10.03)	103.00 (6.19)
WISC Performance IQ	99.85 (5.72)	110.28 (10.24)	88.71 (11.23)
WISC Vocabulary + Similarities subtests (combined) score	20.71 (2.69)	17.14 (3.33)	25.57 (2.22)
WISC Block Design + Object Assembly subtests (combined) score	20.57 (3.35)	25.57 (2.87)	15.00 (3.26)
WRAT Reading (centile)	15.42 (9.03)	21.57 (16.66)	71.71 (28.64)
WRAT Spelling (centile)	13.28 (9.28)	12.71 (5.08)	45.71 (26.68)
WRAT Arithmetic (centile)	15.42 (4.31)	20.42 (12.28)	21.85 (11.36)

Note. Standard deviations appear in parentheses. $n = 7$ in each group.

ADAPTIVE BEHAVIOR OF NPOOD CHILDREN

GENERAL CLINICAL CHARACTERISTICS

The following is a description of our general clinical findings regarding the adaptive behavioral characteristics of children with NPOOD. First, and perhaps foremost, NPOOD children do not typically perform well in novel or otherwise complex situations. Such a child does not usually react well to change and may require much more time and more help in adjusting to even seemingly minor alterations in familiar situations than do most children. Consequently, they frequently avoid particularly troublesome, especially novel, situations.

In general, most NPOOD children appear to be somewhat clumsy and do not perform well in gross motor activities and/or sports, although this is not always the rule. We have found that some boys of this type have managed to develop overlearned basic gross motor skills (e.g., shooting baskets in basketball), and this is actually considered to be one of their strengths. Children who exhibit NPOOD often do not have any close friends, especially among children of their own age. Their parents and others typically report that this type of child seems to get along better with adults than with children. When they do develop friendships with children, these are usually with children much younger than themselves. Because of these and a number of other behavioral characteristics exhibited by NPOOD children, they are often described as being somewhat immature.

LANGUAGE CHARACTERISTICS

Most NPOOD children tend to be quite talkative. In some cases, the tendency toward talkativeness is quite apparent in all situations; in others, the children become talkative in situations in which they are more accustomed to the task requirements. As a group, they do not exhibit obvious difficulties with language syntax. Their vocabularies are typically well developed, and some of the children tend to use lengthy, multisyllabic words as a habit, even when they are uncertain about the correct meaning or usage of the word. There may be a tendency to overuse cliches and other types of jargon, particularly in somewhat unstructured conversations. What is said may not always be related directly to the topic at hand, and there is often a tangential quality to their speech patterns. Run-on sentences are not uncommon in the children's spoken and written verbiage. In many cases, there seems to be an overuse of descriptive terms, given the nature of the subject and the age of the child. Such children seem to imitate adult speech models closely in the form and structure of their spoken language, and, in some cases, in their choice of topics for informal conversations.

A particular emphasis on language as a way of gathering new information and directing one's own actions in virtually any sort of complex situation seems to be exaggerated in NPOOD children as compared to other children. Furthermore, it often appears as though this type of child uses language (talking) as a way of maintaining psychological contact with the listener. In this connection, we have often observed that NPOOD children will use language as a way of manipulating others in (for them) troublesome situations, apparently to avoid anxiety-provoking activities and/or demands or simply to keep others at a distance. These children often use talking as a cathartic mechanism for the immediate relief of their anxiety in situations in which they are confused. The extremely heavy reliance on language as a tool or aid for virtually all forms of (primary) adaptation may very well account for the frequently observed hyperverbal behavior of many children of this subtype. Given this situation, it is not surprising to find that most adults involved with NPOOD children focus on their language characteristics. Unfortunately, the prowess exhibited by such a child in the linguistic realm is often misinterpreted, and he/she is thought to be much "brighter" and more capable than is actually the case.

PSYCHOEDUCATIONAL CHARACTERISTICS

In addition to rather obvious difficulties with mechanical arithmetic, NPOOD children often have problems with all types of written work. In this regard, they may exhibit difficulties in copying from the board, as well as in the speed and neatness of their handwriting, especially their printing. Writing is usually large; letters are poorly formed and spaced, and sometimes do not fit on or between the lines on the paper. With specialized training and appropriate aids (e.g., raised-line paper), we have observed significant improvements with written work.

The facility that these children characteristically exhibit with word recognition (e.g., on the WRAT Reading subtest) after early-occurring grapheme–phoneme matching difficulties have been "cured" is in no way indicative of their reading comprehension abilities. Indeed, reading comprehension has always been observed to be significantly less well developed than are word-recognition skills for this group of children. This may not be obvious to their teachers because the children may score reasonably well on so-called "reading comprehension" tests, mostly because of their memory for verbal detail and their "shotgun" approach to answering the questions. In other words, such children tend to answer all questions that require memory for specific verbal facts, and may sometimes provide an elaborate verbal response; in combination, these response patterns may gain them "reading comprehension" points. However, more often than not, the children do not have a good understanding or general overview of the paragraph or passage. It is only when the number and type of errors that an NPOOD child makes on reading comprehension tests are examined closely that the magnitude of his/her reading comprehension problems becomes apparent.

Qualitative analysis of the NPOOD child's reading and spelling usually reveals a tendency to attend almost exclusively to the phonetic characteristics of the word to be spelled or read. The NPOOD child tends to remember and focus exclusively on the auditory–verbal rather than the visual characteristics of words unless trained intensively to do otherwise. When spelling, for instance, the child's misspellings may be completely accurate from a phonemic standpoint (all the sounds of the word are present), yet the child has failed to appreciate the visual characteristics of the word.

Academic subjects and such activities as art and physical education are obviously problematic for NPOOD children, especially as they become older and the psychomotor and other demands of these areas become greater. Complex subject areas, such as science, may also prove to be particularly difficult for them. Rotary classroom systems, which require frequent class changes during the course of the day, may prove to be more problematic for the NPOOD child than for most other children. The reasons for this range from the child's getting lost to the very probable difficulties that he/she will have in adjusting to the different types of demands of the various teachers met in the daily schedule. These difficulties represent only the most outstanding academic concerns regarding this type of child and by no means illustrate all of the problems that may occur.

SOCIOEMOTIONAL CHARACTERISTCS

Children who exhibit NPOOD do not, as a rule, fare particularly well in novel or unstructured social situations. There are a number of reasons for their social difficulties, some of which have already been mentioned. For example, it is suspected that such children do not attend to or understand the nonverbal gestures and communications of other children. Furthermore, many do not have appropriately developed nonverbal behaviors of their own. Poor posture, a lack of facial and body expression, and general awkwardness are common nonverbal behavioral characteristics of such children.

Another possible reason for the social difficulties of NPOOD children is their tendency to place too much emphasis on the auditory–verbal feedback inherent in social situations. That is, they tend to focus on what other people say without benefiting from the context in which the information is conveyed. This heavy reliance on the receptive aspects of language as a source of feedback in social situations is often coupled with a tendency to talk incessantly and, sometimes, far out of context in these situations. This has the effect of alienating listeners (especially in the case of children) and of further confusing the underlying messages inherent in social situations.

This inability to obtain adequate and appropriate feedback in social situations, and the tendency to give inappropriate messages, may and often do elicit negative feedback from other children (e.g., the NPOOD child may become the butt of other children's jokes); as a result, the child may become extremely anxious in such situations. Secondary anxiety can also hamper the attainment of veridical interpretations of social situations. Furthermore, it should be borne in mind that this type of child does not solve nonverbal problems particularly well under any circumstances, and this too may contribute to social interpretation difficulties.

Finally, it is important to remember that NPOOD children have underdeveloped psychomotor skills, and, as such, are unlikely to participate as often or as well as do their age-mates in unstructured (e.g., playground) games and sports. This complicates their social interpretation difficulties in two ways: (1) They do not receive as much experience as do their age-mates in novel, unstructured social situations because of their inability to compete successfully (for a number of reasons, this is often coupled with a tendency toward "overprotectiveness" on the part of a child's parents); and (2) since they are not participating as much, it leads others (e.g., their parents and other professional persons involved with them) to "explain" their social difficulties simply in terms of a lack of experience or some hypothesized idiosyncratic personality characteristic (e.g., that a child seems to like adults better than children). Such explanations do not enhance the likelihood that parents and other caretakers will seek intervention for NPOOD children for their peer relationship difficulties.

In addition to having social interaction difficulties, children who exhibit NPOOD are often seen as highly dependent, particularly on their elders (especially their mothers) for feedback and direction. Sometimes there is prolonged reliance on adults and others for direct aid for the completion of psychomotor (including "self-help") tasks, such as tying shoelaces. It is sometimes seen, particularly in the case of an NPOOD child who has no siblings, that the outstanding dependency needs of the child become reinforcing for the parent (especially the mother). Naturally, this serves to further the child's tendency toward overdependency and is a hindrance to his/her acquisition of independent living skills.

The important question that must be raised at this point is as follows: What is the significance of the interactions between NPOOD children's neuropsychological strengths and weaknesses and the fairly typical behavioral characteristics that they exhibit? The answers to this question are not obvious and require much more study. It seems clear, however, that there is an interaction between the neuropsychological ability structure of NPOOD children and their personality development. Elsewhere (see Rourke, Bakker, Fisk, & Strang, 1983), we have attempted to explain the systematic interaction among the neuropsychological characteristics of NPOOD children, the general environmental demands placed on them (including the kinds of expectations and treatment afforded them by their parents and others concerned with their development), and the development of their atypical behavioral patterns and other aspects of their personality characteristics. The following account, however, may serve to elucidate further the development of the adaptive personality characteristics and associated behaviors of NPOOD children. This account represents a simulated developmental history of one such child (whom we call Jerry), which we hope will serve to summarize the information derived from the clinical and research follow-ups that we have conducted with children who exhibit these particular neuropsychological problems. It does not represent the developmental history of any one child in particular, and only the outstanding similarities seen among the developmental histories of a large number of children of this type are emphasized. Furthermore, it is assumed that the nonverbal deficiencies that characterize this type of child have been present since birth.

JERRY: A SIMULATED CASE STUDY

During Jerry's infancy, it was noted that he exhibited a lack of exploratory activity. Close scrutiny of the infant's behavior revealed somewhat poor reactions to novel situations. Developmental milestones were delayed, and he appeared to be quite clumsy. However, there was a notable difference between the delay in the development of his verbal expressive skills (talking) and his psychomotor skills (e.g., walking), in that he learned to talk more quickly and more efficiently than he learned to walk.

Jerry's early language was qualitatively different from that typically seen in the "normal" child. From virtually the onset of language, Jerry's words were remarkably clear, and the intonation was quite similar to that of his adult models. Words were frequently repeated without any apparent understanding of their meaning, even after the beginning of his third year.

Overall, his verbal utterances did not always appear to be goal-directed in any obvious way (e.g., communicating a need or want to others), and they were frequently unrelated to the activities at hand.

The reaction of Jerry's parents to the onset of his talking was in many ways more exuberant than that exhibited by most parents. There were clear reasons for this: Jerry was poorly coordinated, clumsy, and did not explore his physical environment well; general developmental milestones were delayed; furthermore, he showed a tendency toward hypoactivity (although in some NPOOD cases there is evidence of hyperactivity). With these findings in mind, Jerry's parents had toyed with the notion that their child was "retarded." This was to some degree reinforced by medical authorities, including the child's pediatrician, who suggested that mental retardation and/or a mild form of cerebral palsy could not be ruled out during the child's early life. Once Jerry had learned to speak, or at least to repeat words, the parents' worst fears were alleviated. Among other things, this had the effect of encouraging the parents to reinforce and promote their child's verbal (even his "echolalic-like") behavior. Furthermore, the parents' impression of the child's general level of intellectual functioning changed dramatically. This child, once considered to be "retarded," was now thought to be quite bright. Casual observers reinforced this opinion by suggesting that Jerry must be bright since he could talk so well.

Jerry's inability to obtain reliable feedback via the tactile and visual modalities was further exacerbated by psychomotor incoordination and a natural tendency to avoid unrewarding situations. Even during his second year (the final stages of Piaget's [1954] "sensorimotor" period), he exhibited a preference for engaging in language rather than in nonverbal activities. In this connection, the following were observed: (1) Jerry did not receive the same amount or quality of sensory–motor experience as did the normal child (this lack of sensory–motor experience eventuated in an impoverished foundation for the later development of "higher-order" problem-solving and related intellectual functions); (2) he tended to rely more heavily than his age-mates on his parents for feedback and direction in virtually any situation in which difficulty was encountered; (3) Jerry's parents tended to be overly concerned with his welfare and protection; and (4) Jerry's language behavior seemed to be developing atypically (the development of his rather automatic verbal expressive capacities was far in excess of the development of any of his other significant neuropsychological abilities).

Closer inspection of Jerry's language revealed that he was learning words without knowledge of their physical and situational referents. Furthermore, the syntactical significance of the word (that is, how it is likely to fit best with other words) was emphasized in word usage. Consequently, even Jerry's early sentences were found to be more typical of his adult models than is usually seen. In this sense, his imitative modeling of adults' verbal behavior was quite advanced. On the other hand, his imitative modeling of the nonverbal behavior of adults and older children was notably poor. This included the full range of nonverbal behaviors—from facial and hand gesturing to simple psychomotor skills (e.g., replicating the hand–eye coordination necessary for hitting a balloon)—that are essential prerequisites for many forms of successful adaptation in later childhood and adulthood.

During roughly the 2- to 5-year-old period (Piaget's [1954] "preoperational" stage for the normal child), Jerry's early-developing deviant language tendencies became more evident. For example, it was observed that he used his verbal expressive skills almost exclusively as a way of obtaining information or simply attention from others. His verbal utterances (including crying) became an increasingly effective way of controlling his environment. Along these lines, his parents and others became accustomed to accommodating the child's needs to an excessive degree.

Parenthetically, it should be noted that the degree to which parents and others tend to reinforce the verbal behavior and other behavioral patterns of the NPOOD child can contribute to a unique pattern of development that seems to result, in part, from overselective experiences of common environmental situations. For example, through watching *Sesame Street* and other "educational" television programs religiously, some NPOOD children develop an appreciation for reading simple words as preschoolers. The sheer amount of practice that such programs afford, coupled with the auditory-based, phonics-type approach to reading used in the programs and the lack of interference from other sources of cognitive activity and concerns—all these factors contribute to this early appreciation for sound–symbol correspondence. This is thought to be especially typical of some NPOOD children whose neuropsychological impairments are particularly outstanding. (Some children who are similar to NPOOD children in their neuropsychological characteristics and their family expectations and demands have been referred to as "hyperlexic.") As is typical of most NPOOD children, Jerry exhibited some difficulty with establishing symbol–sound correspondences during Grades 1 and 2.

Although he had no difficulty with distinguishing or remembering particular sounds, the retention of the visual characteristics of alphabetical letters (graphemes) proved to be problematic for him.

Jerry's early interactions with his age-mates were not particularly productive. An inability to keep up with the psychomotor requirements of situations and to understand the cause-and-effect relationships inherent within games and social interactions contributed to this situation. His use of talking in attempts to control, manipulate, and fend off other children in unstructured play situations caused him to receive negative feedback from them. Jerry did not at first understand this because of his general problems with awareness for such events. However, when he told his mother about what others had said (in effect, repeating what others had said), his mother's protective tendencies were aroused, and play situations that were less challenging were chosen more carefully for him. In addition to having his new experiences closely monitored and chosen carefully for him (it should be noted that there were some realistic concerns here, such as when and how to cross the road), Jerry tended to avoid novel social situations of his own accord. These and some related factors (e.g., internalizing the disparaging remarks of other children) served to further his deprivation of appropriate social and other forms of practical experience.

Without the benefit of feedback from others concerning the appropriateness of one's behavior, even the "normal" child does not learn to modify his/her behavior in socially acceptable ways. It should be kept in mind that this situation was complicated even further for Jerry, in that he did not possess the nonverbal problem-solving and associated abilities necessary for the proper interpretation of feedback in these situations. This resulted in the development of a somewhat distorted view of even elementary cause-and-effect relationships and views of himself in relationship to others.

For the most part, Jerry met the demands of kindergarten, Grade 1, and Grade 2 with a mixed amount of success. On the one hand, the verbal structure of the classroom promoted the development of some better social interactional skills. On the other hand, Jerry's motoric clumsiness and visual–spatial difficulties adversely affected the development of his gross motor and graphomotor skills. In addition, as has been already pointed out, he had problems in recognizing, distinguishing, and remembering the visual characteristics of graphemes. However, it was felt that his gross motor, graphomotor, and grapheme–phoneme matching problems were not particularly significant, especially since he showed some progress in reading. Besides, his teachers were far too busy attempting to meet the needs of those children who were exhibiting outstanding phoneme–grapheme matching difficulties and/or behavioral problems.

By the time Jerry reached Grade 4, his everyday behavior was viewed as immature. Since he could read and spell with great facility by the middle of Grade 4, it was felt that his educational (e.g., mechanical arithmetic) and other difficulties (e.g., he often required some assistance from his Grade 4 teachers in finding his boots when it was time to go home) were the result of motivational problems and a general lack of experience. Jerry's teacher suspected that his parents had helped create this child's apparent overdependency. This was confirmed for the teacher in a parental interview, in which Jerry's mother admitted that she still did many things for her child. It was felt by all concerned that this child would outgrow his immature behavior.

For Jerry, social interactional difficulties, including a marked tendency toward social withdrawal, were quite obvious by the end of Grade 4. Moreover, it was observed that he did not seem to understand mathematical concepts and that he made many "careless" errors when completing mechanical arithmetic assignments. It was at this point that one of his teachers (a special educational consultant) suggested to Jerry's mother that he might benefit from some psychological testing.

Jerry's story does not end here in the real-life situation. It is, however, at this developmental "stage" that many such children (e.g., Laurie) are referred to our department for complete neuropsychological assessment, although it is certainly not clear to all concerned that the children have some seriously deficient neuropsychological abilities.

PROGNOSIS FOR THE NPOOD CHILD

We have recently completed a follow-up study of adults who have undergone complete neuropsychological assessment and who exhibit NPOOD. In this investigation (Rourke, Young, Strang, & Russell, 1985), it was found that, of the eight persons who were selected for study, seven had obtained some form of post-secondary school education. However, none of these persons held a job that was commensurate with their academic qualifications. All of them exhibited emotional and social difficulties and, in general, had a poor understanding of their adaptive limitations. Some of them had carried a diagnosis of schizophrenia at some point in their adult life. In all cases, the prognosis for future adjustment and independent living (without the benefit of involvement from various social agencies) was viewed as quite guarded.

When one considers the particular pattern of neuropsychological strengths and deficiencies exhibited by NPOOD children, their difficulties in benefiting from nonverbal experiences, their lack of experience in these areas, their uncommon reliance on language as a primary tool for adaptation, the confusion of their parents and other caretakers concerning the nature or significance of their condition, and the inappropriate expectations of such children by all concerned, the findings of the Rourke *et al.* (1985) study of NPOOD adults are not at all surprising. In this connection, the incidental behavior exhibited by Laurie in our testing sessions with her and the circumstances surrounding her referral to our department are quite understandable.

Although not all children who exhibit this pattern of neuropsychological strengths and deficiencies have identical developmental histories or behave exactly as outlined in this chapter, we have found that the similarities in behavioral outcome for such children are remarkably similar. At the same time, we have also found that the ability of the family to understand such a child's deficiencies early in life and to hold appropriate expectations for the child is an important factor in determining the degree to which the child will exhibit maladaptive atypical behavior in later childhood. Furthermore, thoughtful guidance from the child's parents and specialized forms of treatment outside the home situation are also important determinants of general prognosis. Finally, the *degree* of neuropsychological impairment would appear to be an important consideration. Children whose abilities are outstandingly impaired and who exhibit the full constellation of neuropsychological difficulties that are the hallmarks of NPOOD are those who are most at risk.

REMEDIATION/HABILITATION FOR THE NPOOD CHILD

The first step in remediation/habilitation usually involves providing the parents with appropriate feedback concerning the nature and significance of their child's neuropsychological disabilities. Often, the child's parents require ongoing counseling and support from the child-clinical neuropsychologist to gear their expectations and their parenting methods and techniques to fit with the child's most salient developmental needs. Remediation and habilitation for such a child on other fronts (e.g., in the school) at this point are difficult. As has been pointed out above, children who exhibit NPOOD are not typically identified as having outstanding educational needs. Consequently, it is seldom found that such children are involved in appropriate educational programs. This is particularly unfortunate, because if treatment is not instituted fairly early in such a child's life, the prognosis, in our experience, is quite bleak. With respect to treatment, we offer the following recommendations:

1. Observe the child's behavior closely, especially in novel or otherwise complex situations. During this potentially informative exercise, focus on what the child does and disregard what the child says. This should help the therapist and/or the teacher to develop a better appreciation of the child's potentially outstanding adaptive deficiencies and to shape their own cognitive "set" for interventions with the child. One of the most frequent criticisms of remedial intervention programs with this particular type of child is that remedial authorities are unaware of the extent and significance of the child's deficiencies. Through direct observation under these conditions, it should become apparent that the child is very much in need of systematic, well-conceived interventions.

2. Be realistic. Once it has been established that the child is quite ineffective, particularly in new or otherwise complex situations, one must then be realistic in assessing the impact of the child's reported neuropsychological strengths ("automatic" language skills) and the child's reported neuropsychological deficiencies. For instance, from an educational standpoint, it should be readily apparent that the child's well-developed word-recognition and spelling abilities are not sufficient for the child to benefit from many forms of formal and informal instruction, especially for those subjects that challenge visual–perceptual–organizational and/or nonverbal problem-solving skills.

3. Teach the child in a systematic, "step-by-step" fashion. Whenever possible, use a parts-to-whole verbal teaching approach. As a rule of thumb, the therapist or teacher should take note that, if it is possible to talk about an idea, concept, or procedure, then the child should be able to grasp that material. On the other hand, if it is not possible to put into words an adequate description of the material to be learned (e.g., as in explaining time concepts), it will probably be quite difficult for this type of child to benefit from the instruction.

It should also be kept in mind that the child will learn best when each of the verbal "steps" is in the correct sequence, because of his/her inadequate problem-solving skills and associated organizational difficulties with novel (even linguistically novel) material. A secondary benefit of this teaching approach is that the child is provided with a set of verbal rules that can be written out and then reapplied whenever it is appropriate to do so. This is particularly important for the teaching of mechanical arithmetic operations and procedures.

4. *Ask for verbal feedback from the child.* This remedial recommendation applies not only to the teaching sessions with the child, but also to any situation in which the child does not seem to appreciate fully the significance of his/her behavior or the behavior of others. For example, when there is an incident on the playground in which this child is "victimized," have the child explain what he/she perceives to be the cause of the incident and its effects. Then, through discussion, help the child to become aware of discrepancies between his/her perceptions (regarding the situation in question) and the perceptions of others. One technique in the teaching of academic subjects is to have the child reteach the teacher or therapist (or in some situations, teach others) the procedure or concept that he/she has been taught. This will ensure that the child has understood the necessary information.

5. *Teach the child appropriate strategies for dealing with particularly troublesome situations that occur frequently.* In some cases, the NPOOD child may not generate appropriate problem-solving strategies independently because he/she is unaware of the actual requirements of the situation. At other times, the child may be unable to generate appropriate strategies simply because this particular type of endeavor (which involves concept-formation and other problem-solving skills) is representative of an area of neuropsychological deficiency for him/her. Therefore, the child should be taught appropriate strategies for handling the requirements of frequently occurring troublesome situations. The teacher or therapist will find that the step-by-step requirements for teaching this type of child are quite similar to those that would be employed effectively for a much younger child.

6. *Promote the generalization of learned strategies and concepts.* While the majority of "normal" children will see how one particular strategy or procedure may apply to a number of different situations, and/or how certain concepts (e.g., equilibrium) may apply to a wide range of topics, the NPOOD child will usually exhibit difficulties with this form of generalization. We have found, for instance, that better visual attention and visual tracking skills have been trained in the laboratory setting, yet the child has failed to employ the skills effectively in everyday

life (e.g., when he/she is required to recall some aspect of a person's physical characteristics). Therefore, one should attempt to teach directly and systematically the possible applications of newly acquired learned strategies and concepts.

7. *Teach the child to refine and use appropriately his/her verbal* (*expressive*) *skills.* As has been pointed out earlier in this chapter, it is quite possible that the NPOOD child may come to use verbal (expressive) skills more frequently and, perhaps, for more reasons than do most children. For example, the child may repeatedly ask questions as a primary way of gathering information about a new or otherwise complex situation. This may be quite inappropriate for situations (e.g., social situations) in which nonverbal behaviors are important for feedback and direction.

The content of the child's verbal responses may also be problematic. We have observed that such children may begin a reply by directly addressing the question asked and then gradually drift into a completely different topic. At the very least, this has the effect of alienating the listener. Furthermore, if the child's verbal responses and other aspects of his/her verbal expressive skills are analyzed systematically, it may be found that problem areas other than the type and/or frequency of questions asked and the general content of the child's overall utterances will emerge. At that point, specific training should be undertaken; this will most likely be concerned with the "what to say," "how to say," and "when to say" aspects of language as these questions apply to the child's problem areas.

8. *Teach the child to make better use of his/her visual–perceptual–organizational skills.* It should always be kept in mind that children tend to "lead with their strong suit" in behavioral situations that are in any way problematic for them. In other words, if a child exhibits an outstanding area of disability (e.g., visual–spatial skills) in combination with relatively intact verbal receptive and verbal expressive skills, we have found that he/she will tend to use his/her better-developed (verbal) skills whenever it is possible, even when it is quite inappropriate to do so. This promotes a situation in which the poorly developed skills (e.g., visual–spatial skills) are not challenged or "exercised," so that optimal development may not be realized. The tendency to "play one's strong suit" also encourages the NPOOD child to develop other ways to use his/her language-related skills, many of which are clearly maladaptive.

To increase the likelihood that the child's visual modality and associated perceptive and analytic abilities will be developed and used optimally, a younger child of this type could be taught to name visual details in pictures as a way of encouraging him/her to pay attention to these details. In conjunction with this exercise, the child could be asked to talk about the relationship between various details in a picture (e.g., intersecting lines) as a way of drawing his/her attention to the complexity, importance, and significance of visual feedback.

When the child is older, remedial suggestions and exercises should be more "functional" or practical in nature, and at the same time should directly address the child's outstanding areas of difficulty. For example, it is necessary to decipher the nonverbal behavior of others in social settings to interpret them properly, and children of this type are deficient in nonverbal social-analytic skills. Therefore, one might create "artificial" social situations that require the child to rely only on his/her visual-receptive and other nonverbal skills for interpretation. This could be done with pictures, films, or even real-life situations (that are contrived) for which there is no verbal feedback available. After an exercise of this type, one should discuss the child's perception of the social situation and of his/her most appropriate role in the situation. At the same time, one might provide the child with strategies for deciphering the most salient nonverbal cues inherent in these contrived social situations.

9. Teach the child to interpret visual information when there is "competing" auditory information. This type of training is usually more complex than the suggested remedial interventions already mentioned. This remedial recommendation is particularly important when attempting to teach the child to deal more effectively with novel social situations. In these situations, it is important not only to interpret others' nonverbal behavior correctly, but also to interpret what is being said in conjunction with these nonverbal cues. In most cases, this type of training should be undertaken only when there has been adequate work and progress in the previously mentioned areas.

10. Teach appropriate nonverbal behavior. Many NPOOD children do not appear to have adequately developed nonverbal behavior. For example, such children often present with a somewhat "vacant look," especially those individuals who are found to be significantly impaired from a neuropsychological standpoint. At the same time, a child might smile in situations in which that behavior is quite inappropriate (e.g., when he/she is experiencing failure with a task). One might attempt to teach more appropriate nonverbal behavior, keeping in mind the concepts introduced in association with the refinements of the child's verbal expressive skills. In this connection, teaching the child "what to do" and "how and when to do it" should be the focus of concern. For example, some children may not know how or when to convey their feelings in a nonverbal manner. The use of informative pictures, imitative "drills," work with a mirror, and other techniques and concrete aids can prove to be invaluable in this type of training. This sort of intervention may also serve to make the child more aware of the significance of the nonverbal behavior of others.

11. Facilitate structured peer interactions. It is not always possible to promote social training in unstructured social situations, because these are largely beyond the reach of the remedial therapist or teacher. For instance, when the child is on the playground, it is not often possible to regulate his/her play in any way (at least to the extent that it promotes positive social growth for the socially impaired youngster). However, intramural activities of one sort or another, clubs, and formal groups (e.g., Boy Scouts and Girl Scouts or Guides) can provide a forum for social training if exploited in a proper manner. Unfortunately, because many children of this type tend to be somewhat socially withdrawn, they may not be encouraged to join their peers in social activities of any kind as a "protective" maneuver on the part of parents and other caretakers. This attitude needs to be addressed and dealt with as early as possible in the remedial program (see above).

12. Promote, encourage, and monitor "systematic" explorative activities. One of the most potentially harmful tacks that a well-meaning therapist can take with the NPOOD child is to leave the child to his/her own devices in already unstructured activities. On the other hand, it is quite worthwhile to design specific activities through which the child is encouraged to explore his/her environment. For example, exploratory activity may be encouraged within the structure of a gross motor program. In this setting, the child could be provided with the opportunity to explore various types of apparatus and the exercises that would suit each apparatus. In this situation, it is important that the child does not feel as if he/she is competing with his/her peers. In addition, following the lesson, the child should be required to give the instructor some verbal feedback and, perhaps, accompanying demonstrations regarding his/her activities.

13. Teach the "older" child (at least 10 years of age) how to use available aids to reach a specific goal (e.g., completing a mechanical arithmetic assignment correctly). One potential "aid" is a hand calculator, which could be used to provide the child with a way of checking the accuracy of his/her mechanical arithmetic work. After the child has completed a question independently, allow him/her to redo the same question with a hand calculator. This gives the child a way of checking the accuracy of the answer (as long as the hand calculator is used correctly). If it is found that the solution is incorrect, the child should then be encouraged to rework the question with pen and paper. At the high-school level, hand calculators should probably be used whenever possible, so that the adolescent or young adult will develop at least a functional grasp of common mathematical operations and their applications in everyday life situations.

Another aid that could be used, especially for the younger child of this type, is a digital watch. We have found that many such children have difficulty in reading the hands of a traditional type of watch, and that this imposes further limitations on their already impoverished appreciation of time concepts. A digital watch is more easily read and can serve as a concrete tool for the teaching of elementary time concepts.

14. Help the child to gain insight into situations that are easy for him/her and those that are potentially troublesome. It is important for older children and adolescents of this type to gain a reasonably realistic view of their capabilities. This is certainly more easily said than done. In this regard, the therapist's expectations always need to be in concert with the child's abilities, since gains in this area may prove to be marginal at best. For instance, it may be that the child's practical insight may be limited to "I am good at spelling and have problems with math." However, if he/she is given consistent and appropriate feedback from concerned and informed adults regarding his/her performances in various kinds of situations, he/she may develop fairly sophisticated insights, which would help him/her to perceive the need for the utilization of prelearned strategies in appropriate situations. Furthermore, it is important that NPOOD children learn that they do have some cognitive strengths and that these strengths can be used to advantage in specific situations.

15. Work with the child's parents to help them gain insight and direction regarding the child's most salient developmental needs. In this regard, virtually all of the recommendations that have been made above can apply to the style and emphasis that parents could incoporate within their relations with their child. We have found that those well-motivated parents who have an intuitive or learned appreciation of their child's adaptive strengths and weaknesses most often create a milieu at home in which the child prospers and adaptive deficiencies are minimized. Unfortunately, this ideal parent–child relationship is not often found; in consequence, the psychologist must assume a major responsibility for guiding the child's parents. In some cases, it may be advisable and/or necessary to employ highly structured "parenting" programs (e.g., Directive Parental Counselling; see Holland, 1983) to assist parents in their role in the habilitational process.

16. Other specific educational recommendations. Among the other specific educational recommendations for this type of child are the following: (a) Teach and emphasize reading comprehension skills as soon as the child has gained a functional appreciation of sound–symbol correspondence; (b) institute regular drills early in the child's educational career to help further the development of his/her handwriting skills; (c) before any copying task, teach the child to read the material to be copied carefully; (d) teach the child (verbal) strategies that will help him/her to organize his/her written work; (e) teach mechanical arithmetic in a systematic, verbal, step-by-step fashion, as outlined in some detail elsewhere (see Chapter 8, this volume).

17. Be cognizant of the therapist's/remedial specialist's role in preparing the NPOOD child for adult life. Special educators, in particular, should assume a major role in preparing this type of child for adult life. Unlike most educational programs, in which it would appear that the primary goal is to help the child to master a particular curriculum, the program required by NPOOD children is one that focuses primarily on the development of life skills. The child's mastery of the standard academic curriculum is insignificant if the child is not prepared to meet the social and other adaptive demands of independent living. Indeed, we have found through longitudinal follow-up that some NPOOD children as adults have developed rather seriously debilitating forms of psychopathology (Rourke *et al.*, 1985). This being the case, it is clear that remedial/habilitational interventions with such children should always be consonant with their short- and long-term remedial needs and remediable capacities.

REFERENCES

Benton, A. L. *Sentence Memory Test.* Iowa City, Iowa: Author, 1965.

Dunn, L. M. *Expanded Manual for the Peabody Picture Vocabulary Test.* Minneapolis: American Guidance Service, 1965.

Holland, C. J. *Directive Parental Counselling: The counsellor's guide.* Bloomfield Hills, Mich.: Midwest Professional Publishing, 1983.

328 / *Personality and Socioemotional Dimensions*

Jastak, J. F., & Jastak, S. R. *Wide Range Achievement Test.* Wilmington, Del.: Guidance Associates, 1965.

Kass, C. E. Auditory Closure Test. In J. J. Olson & J. L. Olson (Eds.), *Validity studies on the Illinois Test of Psycholinguistic Abilities.* Madison, Wisc.: Photo Press, 1964.

Kløve, H. Clinical neuropsychology. In F. M. Forster (Ed.), *The medical clinics of North America.* New York: Saunders, 1963.

Piaget, J. *The construction of reality in the child.* New York: Basic Books, 1954.

Reitan, R. M., & Davison, L. A. (Eds.). *Clinical neuropsychology: Current status and applications.* Washington, D.C.: V. H. Winston & Sons, 1974.

Rourke, B. P., Bakker, D. J., Fisk, J. L., & Strang, J. D. *Child neuropsychology: An introduction to theory, research, and clinical practice.* New York: Guilford Press, 1983.

Rourke, B. P., & Finlayson, M. A. J. Neuropsychological significance of variations in patterns of academic performance: Verbal and visual disabilities. *Journal of Abnormal Child Psychology,* 1978, *6,* 121–133.

Rourke, B. P., & Strang, J. D. Neuropsychological significance of variations in patterns of academic performance: Motor, psychomotor, and tactile–perceptual abilities. *Journal of Pediatric Psychology,* 1978, *2,* 62–66.

Rourke, B. P., Young, G. C., Strang, J. D., & Russell, D. L. Adult outcomes of central processing deficiencies in childhood. In I. Grant & K. M. Adams (Eds.), *Neuropsychological assessment in neuropsychiatric disorders: Clinical methods and empirical findings.* New York: Oxford University Press, 1985.

Strang, J. D., & Rourke, B. P. Concept-formation/non-verbal reasoning abilities of children who exhibit specific academic problems with arithmetic. *Journal of Clinical Child Psychology,* 1983, *12,* 33–39.

Strang, J. D., & Rourke, B. P. *Personality dimensions of learning-disabled children.* Manuscript in preparation, 1985.

Wechsler, D. *Wechsler Intelligence Scale for Children.* New York: Psychological Corporation, 1949.

Wirt, R. D., Lachar, D., Klinedist, J. K., & Seat, P. D. *Multidimensional description of child personality: A manual for the Personality Inventory for Children.* Los Angeles: Western Psychological Services, 1977.

VI
Summary and Conclusions

15

Major Findings and Future Directions for Learning Disability Subtype Analyses

JOHN L. FISK
RHEA FINNELL
BYRON P. ROURKE

It is generally agreed that classification of relevant phenomena constitutes a basic step that is crucial for the meaningful development of a scientific discipline. The role of the periodic table of elements in physical chemistry and the systematic taxonomies of modern botany and zoology spring to mind as obvious examples of scientifically useful classification schemes. In the behavioral sciences, the utilization of taxonomic principles to develop classification schemes is clearly at a very early developmental stage. The relative absence of this effort and its attendant results heretofore may very well have been responsible for the view of some lay persons, as well as many investigators in the so-called "hard" sciences, that behavioral sciences are not "real" sciences at all, or, at best, only "soft" sciences.

Historically, psychology (at least in the Western world) has come to view favorably only specific models of methodology—namely, those that involve empirical hypothesis testing. For the most part, the role of description in scientific psychology has been accorded much less respect—a kind of "back seat," so to speak. Within this empirical psychology tradition, considerable emphasis is given over to the quantification of the

John L. Fisk. Department of Neuropsychology, Windsor Western Hospital Centre, Windsor, Ontario, Canada.

Rhea Finnell. Division of Neuropsychology, North Shore University Hospital, Manhasset, New York, USA.

Byron P. Rourke. Department of Psychology, University of Windsor, and Department of Neuropsychology, Windsor Western Hospital Centre, Windsor, Ontario, Canada.

constructs and variables utilized in research endeavors. However, it is very often the case that the careful specification of the experimental subjects is either overlooked or treated in a far less precise, even cavalier, manner. This state of affairs can, and often does, detract substantially from the reliability and validity of empirical investigations, in spite of the precise operationalization of their salient constructs and variables.

We would maintain that the clarification and precise description of relevant taxonomic categories and the proper identification of subjects for inclusion within them can contribute substantially to the operationalization of empirical investigations of human behavior, including those that focus on learning disabilities in children. Failure to do this will, quite simply, do little more than confuse this already muddled area of scientific scrutiny.

A perusal of the literature on learning disabilities reveals that the most common research strategy employed is one of the contrasting groups of disabled learners with so-called "normals" on the basis of some variable thought to represent an underlying construct. When differences between the groups are discovered, the construct is often accorded the status of an "explanation" for why children fail to learn in the expected fashion. However, as has been illustrated in a number of reviews (Benton, 1975; Fletcher, 1981; Rourke, 1978a), a rather vast catalogue of variables can be used to differentiate the performances of learning-disabled children from those of controls.

As Fletcher and Satz (see Chapter 3, this volume) point out, there are two large sources of variability inherent in studies of learning-disabled children: the construct validity of the dependent variables, and the heterogeneity of the population under investigation. This being the case, one would hardly expect reliable scientific findings to emerge through the use of complex, poorly understood measures applied to some ill-defined set or grouping of learning-impaired children. For some time it has been recognized (Applebee, 1971; Rourke, 1978b; Taylor & Fletcher, 1983) that children with learning disabilities need to be classified into relatively homogeneous subgroups if the results of empirical investigations in this area are to have any theoretical or applied significance.

The use of formal taxonomic methods to accomplish this is a fairly recent phenomenon in psychology. Indeed, it would not be totally unfair to characterize most psychologists as neophytes in terms of their understanding of taxonomic principles. If the reader, after having perused the foregoing chapters in this volume, feels some sense of disquiet because of a vague feeling that he/she either does not comprehend the principles described or cannot incorporate the data presented into any conceptual framework, then this volume has, at least in part, met its basic objective. This is so because objectivity and precision in taxonomical classification remain fleeting goals, even for those disciplines wherein they have been pursued for many years (e.g., many areas of contemporary biology). In short, the classification of naturally occurring phenomena is a complex and challenging enterprise, open to many subjective and arbitrary choices, both in philosophical (theoretical) as well as practical (technical) terms (see Adams, Chapter 2; Fletcher & Satz, Chapter 3).

Classification serves a variety of purposes, not the least of which is the provision of an articulated context and background that serves to enhance the organization and integration of knowledge. Furthermore, classification systems serve a heuristic purpose by generating hypotheses and by stimulating research regarding the underlying structure of the observed phenomena. More basically, with respect to the classification of learning-disabled children, one would hope that an appropriate classification scheme would facilitate communication among scientists and clinicians who are concerned with this group of clinical disorders (see Fletcher, Chapter 9). From an applied perspective, one would hope that a cogent, rational classification system would provide new and more productive directions for generating distinct modes of intervention with this particular population (see Strang & Rourke, Chapters 8 and 14). These are only some of the reasons relating to issues of both theoretical and practical concern that motivate researchers to pursue this taxonomic enterprise.

In distinguishing between the phyletic and phenetic perspectives, Adams (see Chapter 2) stresses the need for an adequate theoretical framework to guide the utilization of mathematical procedures associated with numerical taxonomy. Indeed, one must view with dismay the unfortunate tendency of some investigators who, dazzled by the "number-crunching" capacities of modern digital computers, have opted to apply multivariate mathematical procedures to data sets in what can only be described as a facile and almost random fashion. Even when some sort of theoretical rationale or expectation has been developed, it is often the case that procedures are applied until results emerge that fit the particular theoretical proclivities of the investigator. This is not the sort of strategy that is likely to contribute to a meaningful classification system.

Unfortunately, there exists no specific set of procedures or rules to which one can refer in order to guarantee a cogent and rational outcome in this endeavor. Rather, one must evaluate carefully a variety of parameters prior to making decisions regarding the form of statistical analysis to be used (see Joschko & Rourke, Chapter 4; Del Dotto & Rourke, Chapter 5). When results do not conform to predictions, it is not sufficient to insert (say) algorithm B for algorithm A, based on the fact that the statistical procedure did not illustrate what one had hoped it would. In such cases, the investigator is faced with the tedious and painstaking task of re-examining in detail the characteristics of the data set, the mathematical assumptions underlying the statistical procedure used, and the rationale for the hypotheses tested. Furthermore, there is no compelling objective reason for one to believe that a particular multivariate procedure (e.g., Q-type factor analysis) is any more or less superior to an alternative (e.g., cluster analysis). This point is illustrated in rather dramatic fashion in the study carried out by Del Dotto and Rourke (see Chapter 5), in which left-handed learning-disabled children were classified into virtually identical subtypes utilizing, on the one hand, a Q-type factor-analytic procedure and, on the other, two clustering algorithms. This sort of concurrence is rare in taxonomic research, but does suggest that a variety of mathematical techniques might be profitably utilized as a means of validating findings (see Adams, Chapter 2).

To return to a more general consideration, Fletcher and Satz (see Chapter 3), in their discussion of the Florida Longitudinal Project, illustrate the emergence of a problem in classification that resulted from the initial acceptance of a standard definition of reading disability that did not reflect the heterogeneous nature of the experimental group under investigation. Had these investigators not been alert to, or had they chosen to ignore, signs of a major problem with this fundamental assumption, the results of their study would indeed have been trivial. As they relate, the presence of a relatively high incidence of reading problems, and the observation that many subjects under investigation were encountering academic difficulties in addition to reading, led to a dramatic alteration in the focus of their investigation. While one should recognize that there is no one specific method for conducting such research, this study illustrates the sort of careful evaluation needed in order to develop an appropriate rationale for decisions regarding, for example, (1) investigative approach (clinical vs. statistical), (2) statistical method (cluster analysis vs. Q-type factor analysis), and (3) selection of similarity coefficients (that emphasize shape, scatter, and/or elevation). Whether or not these and other investigators whose work appears in this volume have been judicious in their utilization of statistical techniques remains for the reader to decide. The important point is that the conceptual and methodological problems encountered in the Florida Longitudinal Project are well documented by Fletcher and Satz. In addition, they shed considerable light on the relevant decision points and the sort of careful, considered thinking that is needed in conducting this type of research.

Any involved discussion of such constructs as reliability and validity is obviously beyond the scope of this chapter. The reader is referred to any standard text dealing with research design and statistics (e.g., Kerlinger, 1973) and a presentation that deals with these issues within the context of subtyping research (Rourke & Adams, 1984) for a more complete evaluation of these complex and sometimes controversial topics. At the same time, we would be remiss in the present context were we not to offer some observations with respect to validation, particularly as this applies to the subtyping of learning-disabled children.

We are concerned here with what is referred to as "external validity" (see Fletcher, Chapter 9). As Fletcher points out. the development of a typology is not the endpoint of subtyping investigations. Rather, the typology allows for the systematic investigation of hypotheses concerning subtype similarities and differences. In this context, he suggests that one should focus on the evaluation of relationships between neuropsychological profiles of learning-disabled children on the one hand and various biological measures, known clinical syndromes, behavioral indices (such as response to treatment), and academic performances on the other.

Although there are no hard-and-fast criteria by which to judge the validity of various typologies, one very obvious and reasonable approach is to determine how subtypes predict differences on measures not used to establish the typology. Several chapters in this volume (see Doehring, Chapter 6; Sweeney & Rourke, Chapter 7; Strang & Rourke, Chapter 8; Lyon, Chapter 11) illustrate how, for example, academic measures might be utilized to validate an existing, albeit tentative, classification. Furthermore, within the context of learning disabilities research, some would maintain that a classification scheme should also enhance the generating of hypotheses regarding differences in subtypes associated with different patterns of CNS function and dysfunction. In this way, one would not only enhance the validity of a potentially meaningful typology, one might also generate additional data that would shed light on the interactions of CNS function and dysfunction and behavior. Electrophysiological studies, such as those reviewed by Fletcher (see Chapter 9), constitute a potentially important contribution to our understanding of brain–behavior relationships in this connection. Future studies that utilize more advanced technology, such as cerebral blood flow, positron emission tomography, and nuclear magnetic resonance imaging, offer even more exciting possibilities.

The ultimate aim of any science is predictability. In the case of child neuropsychology, and, in particular, the subtype classification of learning-disabled children, one ultimate issue must be the predictive utility of these classifications with respect to the differential effect of various intervention strategies. Evidence of such an interaction has been found in academic and other interventions with reading-disabled children (Bakker, Licht, Kok, & Bouma, 1980; Bakker, Moerland, & Goekoop-Koefkens, 1981; Lyon, Chapter 11). Such research is the hallmark of the predictive validity of these classifications within the academic domain; their application to the "nonacademic" realm is a frontier under current exploration (Strang & Rourke, Chapter 14). It may be instructive at this point to address the importance of continued investigation of the "nonacademic" dimensions of adaptational behavior in learning-disabled children within the socio-historical context of modern behavioral science.

Historically, psychology has tended to emphasize environmental factors almost exclusively as determinants of individual personality dimensions. While it is abundantly clear that the contribution of factors associated with culture, social class, family, and early experiences are extremely important, it would appear that insufficient attention has been paid to the role that constitutional factors play in personality development, especially those associated with the adaptive ability structure of the individual child. Indeed, one has only to spend a short time in the careful observation of learning-disabled children to appreciate that the weaknesses that interfere with their academic learning also intrude upon their extracurricular lives. A learning-disabled child who has difficulty in acquiring academic skills may also have problems with social interactions. While the effect is readily discernible, the relationship is, for most, not intuitively obvious. In short, the particular pattern of adaptive strengths and weaknesses that learning-disabled children exhibit may well be a crucial determinant of important social, emotional, and other behavioral characteristics. What is clearly needed is the elucidation of the abilities and deficits that play an important role in social interactions in order to understand better why these children have difficulty in any number of everyday situations.

Attempts to investigate and deal with the implications of such "nonacademic" behavior in this volume are the presentations of Ozols and Rourke (Chapter 13) and Strang and Rourke (Chapter 14). These investigators were able to demonstrate some fairly clear relationships between the subtypal classification of learning-disabled children and socioemotional behaviors. A companion endeavor relates to the rather more basic consideration of distinct personality subtypes among learning-disabled children (see Porter & Rourke, Chapter 12). Ideally, further investigation of these parameters will eventuate in the determination of specific interventions for these subtypes of learning-disabled children that are based on their particular pattern of abilities and disabilities. The promise of such research is predictability; its hope will be in serving as a fresh warrant for an ecological approach to intervention. Central processing deficiencies that eventuate in various types of learning disabilities would be expected to have wide-ranging effects on a child—effects that can be understood only by understanding the child's interactions with his/her environment. Ideally, intervention programs would incorporate the implications of such an awareness. The challenge posed to the researcher–clinician in this context is to explain and deal with the manifold nature of the child's adaptational requirements. To do less would be to shirk responsibility for the total, unified explanation that is required in this complex endeavor (Rourke, 1982a).

The science of ecology, which maps the interdependence of living forms and their environments, would seem to provide a desirable framework for the treatment of the learning-disabled youngster. An ecological approach to intervention would allow not only for the consideration of the developing nervous system of the child, but also for the relational aspects of the disability. Both are critical considerations. The child's particular state of development in terms of cerebral organization may very well increase the therapeutic potential of particular remedies. For example, visual–perceptual and psychomotor deficiencies that may affect a child's sensory–perceptual mode of development rather generally are often regarded as "immaturity" and are rarely singled out as disabilities. However, as is hypothesized by Strang and Rourke (Chapter 14), these inefficiencies may be expected to intrude later upon the youngster's nonverbal functioning and to jeopardize his/her social interactions, thus rendering this apparent "delay" a seriously disabling condition. Thus, quite different insights flow from an understanding of how the limiting effects of an impairment vary over time and with changes in the environment.

In line with the foregoing, it would seem reasonable to suggest that the course of effective intervention for a learning-disabled child will need to be quite specific and tailored precisely to the child. Indeed, there is much to recommend such specificity. The classic remediational caveat that intervention must be "child-based" and not "classroom-based" has great value. However, failures in the remediation of learning-disabled children far outweigh the successes. Although an analysis of the effectiveness of intervention is beyond the scope of this chapter, a few thoughts about the issue as it pertains to subtype classification follow.

In the absence of a cure or prophylactic treatment, rehabilitation/ habilitation has been the most favored form of intervention with learning disabled children. The traditional focus of rehabilitation has been the treatment of task-related functional skills. This begins with an analysis of the task, which is thought to yield information regarding the degree and kinds of assistance that are needed to perform the task. The results of studies that have employed this mode of approach with learning-disabled children seem to mimic those found with adults (Diller, Ben-Yishay, Gerstman, Goodkin, Gorden, & Weinberg, 1974); that is, while improvement may be seen on a specific task, the processing aspects of the performance very often remain essentially unchanged. Efforts aimed at teaching the competence aspects of performance have yielded little or no generalization of the skill. Moreover, most programs that have been designed to remediate particular processes have been less than successful (Hammill & Larson, 1974, 1978). At the same time, it is clear that well-articulated intervention programs that address the remediation of processing skills can have discernible impacts upon functional incapacities (e.g., Young, Collins, & Hren, 1983).

A systematic, theoretically based approach to the remediation of learning-disabled children would seem to be the most useful way of proceeding at this time. Couching intervention studies, as well as other attempts to determine the concurrent, predictive, and construct validity of learning disability typologies, within a hypothesis-testing framework with clearly articulated and falsifiable expectations would seem eminently desirable (see Fletcher, Chapter 9). Indeed, the need to determine subtype × treatment modality interactions, as well as to establish validity in any number of other ways, is the most pressing need in this field today (Fisk & Rourke, 1983).

Classifications of learning-disabled children that are based upon a more comprehensive understanding of brain–behavior relationships (e.g., Rourke, 1982a) are now available and thus may provide a more appropriate model from which to deduce remediation programs (Rourke, 1982b). In this vein, Das, Snart, and Mulcahy (1982) are currently investigating the effectiveness of intervention strategies based on a successive–simultaneous processing model. Research by Bakker *et al.* (1981) and Lyon (see Chapter 11) would suggest that there is reason for cautious optimism regarding the fruitfulness of the hypothesis-testing approach, at least with respect to effective intervention for some reading problems. Some research currently being conducted (e.g., along the lines suggested by Ozols & Rourke, Chapter 13, and by Strang & Rourke, Chapters 8 and 14) would seem to hold promise for elucidating the relationship between neuropsychological patterns of performance on the one hand and both academic and "nonacademic" behavior on the other. Such research is geared quite precisely toward the goal that we feel is of central importance: namely, the ecological validity of interventions for the learning-disabled child.

In this volume, a number of arguments have been marshalled to support the view that the identification and description of subtypes constitutes a crucial and necessary step in the development of theoretical and applied knowledge regarding learning-disabled children. The investigations described by Joschko and Rourke (Chapter 4), Del Dotto and Rourke (Chapter 5), Doehring (Chapter 6), Sweeney and Rourke (Chapter 7), and Strang and Rourke (Chapter 8) are examples of this orientation. Moreover, progress in this taxonomic enterprise will, in addition, be quite dependent upon the ability of investigators to integrate and synthesize current theories of development, cognition, and brain–behavior relationships to serve as a guide for the utilization of appropriate statistical procedures and the interpretation of findings within the proposed ecological perspective. There is obviously a need to explore in a much more systematic and detailed manner than has heretofore been done the implementation of various multivariate algorithms within a variety of settings and with a number of different populations (e.g., van der Vlugt & Satz, Chapter 10). Methodological research of this type is often tedious and time-consuming, but is necessary if we are to establish a rational classification scheme that will address our theoretical and applied concerns in an adequate fashion.

Finally, if this volume illustrates nothing else, it should be abundantly clear that the univariate contrasting-groups methodology so typical of much of the learning disabilities research of the past is no longer justified on either theoretical or applied grounds. It is our considered opinion that investigations that fail to recognize the value of identifying homogeneous subtypes in this population will produce, at the very best, only trivial results. Indeed, continuation of this sort of research methodology, in addition to retarding the growth of real knowledge in the field, constitutes a serious waste of time, effort, and economic resources.

REFERENCES

Applebee, A. N. Research in reading retardation: Two critical problems. *Journal of Child Psychology and Psychiatry and Allied Disciplines*, 1971, *12*, 91–113.

Bakker, D. J., Licht, R., Kok, A., & Bouma, A. Cortical responses to word reading by right- and left-eared normal and reading disturbed children. *Journal of Clinical Neuropsychology*, 1980, *2*, 1–12.

Bakker, D. J., Moerland, R., & Goekoop-Hoefkens, M. Effects of hemisphere-specific stimulation on the reading performance of dyslexic boys: A pilot study. *Journal of Clinical Neuropsychology*, 1981, *2*, 155–159.

Benton, A. L. Developmental dyslexia: Neurological aspects. In W. J. Friedlander (Ed.), *Advances in neurology* (Vol. 7). New York: Raven Press, 1975.

Das, J. P., Snart, F., & Mulcahy, R. F. Information integration and its relationship to reading disability. In J. P. Das, R. F. Mulcahy, & A. P. Wall (Eds.), *Theory and research in learning disabilities*. New York: Plenum, 1982.

Diller, L., Ben-Yishay, Y., Gerstman, L., Goodkin, R., Gorden, W., & Weinberg, J. *Studies in cognition and rehabilitation in hemiplegia* (Rehabilitation Monograph No. 50). New York: Institute of Rehabilitation Medicine, New York University Medical Center, 1974.

Fisk, J. L., & Rourke, B. P. Neuropsychological subtyping of learning disabled children: History, methods, implications. *Journal of Learning Disabilities*, 1983, *15*, 529–531.

Fletcher, J. M. Linguistic factors in reading acquisition: Evidence for developmental changes. In F. Pirozzolo & M. C. Wittrock (Eds.), *Neuropsychological and cognitive processes in reading*. New York: Academic Press, 1981.

Hammill, D., & Larson, S. The effectiveness of psycholinguistic training. *Exceptional Children*, 1974, *41*, 5–14.

Hammill, D., & Larson, S. The effectiveness of psycholinguistic training: A reaffirmation of position. *Exceptional Children*, 1978, *44*, 402–414.

Kerlinger, F. N. *Foundations of behavioral research* (2nd ed.). New York: Holt, Rinehart & Winston, 1973.

Rourke, B. P. Neuropsychological research in reading retardation: A review. In A. L. Benton & D. Pearl (Eds.), *Dyslexia: An appraisal of current knowledge*. New York: Oxford University Press, 1978. (a)

Rourke, B. P. Reading, spelling and arithmetic disabilities: A neuropsychological perspective. In H. R. Myklebust (Ed.), *Progress in learning disabilities* (Vol. 4). New York: Grune & Stratton, 1978. (b)

Rourke, B. P. Central processing deficiencies in children: Toward a developmental neuropsychological model. *Journal of Clinical Neuropsychology*, 1982, *4*, 1–18. (a)

Rourke, B. P. Child-clinical neuropsychology: Assessment and intervention with the disabled child. In J. deWit & A. L. Benton (Eds.), *Perspectives in child study: Integration of theory and practice*. Lisse, The Netherlands: Swets & Zeitlinger, 1982. (b)

Rourke, B. P., & Adams, K. M. Quantitative approaches to the neuropsychological assessment of children. In R. E. Tarter & G. Goldstein (Eds.), *Advances in clinical neuropsychology* (Vol. 2). New York: Plenum, 1984.

Taylor, H. G., & Fletcher, J. M. Biological foundations of "specific developmental disorders": Methods, findings, and future directions. *Journal of Clinical Child Psychology*, 1983, *12*, 46-65.

Young, G. C., Collins, D., & Hren, M. Effects of pairing scanning training with block design training in the remediation of perceptual problems in left hemiplegics. *Journal of Clinical Neuropsychology*, 1983, *3*, 201-212.

Author Index

343

Subject Index

Italicized numbers denote material in tables and figures.

phenetic, 22-25, 28
phyletic, 21-30
Token Test, 233-236, *242*, 244, 245
Toward Affective Development Kit, 290,
292-295
Trail Making Test for Children, *70*, 80, *95*

Validity
external, 26, 27, 48, 54, 55, 58, 61, 76-
86, 188-193, 205-208
internal, 26-28, 47, 54, 57, 61, 72-75,
81-86, 188-190
Verbal Fluency Test, 48, 52-54, 56, *70*, 78,
81, 149, *150*, 153, 221-223
Visual Memory Test, 159-161
VMI (*see* Beery Test of Visual-Motor
Integration)

Wechsler Intelligence Scale for Children
(WISC), 5, 65-68, *70*, 79, 85, 94, 109,
112, 114, 116-119, 135, 136, 148-150,
151, 170, *175*, 201, 202, 262, 263, 266,
274, 275, *290, 291*, 306
ACID pattern, 7, 30, 31, 66-69, 71-86
Arithmetic subtest, 7, 66, 69, *70*, 79, *95*,
149, *151*, 153, 155, 156, 289, *290, 291*,
293
Block Design subtest, *70*, 78, *95, 175*,
306
Coding subtest, 7, 66, 69, *70*, 79, 119,
289, *290, 291*, 293
Comprehension subtest, 69, *70, 95*, 149,
151, 153-155
Digit Span subtest, 7, 66, 69, *70*, 79, 80,
95, 136, 149, *151*, 153, *175*
Information subtest, 7, 66, 69, *70, 95*,
149, *151*, 153-155, *175*
Object Assembly subtest, *70*, 78, *95, 175*,
289, *290, 291*, 293, 295, 306
Picture Arrangement subtest, *70, 175*,
289, *290, 291*, 293

Picture Completion subtest, *70*, 78, *95,
175*
Similarities subtest, 69, *70*, 149, *150*,
153, *175*
Verbal IQ-Performance IQ
discrepancies, 5, 79-81, 114, 116, 117,
148, 201, 202, 275, 289
Vocabulary subtest, 69, *70*, 149, *151*,
153-155, *175*, 289, *290, 291*, 203, 306
Wechsler Intelligence Scale for Children—
Revised (WISC-R), 65, 66, 194, 288
Block Design subtest, 288
Coding subtest, 288
Comprehension subtest, 288
Digit Span subtest, 288
Object Assembly subtest, 288
Picture Completion subtest, 288
Similarities subtest, 48, 52, *53*, 56, 221-
224, 288
Vocabulary subtest, 288
Wepman Test (*see* Auditory
Discrimination Test)
Wide Range Achievement Test (WRAT),
48-52, 60, 68, *70*, 77, 79-81, 84, 112,
114-119, 124, 170, 171, 173, 193-197,
205, 213-221, 225, 262, 263, 266, 274,
289, *290, 291*, 293, 302, 304-307, 312
Arithmetic subtest, *51, 151*, 168-171,
174-177, 193-196
Reading subtest, *51, 151*, 155, 156, 193-
196
Spelling subtest, *51*, 148, 149, *150*, 193-
196
WISC (*see* Wechsler Intelligence Scale for
Children)
WISC-R (*see* Wechsler Intelligence Scale
for Children—Revised)
Woodcock Reading Mastery Tests, 243-
246
WRAT (*see* Wide Range Achievement
Test)